Neurofibromatosis

Neurofibromatosis

A Handbook For Patients, Families, and Health-Care Professionals

Allan E. Rubenstein, M.D.
Associate Professor of Neurology
Director, Mount Sinai Neurofibromatosis Center
Mount Sinai School of Medicine
New York, New York

Bruce R. Korf, M.D., Ph.D.
Assistant Professor of Neurology
Harvard Medical School
Director, Clinical Genetics Program
Children's Hospital, Boston, Massachusetts

NF™
THE NATIONAL NEUROFIBROMATOSIS FOUNDATION, INC.

1990
Thieme Medical Publishers, Inc., New York
Georg Thieme Verlag, Stuttgart • New York

Thieme Medical Publishers, Inc.
381 Park Avenue South
New York, New York 10016

NEUROFIBROMATOSIS: A HANDBOOK FOR PATIENTS, FAMILIES, AND HEALTH-CARE PROFESSIONALS
Allan E. Rubenstein and Bruce R. Korf

Library of Congress Cataloging-in-Publication Data

Neurofibromatosis: a handbook for patients, families, and health-care professionals / edited by Allan E. Rubenstein and Bruce R. Korf.
p. cm.
ISBN 0-86577-154-5
1. Neurofibromatosis. I. Rubenstein, Allan E., II. Korf, Bruce R. 1944-
RC280.N4N488 1990
616.99'383—dc20 90-10744
CIP

Important note: Medicine is an ever-changing science. Research and clinical experience are continually broadening our knowledge, in particular our knowledge of proper treatment and drug therapy. Insofar as this book mentions any dosage or applications, readers may rest assured that the authors, editors, and publishers have made every effort to ensure that such references are strictly in accordance with the state of knowledge at the time of production of the book. Nevertheless, every user is requested to carefully examine the manufacturers' leaflets accompanying each drug to check on his own responsibility whether the dosage schedules recommended therein or the contraindications stated by the manufacturers differ from the statements made in the present book. Such examination is particularly important with drugs that are either rarely used or have been newly released on the market.

Printed in the United States of America.

5 4 3 2 1

TMP ISBN 0-86577-154-5
GTV ISBN 3-13-665101-4

Dedicated to all those affected with neurofibromatosis, their families, and to the officers and members of the National Neurofibromatosis Foundation, whose courage and dedication have given hope to everyone.

A.E.R.

Contents

CONTRIBUTORS

Alan M. Aron, M.D.
Mount Sinai School of Medicine
New York, New York

Peter R. W. Bellermann
Executive Director
National Neurofibromatosis Foundation
New York, New York

Barbara Bernhardt, M.S.
Sinai Hospital of Baltimore
Baltimore, Maryland

John C. Carey, M.D., M.P.H.
University of Utah School of Medicine
Salt Lake City, Utah

Roswell Eldridge, M.D.
NINDS—National Institutes of Health
Bethesda, Maryland

Sarah A. Ellis, Ph.D.
NYU Medical Center
New York, New York

Thomas B. Fitzpatrick, M.D., Ph.D.
Harvard Medical School
Massachusetts General Hospital
Boston, Massachusetts

Jane C. Halperin, M.S.
Mount Sinai School of Medicine
New York, New York

Steven Handler, M.D.
Children's Hospital of Philadelphia
Philadelphia, Pennsylvania

Dan F. Konkle, Ph.D.
Children's Hospital of Philadelphia
Philadelphia, Pennsylvania

Bruce R. Korf, M.D., Ph.D.
Harvard Medical School
Children's Hospital, Boston
Boston, Massachusetts

Ilene B. Lefkowitz, M.D.
Children's Hospital of Philadelphia
Philadelphia, Pennsylvania

Richard A. Lewis, M.D.
Cullen Eye Institute
Baylor College of Medicine
Houston, Texas

G. Dean MacEwen, M.D.
Children's Hospital
New Orleans, Louisiana

Robert L. Martuza, M.D.
Harvard Medical School
Massachusetts General Hospital
Boston, Massachusetts

Anna T. Meadows, M.D.
University of Pennsylvania School of Medicine
Children's Hospital of Philadelphia
Philadelphia, Pennsylvania

John B. Mulliken, M.D.
Harvard Medical School
Children's Hospital, Boston
Boston, Massachusetts

John J. Mulvihill, M.D.
Clinical Epidemiology Branch
National Cancer Institute
Bethesda, Maryland

Angela C. Obringer, Ph.D.
Hospital of The University of Pennsylvania
Philadelphia, Pennsylvania

Allan E. Rubenstein, M.D.
Mount Sinai School of Medicine
New York, New York

R. Neil Schimke, M.D.
University of Kansas
Kansas City, Kansas

Cynthia B. Solot, M.A., C.C.
Children's Hospital of Philadelphia
Philadelphia, Pennsylvania

Arthur K.F. Tong, M.D., B.S. (Lond.)
Harvard Medical School
Massachusetts General Hospital
Boston, Massachusetts

Sibylle A. Wallace, M.D.
Mount Sinai School of Medicine
New York, New York

Barbara Wellman, M.S.W.
Former NNFF Chapter President

Mary Ann Wilson
Former NNFF Chapter President

Felice Yahr, M.S.
Former Executive Director, NNFF

Elaine H. Zackai, M.D., Ph.D.
University of Pennsylvania School of Medicine
Children's Hospital of Philadelphia
Philadelphia, Pennsylvania

Foreword

Despite some remarkable insights, until recently the genetic analysis of human beings has been an intractable problem. It is true that in 1908 Archibald Garrod showed that a human inherited disease, alkaptonuria, resulted from a deficiency in an enzyme, but this was an isolated incident. The lack of progress in succeeding years is shown by the fact that the double helical nature of the DNA molecule was discovered three years before the number of human chromosomes was determined correctly by Tjio and Levan in 1956! And while sex-linked diseases such as hemophilia had long been recognized, it was not until 1967 that the first human gene was assigned to an autosome (thymidine kinase to chromosome 17 by Weiss and Green).

Human beings are not satisfactory subjects for experimental genetic analysis. Instead, genetics advanced through work on "simpler" organisms beginning with Mendel's pea plants and progressing through *Drosophila, Neurospora,* and *E. coli* to viruses. This approach was tremendously successful, but there seemed to be no way these advances in bacterial and viral genetics could be translated into human genetics. In 1966, Sir Macfarlane Burnet even went so far as to write that molecular biology was "very largely a laboratory artefact" and that "as far as the advance of medicine is concerned molecular biology may be an evil thing." This was no doubt said provocatively but it was no less true for that. It required the development of means for the direct analysis and manipulation of the genes of higher organisms to propel human genetics into the molecular age.

These technical advances came about in the early 1970's when it became possible to clone genes and the recombinant DNA era began. It was not until 1976 that the first eukaryotic gene—the rabbit β-globin gene—was cloned. That same year Kan, Globus and Dozy showed that Macfarlane Burnet was wrong and that molecular genetics could be applied to human diseases. Gene cloning together with DNA sequencing and linkage analysis using restriction fragment length polymorphisms (RFLPs), has led to a revolution in human genetics.

What does this mean for neurofibromatosis? It is clear that those striving to clone the NF genes have made good use of lessons learned from cloning other genes, especially those for Duchenne musclar dystrophy and cystic fibrosis. Under the auspices of the National Neurofibromatosis Foundation there has been an exemplary blend of competition and cooperation between the groups involved, such that success is near. The chromosomal locations of both NF1 and NF2 have been determined, and there are probes sufficiently close to the genes that they can be used for family diagnosis. Cytogenetic abnormalities have been found that are being used to narrow down the region containing the genes. But while we have every reason to be optimistic, it may be many years before the research on the molecular genetics of neurofibromatosis can be translated into remedial action for patients. It is entirely right and appropriate that a handbook on neurofibromatosis should concentrate on what can be done for patients while the laboratory research is pursued.

Inherited disorders are rare, and their scarcity together with the fact that they are genetic can lead to unnecessary fears among patients and their families. These fears may be compounded by lack of experience of such rare disorders among health care professionals. Handbooks of this kind have a tremendous potential for doing good simply by explaining in clear, straightforward terms the nature of a genetic disorder and its consequences for patients and families. Drs. Rubenstein and Korf and those who contributed to the book deserve, and will receive, the grateful thanks of all who take up and use this handbook.

James D. Watson, M.D.
Director
Cold Spring Harbor Laboratory

Preface

Coping with neurofibromatosis is a challenge for both affected individuals and health-care professionals alike. For those with neurofibromatosis 1 or 2 this begins with the medical burdens of the disorder and uncertainty about future medical problems. Many affected individuals and their family members also face burdens of stigmatization, guilt, and financial hardship that accompany a genetically determined, variable medical condition. Worst of all, many feel that they must endure in isolation, and are frustrated by the fact that for many critical medical issues, no two physicians may give the same advice.

From the perspective of the health professional, neurofibromatosis can be equally daunting. Neurofibromatosis is common for a rare disorder, which means that most will encounter at least a few with the condition during their careers, sufficient to make one uncomfortable, but not to make one expert. Moreover, the variability of expression of the neurofibromatosis genes can lead to imposingly long differential diagnoses, cutting across multiple medical specialties, and each patient may present unique challenges. Finally, there may be little guidance from the medical literature, or from colleagues, as there is no true consensus on how to deal with some of the more difficult medical problems.

It is with this background that we have assembled this book, which is directed at individuals affected with neurofibromatosis, their family members, and the health professionals who provide their care. It is our hope that this book will serve as a source for patients to learn more about their condition, and to better understand medical problems with which they might be affected. Health professionals may use it to help them better care for their patients, or to become familiar with neurofibromatosis-related problems outside their primary area of specialization. It is very difficult to write in a manner that is equally informative to both laypersons and professionals. To aim for the mean risks missing both marks. In this book we have sought to explain major concepts as thoroughly as possible, with minimal reliance on prior medical background. On the other hand, sufficient detail has been included on most topics to go well beyond standard medical texts. A glossary of terms provided in an appendix may help nonmedically trained readers to follow the more technical discussions.

The major handicap facing those who deal with neurofibromatosis is lack of knowledge about the condition. In more than 100 years since neurofibromatosis was described by von Recklinghausen, we have learned very little about its basic pathogenesis. It is this lack of information that is at the root of apparent disagreements in the medical community about how to deal with some of the complications of neurofibromatosis. There is simply no single "correct" approach to the care of affected individuals. Such diversity is reflected in the chapters of this book, in which different points of view on the same problem are often presented. We have not sought to present a consensus approach here, because on many topics there are too few data to achieve consensus. We have asked authors to explain their reasons for the approach they take, however, and take stock of alternative viewpoints for some of the more controversial areas. This may help both patients and their caretakers to understand the available choices, and identify clinical questions on which further research is needed.

Given the great need for more information about neurofibromatosis, it is gratifying to report that research into the disorder has recently entered an exponential phase. This is largely due to application of the techniques of molecular genetics, with the hope that in the near future the genes responsible for NF1 and NF2 will be identified and will provide the keys to studying the basic mechanisms of these disorders. Already this research has borne fruit for clinical practice by providing tools for presymptomatic and prenatal diagnosis. The ultimate goal of developing a treatment for neurofibromatosis, though still elusive, seems increasingly realistic. This rapid progress to some degree accounts for the long gestational period of this book, which was conceived several years ago and would already be out-of-date had it come out when originally planned. It would be surprising if additional significant progress, possibly including the cloning of the NF1 gene, is not made by the time this book completes production. Yet at some point the decision must be made to capture the state of our knowledge, like a snapshot, as it exists at a point in time. We have chosen to do that now, providing as much background as possible to anticipate the advances likely to occur in the near future. One can only hope that our foresight proves myopic, and that progress renders this book obsolete rapidly.

Most of the authors are clinicians with a special interest in neurofibromatosis; some are lay people who have neurofibromatosis themselves or in their family. Most, at one time or other, have been affiliated with the National Neurofibromatosis Foundation, in some cases serving as Chapter officers, on its Board of Directors, Research Advisory Board, or Clinical Care Advisory Board. We are grateful to all those who have shared their approaches to neurofibromatosis and hope that this demonstrates that no one need deal with the condition alone.

Allan E. Rubenstein, M.D.
Bruce R. Korf, M.D., Ph.D.

Neurofibromatosis

1

Introduction and History

John J. Mulvihill, M.D.

Neurofibromatosis (NF) is a term applied to two clinical genetic disorders with a few overlapping features, but on the whole with very distinctive clinical manifestations and genetic origins. The more common is called neurofibromatosis type 1 (NF1, von Recklinghausen neurofibromatosis), and the rarer is called neurofibromatosis type 2 (NF2, bilateral acoustic neurofibromatosis). This chapter will provide definitions of these disorders, a brief review of their histories, and an overview of current research.

Definitions

The nomenclature and definitions of NF1 and NF2, as well as recommendations for clinical care and research, were addressed at a National Institute of Health Consensus Development Conference held in Bethesda, Maryland, in July 1987 (Fig. 1–1) (1). The major features of NF1 and NF2 are compared in Table 1–1 and diagnostic criteria are described in Chapter 2 of this book. NF1 is characterized by prominent cutaneous manifestations such as café au lait spots, skin-fold freckles, and neurofibromas. Other features include iris Lisch nodules, dysplasia of long bones, optic glioma, and plexiform neurofibroma. NF2 is characterized by the occurrence of acoustic neuromas, usually bilaterally. In addition, meningiomas, schwannomas, gliomas, and juvenile posterior subcapsular cataracts occur in this disorder.

The two disorders are very distinct in their clinical features and are caused by mutation of genes on two different chromosomes. The gene for NF1 is located on the long arm of chromosome 17 (2–5), and the gene for NF2 is located on the long arm of chromosome 22 (6,7). There is very little overlap. An argument can be made that more harm than good is done by applying the term neurofibromatosis to both. For example, individuals with NF1 do not have sufficient risk of acoustic neuromas to warrant routine hearing tests. Likewise, pheochromocytoma (a tumor of the adrenal gland) does not occur in NF2. There are other syndromes (multiple endocrine neoplasia type 3, or multiple mucosal neuroma syndrome and the NAME [*n*evi, *a*trial myxoma, *m*yxoid

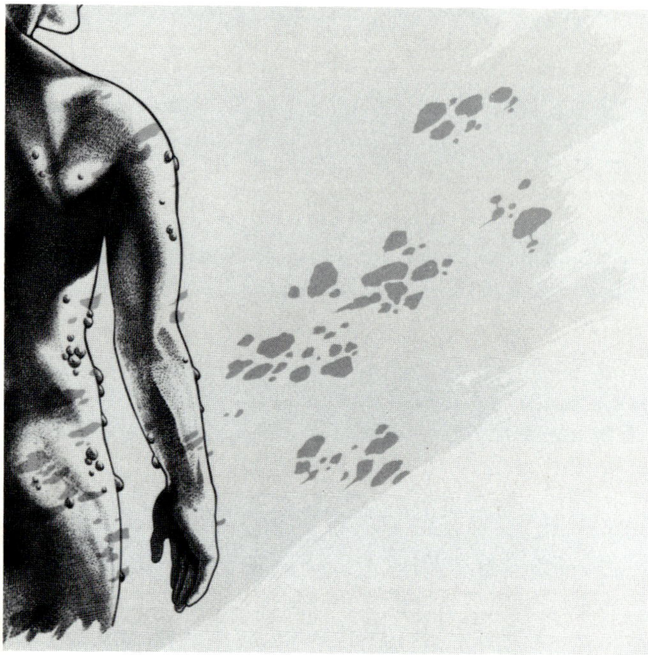

Figure 1–1. Logo for the 1987 National Institutes of Health Consensus Development Conference on NF, designed and executed by graphic artists Scott Pollard and Trudy Nicholson, with consultation by Dr. N. Myrianthopolous.

neurofibromata, and *e*phelides] syndrome) that have more overlap with NF1 than does NF2. Moreover, NF still evokes the image of "Elephant Man," and, when applied to NF2, may stigmatize individuals who may be denied health and life insurance because of the confusion with NF1. Finally, as pointed out in

Table 1–1. Comparison of Major Characteristics of Neurofibromatosis Type 1 (NF1) and Type 2 (NF2)

	NF1	NF2
Frequency	1/4000	1/40,000
Inheritance	Autolomal dominant	Autolomal dominant
Chromosomal location	17	22
Skin	Café au lait spots, skin-fold freckles, neurofibromas	Rare café au lait spots and neurofibromas
Tumors	Neurofibromas, optic gliomas, gliomas	Acoustic neuromas, schwannomas, meningiomas
Eye	Lisch nodules	Posterior subcapsular cataract
Cognitive impairment	Learning disabilities	None

Chapter 3, the term acoustic neuroma is technically wrong, because the tumor is actually a schwannoma of the vestibular nerve.

History

Just a few books have been written exclusively about NF (Table 1–2), but the pace of research and writing is quickening.

The earliest recognized portrayal of a man with NF is possibly in a nearly 13th century Syrian illustration, attributed to a scribe named Heinricus, in a Cistercian abbey in Austria. To diagrams of amphibia, a different hand, probably working at a later time, added a man with skin nodules suggestive of NF1. In a 1785 article entitled, "Observations on Cancers" (8), British physician Mark Akenside noted a man of some 60 years who had

> a constant succession of wens that shot out in several places, on his head, trunk, arms, and legs; which indisposition he inherited from his father. As often as one

Table 1–2. Books on Neurofibromatosis

YEAR	AUTHORS	TITLE	REFERENCE
1882	Recklinghausen, F.V.	Ueber die multiplen Fibrome der Haut und ihre Beiehung zu den multiplen Neuromen.	10
1900	Thomson, A.	On neuroma and neurofibromatosis.	11
1951	Borberg, A	Clinical and genetic investigations into tuberous sclerosis and Recklinghausen's neurofibromatosis.	30
1956	Crowe, F.W., Schull, W.J., Neel, J.V.	A clinical, pathological, and genetic study of multiple neurofibromatosis.	31
1972	Savitzky, V.A., Chereponov, A.N.	Recklinghausen's neurofibromatosis.	32
1981	Riccardi, V.M., Mulvihill, J.J.	Neurofibromatosis (von Recklinghausen's disease): Genetics, cell biology, and biochemistry.	33
1981	Samuelsson, B.	Neurofibromatosis (von Recklinghausen's disease). A clinical-psychiatric and genetic study.	34
1986	Rubenstein, A.E., Bunge, R., Housman, D.E.	Neurofibromatosis.	35
1986	Richardi, V.M., Eichner, J.E.	Neurofibromatosis: Phenotype, natural history and pathogenesis.	36

> of these wens became inconvenient from their size, his method was to cut them off with a razor; at which times, he constantly found that they grew upon the part by five or six suckers, as he called them.[8]

An additional 18th century report (in Latin and German) was made by Tilesius (9), in 1793, on a patient, called the Wart Man, with multiple fibrous tumors of the skin, under the title, "Case History of Extraordinarily Unsightly Skin" (Fig. 1–2).

Just over a century ago, Frederich Daniel von Recklinghausen (Fig. 1–3) released his memorial monograph (10) on the 25th anniversary of the founding of the Berlin Pathologic Institute, established by his mentor Rudolf Virchow, the father of pathology. The 125-page volume was based on two new cases, but has 168 citations of prior publications. Von Recklinghausen's contribution that attached his name to the disorder was in correctly identifying the intense comingling of nerve cells with fibrous tissue in the multiple cutaneous and deeper neurofibromas (which, incidentally, he sometimes called "fibroneuromas"!).

The case report literature had grown so that by 1900, Thomson (11), in the first English language monograph on the disease, said the bibliography was truly "an embarrassment of riches." Additional authors given pioneering credit for various observations are enumerated in Table 1–3.

The history of NF2 mingled with that of NF1, until just recently. If one wanted to suggest an eponymic designation, one could choose the term Wishart-Gardner-Young syndrome: Wishart in 1822 (12) had a patient with multiple intracranial meningiomas and cranial nerve tumors, including acoustic neuromas; Gardner and Frazier in 1930 (13) reported five generations of a family

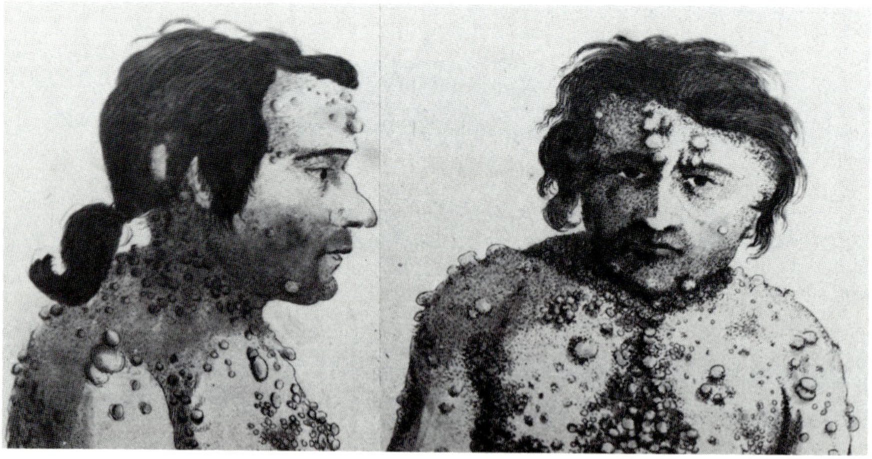

Figure 1–2. Detail of drawings of Johann Gottfried Rheinhard, who was called Wart Man by Professor Christian Friedrech Ludwig. Original drawings are in color in the 1793 report by Tilesius, a student of Ludwig's.

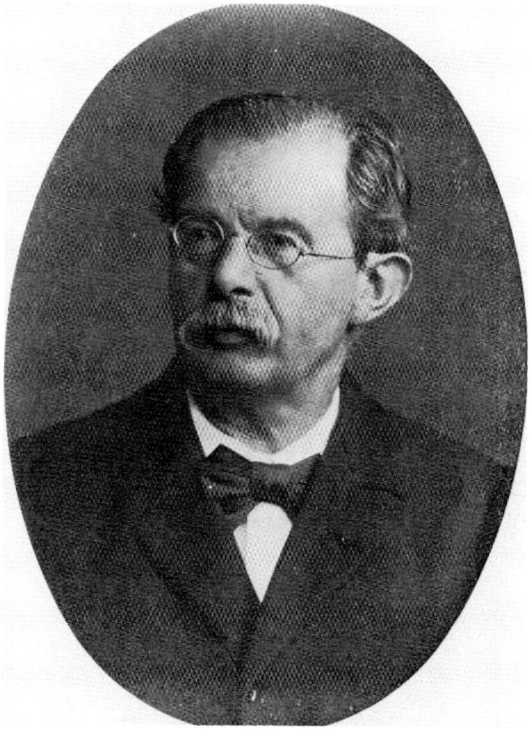

Figure 1–3. Friedrich Daniel von Recklinghausen (1833–1910, Professor of Pathology, Strassburg), around the time when he wrote his monograph, *On Multiple Neurofibromas of the Skin and Their Relationship to Multiple Neuromas.* (Courtesy of the National Library of Medicine.)

Table 1-3. Landmarks in Neurofibromatosis

DATE	NAME	LANDMARK
1200s	Heinricus	A Cistercian monk who illustrated amphibians, and, perhaps as a later addition, included a man possibly with NF1.
1592	Aldrovandi	Observed a case of elephantiasis neuromatosa in an Indian man of short stature.
1768	Akenside	Published first English-language description of NF1.
1793	Tilesius	In Latin and German, described a patient with multiple fibrous tumors on the skin.
1822	Wishart	Reported a patient with multiple intracranial meningiomas and cranial nerve tumors, including acoustic neuromas.
1830	Schwann	Described the nerve sheath cell that later was appreciated as the predominant cell in the tumors of NF.

(*Cont.*)

Table 1-3. *Continued*

DATE	NAME	LANDMARK
1847	Virchow	Reported NF in multiple family members.
1863	Virchow	Described the pathology of peripheral nerve tumors, differentiating between nerve sheath tumors and nerve tumors.
1870	Genersich	Reported a patient with kyphoscoliosis.
1873	von Michel	Reported a patient with optic glioma.
1882	von Recklinghausen	Recognized the relationship of multiple "false neuromas" with tumors of the skin; coined the term neurofibroma; believed that skin tumors arose from fibrous connective tissue sheath of small nerves; said NF was not acquired.
1896	Chauffard, Marre, Bernard	Identified pigmentary changes as a primary aspect of the disease.
1900	Thomson	Assembled reports of familial instances.
1901	Adrian	Noted high incidence of skeletal changes, such as atrophy, hypertrophy, and scoliosis.
1909	Suzuki	Reported a patient with pheochromocytoma.
1910	Verocay	Found that the nerve sheath proliferated; postulated that it was this cell that provided tumors in NF.
1916	Henshen	Identified the high incidence of bilateral acoustic neuromas associated with NF.
1918	Prieser, Davenport	Established that NF is not sex-linked and followed mendelian law as dominant trait.
1924	Harrison	Identified the neural crest origin of Schwann cells.
1931	Hosoi	Identified the association of malignant nerve sheath tumors with NF.
1937	Lisch	Put description by Goldstein and Wexler of iris nodules (Lisch spots) in patients with NF1 into proper perspective.
1940	Davis	Established optic glioma as a part of NF.
1945	Reubi	Identified large and small arteriovascular pathology as part of NF.
1956	Crowe, Schull, Neel	Determined the diagnostic importance of café au lait macules in NF.
1971	Fialkow	Proved multiple cell origin of neurofibromas.
1978	Rubenstein, Courtemanche	Formally established the National Neurofibromatosis Foundation.
1982	National Neurofibromatosis Foundation	Awarded its first research grants for the study of NF.
1987	Barker et al., Seizinger, et al.	NF1 gene assignment to chromosome 17 by linkage to DNA marker in family studies; NF2 gene assigned to chromosome 22 by analysis of tumor DNA and family study.
1989	National Neurofibromatosis Foundation	Support of first project to provide prenatal and presymptomatic diagnosis of NF1.

with bilateral deafness in 38 members; and Young et al. in 1971 (14) updated the kindred and added new observations.

THE ELEPHANT MAN, JOSEPH MERRICK

The Elephant Man has long been the epitome of NF1 (Table 1–4). This infamous example, now known to be wrong, has served patients with the disorder and their relatives well by being a focus for new attention by the public and biomedical researchers on this much neglected disorder. What an irony that it seems certain that, as discussed below, he did not have NF1! Sir Frederick Treves believed that at age 50 years surgeons should put down their scalpel, and he took up the pen to record some of his memorable patients. One (15) was that of a man he placed in London Hospital for 3 years, having discovered him as a freak in the back room of a green grocer. Recounting his story some 30 years after the patient's death (16), Sir Frederick erroneously called his patient John, not Joseph Merrick, as is known from his birth certificate. Regardless, his account was the basis for an extended essay by Ashley Montague (17), who dwelt on the human splendor and dignity that radiated from the deformed by spirited Joseph Merrick.

The celebrated British dermatologist, F. Parkes Weber, first suggested that the Elephant Man had von Recklinghausen disease (18), a suggestion never made by Treves. Weber listed Treves' case last in a miscellaneous category of

Table 1–4. The Story of Joseph Merrick

YEAR	AUTHORS	TITLE	REFERENCE
1885	Treves, F.	A case of congenital deformity.	15
1909	Weber, F.P.	Cutaneous pigmentations as an incomplete form of Recklinghausen's disease, with remarks on the classification of incomplete and anomalous forms of Recklinghausen's disease.	18
1923	Treves, F.	The Elephant Man and other reminiscenses.	16
1979	Montague, A.	The Elephant Man. A study in human dignity.	17
1979	Pomerance, B.	The Elephant Man.	37
1980	Howell, M., Ford, P.	The true history of the Elephant Man.	38
1982	Felson, B., Bean, W.B., Dolan, K.D.	A nonletter from the editor and a case for all seasons.	19
1986	Tibbles, J.A.R., Cohen, M.M., Seward, G.R.	The Porteus syndrome: The Elephant Man diagnosed.	20

incomplete and anomalous forms of von Recklinghausen disease. None of the records indicate that Merrick had pigmentary changes, almost universal in NF1, and his deformities were certainly greater than ever seen by clinicians involved with current patients. Nonetheless, the suggestion was unchallenged until 1982, when a senior American physician and two radiologists examined the record and the skeleton (19). They made the suggestion that Joseph Merrick had, in fact, three diseases: NF; mono-ostotic fibrous dysplasia, to account for the great scalp deformity; and tuberculosis of the hip, resulting in severe hip deformity and limp.

Independently, two geneticists working in Canada saw the great parallels between the newly recognized multiple malformation syndrome, called the Proteus syndrome, and the case of Joseph Merrick (20), although reservation about that diagnosis has been raised. In any case, newly diagnosed patients and their families should know that respected diagnosticians feel that Merrick did not, in fact, have just NF, if he had it at all. There is no reason to fear that their disorder, NF1, could result in such severe and lethal deformities as the Elephant Man's.

THEORIES OF PATHOGENESIS

How does one mutant gene cause NF1 and another NF2? By what route does a mutant gene on chromosome 17 result in café au lait macules of the skin, plexiform neurofibromas of large nerves, large head, pheochromocytoma, fibrous dysplasia of bone, and optic glioma? How does a mutation on chromosome 22 give rise to independent tumors of the eighth cranial nerve, multiple neurofibromas of the cervical spine, and juvenile posterior cataracts?

Trying to bring all the facets of just NF1 into a unified hypothesis has been frustrating, but nonetheless worthwhile as a way to focus research efforts. Many areas of active basic biological research relate to the NFs, but exactly which field will contribute a fundamental insight and when it will come remain uncertain. Areas of investigation involve the embryonic neural crest, Schwann cell biology, nerve growth factors and receptors, mast cell biology, oncogenes, bone formation, melanin regulation, and potential animal models.

Robert Bolande, a pediatric pathologist, termed NF "the quintessential neurocristopathy" (21). Specifically, many features of NF seem to represent abnormal development of body organs and tissues that develop from the transient collection of cells called the embryonic neural crest. Such cells are seen as a discrete tissue only in the embryo where they arise from the lateral ridges of the early neural plate. They can be recognized under the microscope by their peculiar reactions to various stains that indicate they have many chemicals relating to nerve cell communication and neuroendocrine function. Through basic embryological research on quail and chickens (and with confirmatory, although limited observations in human beings), these cells are known to disperse in fetal life and migrate to multiple organs throughout the adult body. They become pigmented cells in the skin and neurosecretory cells of the adrenal medulla and other endocrine organs. They help form the bones and the connective tissue of the head and face. They infiltrate the peripheral nervous system and become, among other things, Schwann cells of the nerves and neurons of the autonomic nervous system. Because many features of NF seem to derive from the neural crest, the neurocristopathy hypothesis is attractive: the occurrence of café au lait macules, pheochromocytoma, schwannomas, and skull defects. Apparent contradictions to the theory deserve exploration, such as the excess of rhabdomyosarcoma and nonlymphocytic leukemias (malignancies not thought to be derived from the neural crest), osseous dysplasia of long bones, and scoliosis.

Neurofibromas are known to be a mixture of fibroblasts, Schwann cells, and perineurial cells, and may well result from abnormal interaction of Schwann cells with their environment. Various laboratories using in vitro systems have explored the control of Schwann cell proliferation and have identified cells and chemicals that modulate their behavior. As a generalization, neurofibromas grown in tissue culture tend to polarize toward fibroblast-like cells (22). The Schwann cell cultures produce laminin and the various collagens (23), some of which stimulate Schwann cell proliferation.

One specific substance that has been of enduring interest is nerve growth factor, a protein normally involved in the development, maintenance, and regulation of the nervous system. Early quantification of nerve growth factor in sera showed that it was increased in patients with NF1 according to a functional bioassay (24) and in those with NF2 by an antigenic immunoassay (25). Schwann cells have been shown to have receptors for nerve growth factor. Genetic linkage studies proved that the NF1 gene is not near the beta nerve growth factor gene on chromosome 1 (5). It is located near the receptor for nerve growth factor on chromosome 17, but genetic linkage studies showed that this gene is distinct from that responsible for NF1 (3).

At present, it seems most likely that insights into the pathogenesis of both forms of NF will follow from identification and study of the genes responsible for the disorders. The current status of that work is described in detail in Chapter 16.

The research summarized depends on analysis of samples from NF patients. An alternate strategy emphasizes the development of an animal model for NF. In cattle, multiple neurofibromas are seen but are not known to be hereditary. A colony of goldfish in a pond on the campus of Western Reserve University, Cleveland, was found to have neurofibromas and schwannomas. In coral reefs off the Florida Keys, some, but not all, colonies of bicolor damselfish have high rates of pigmented and nonpigmented Schwann cell tumors, up to 20% in certain populations (26). Minute doses of ethylnitrosourea given to pregnant rats or newborn pups results in many adolescent rats with schwannomas, especially of the trigeminal nerve (27). Recently, the *tat* gene of human lymphotrophic virus 1 (HTLV1) was experimentally introduced into mice. A dominantly inherited transgenic animal line was established with a high frequency of perineurial fibromas (28) (Fig. 1–4).

CONCLUSION

In conclusion, no single theory of pathogenesis seems sufficient to explain all manifestations of the two common syndromes of NF. Current strategies depend on progress in diverse fields of very active biomedical research. Many of these approaches depend on the availability of fresh tumor specimens, both benign and malignant, from patients with NF. Hence, whenever a NF patient is undergoing surgery, the question should be asked before the operation about

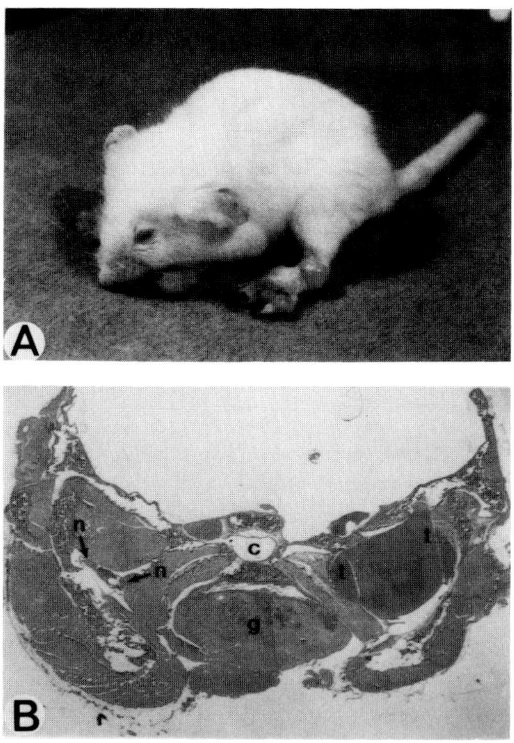

Figure 1–4. **(A)** Four-and-one-half-month old male mouse with multiple tumors of the front and hind legs, ears, and tail. **(B)** Cross section from a female mouse from the same line with large tumors (t), on the right, replacing normal nerve trunks and, on left, compressing surrounding muscles. c = nose, g = tongue, n = mouth. (Reprinted from Science 237:1341, 1987, Copyright 1987 by the American Association for the Advancement of Science, with author's and publisher's permission.)

whether or not part of the operative specimen could be obtained for research purposes.

REFERENCES

1. D.A. Stumpf, J.F. Alksne, J.F. Annegers, et al. Neurofibromatosis. Arch Neurol 1988;45:575–578.
2. D. Barker, E. Wright, K. Nguyen, et al. Gene for von Recklinghausen neurofibromatosis is in the pericentromeric region of chromosome 17. Science 1987;236:1098–1102.
3. R.R. Seizinger, G.A. Rouleau, L.J. Ozelius, et al. Genetic linkage of von Recklinghausen neurofibromatosis to the nerve growth factor receptor gene. Cell 1987;49:589–594.
4. F.S. Collins, B.A.J. Ponder, B.R. Seizinger, and C.J. Epstein. The von Recklinghausen neurofibromatosis region on chromosome 17—Genetic and physical maps come into focus. Am J Hum Genet 1989;44:1–5.
5. D.E. Goldgar, P. Green, D.M. Parry, and J.J. Mulvihill. Multipoint linkage analysis in neurofibromatosis type I: An international collaboration. Am J Hum Genet 1989;44:6–12.
6. G.A. Rouleau, W. Wertelecki, J.L. Haines, et al. Genetic linkage of bilateral acoustic neurofibromatosis to a DNA marker on chromosome 22. Nature 1987;329:246–248.
7. W. Wertelecki, G.A. Rouleau, D.W. Superneau, et al. Neurofibromatosis 2: Clinical and DNA linkage studies of a large kindred. N Engl J Med 1988;319:278–283.
8. M. Akenside. Observations on cancers. Med Trans Coll Physicians London 1785;1:64–92.
9. W.G. von Tilesius. Historia Pathologica Singularis Cutis Turpitudinis J. Godofredi Rheinhardi Viri 50 Annorum. Leipzig, S.L. Crusius, 1793.
10. F.D. von Recklinghausen. Ueber die multiplen Fibrome der Haut und ihre Beziehung zu den multiplen Neuromen. Berlin, Hirschwald, 1882.
11. A. Thomson. On neuroma and neurofibromatosis. Edinburgh, Turnbull & Spears, 1900.
12. J.H. Wishart. Case of tumours in the skull, dura mater, and brain. Edinburgh Med Surg J 1822;18:393–397.
13. W.J. Gardner and C.H. Frazier. Bilateral acoustic neurofibromatosis: A clinical study and field survey of a family of five generations with bilateral deafness in thirty-eight members. Arch Neurol Psychiatry 1930;23:266–302.
14. D.F. Young, R. Eldridge, G.T. Nager, et al. Hereditary bilateral acoustic neuroma (central neurofibromatosis). Birth Defects 1971;7:73–86.
15. F. Treves. A case of congenital deformity. Trans Pathol Soc London 1885;36:494–498.
16. F. Treves. The Elephant Man and other reminiscences. London, Cassell, 1923.
17. A. Montague. The Elephant Man. A study in human dignity. London, E.P. Dutton, 1979.
18. F.P. Weber. Cutaneous pigmentations as an incomplete form of Recklinghausen's disease, with remarks on the classification of incomplete and anomalous forms of Recklinghausen's disease. Br J Dermatol 1909;21:49–53.
19. B. Felson, W.B. Bean, and K.D. Dolan. A nonletter from the editor and a case for all seasons. Sem Roentgenol 1982;17:153–162.
20. J.A.R. Tibbles and M.M. Cohen. The Proteus syndrome: The Elephant Man diagnosed. Br Med J 1986;293:683–685.
21. R.P. Bolande. 1981. Neurofibromatosis—The quintessential neurocristopathy: Pathogenic concepts and relationships. Adv Neurol 1981;29:67–75.

22. J. Peltonen, H. Aho, U.K. Rinne, and R. Penttinen. Neurofibromatosis tumor and skin cells in culture. Acta Neuropathol 1983;61:275–282.
23. J. Peltonen, S. Jaakkola, M. Lebwohl, et al. Cellular differentiation and expression of matrix genes in type 1 neurofibromatosis. Lab Invest 1988;59:760–771.
24. R.N. Fabricant and G.J. Todaro. Increased serum levels of nerve growth factor in von Recklinghausen's disease. Arch Neurol 1981;38:401–405.
25. R.N. Fabricant, G.J. Todaro, and R. Eldridge. Increased levels of a nerve-growth-factor cross-reacting protein in "central" neurofibromatosis. Lancet 1979;1:4–7.
26. M.C. Schmale, G. Hensley, and L.R. Udey. Animal model of human disease: Neurofibromatosis, von Recklinghausen's disease, multiple schwannomas, malignant schwannomas. Am J Pathol 1983;112:238–241.
27. A. Koestner, J.A. Swenberg, and W. Wechsler. Transplacental production with ethylnitrosourea of neoplasms of the nervous system in Sprague-Dawley rats. Am J Pathol 1971;63:37–50.
28. S.H. Hinrichs, M. Nerenberg, R.K. Reynolds, et al. A transgenic mouse model for human neurofibromatosis. 1987;237:1340–1344.

SECTION I

MEDICAL ASPECTS

2

Diagnosis of Neurofibromatosis and Clinical Overview

Bruce R. Korf, M.D., Ph.D.

The care of persons with neurofibromatosis (NF) is made complex by the wide range of expression of the disorder. First, there are at least two forms of NF, each of which affects the body in a wide variety of ways. Even among those with the same form of NF it is difficult to predict the specific problems that will occur in a particular individual. Moreover, ignorance about the basic pathogenetic mechanisms of NF has so far left us unable to prevent or reverse significant medical complications. Instead, patient management focuses on accurate diagnosis and medical surveillance to detect and manage complications as early as possible.

This chapter will provide an overview of the clinical approach to NF. It will attempt to summarize some areas of general agreement among clinicians, and place into perspective some areas of controversy. It is hoped that this will provide a basis for making some of the very complex choices which face both care providers and patients in dealing with NF.

Diagnosis of Neurofibromatosis

Classification

As described in Chapter 1, there are at least two distinct forms of NF, now called NF1 and NF2, according to recommendations made by the National Institutes of Health (NIH) Consensus Development Conference in July 1987 (1). NF1 has also been referred to as von Recklinghausen NF, or peripheral NF, and NF2 has been called central NF or bilateral acoustic NF. In spite of some overlap in their manifestations, the two disorders are known to be different because the responsible genes are on two different chromosomes: chromosome 17 for NF1 and chromosome 22 for NF2.

It has been proposed that in addition to NF1 and NF2, there exist a number of other forms of NF (2,3). Some of these forms may be "allelic variants" of NF, in which the alteration of the gene for NF1 or NF2 differs from that which occurs in most people with NF. Others may simply represent rare manifestations of one of the common forms of NF. Proof that there are additional distinct genetic loci which can result in NF-like disorders will require additional research to define the genetic basis of these disorders. Most people with NF fit fairly well into the NF1 and NF2 categories; those who do not should be followed closely without being forced into inappropriate descriptive labels until more powerful diagnostic tools are available.

Two proposed variants of NF deserve special mention. One has been referred to as segmental neurofibromatosis. This label has been applied to individuals who have features of NF1 confined to a single body region such as a limb or a portion of the trunk (4–7). The affected segment may have only multiple neurofibromas, or pigmentary manifestations of NF as well. It has been speculated that segmental NF represents somatic mutation of the NF gene; that is, the NF mutation occurred after fertilization and involves only a portion of the body. Alternatively, some persons with NF1 may, by chance, have involvement limited to a small region of the body. It is currently impossible to decide between these hypotheses. Although most cases of segmental neurofibromatosis have been sporadic, as would be expected for a somatic mutation, one cannot be so sure that this will invariably be the case as to counsel an affected individual that there is no risk of transmitting NF to a child.

The other entity that may represent a distinct form of NF is the neurofibromatosis-Noonan syndrome. Noonan syndrome is a separate genetic disorder characterized by short stature, congenital heart disease, and distinctive facial features. A number of people have been reported recently in whom features of NF and Noonan syndrome coexist (8–12). It is not known whether this represents a coincidental occurrence of two disorders in the same individuals or a distinct new disorder that combines features of both. It is also possible that genes for the two conditions are somehow simultaneously disrupted by a single mutation.

Diagnostic Criteria

The diagnosis of NF is based on clinical criteria. So far no laboratory test can provide a definite diagnosis, although in some instances x-ray or biopsies may be suggested to provide information that may help in establishing a diagnosis. The diagnostic criteria for NF1 and NF2 recommended by the NIH Consensus Conference are presented in Tables 2–1 and 2–2. It should be stressed that these are not intended to strictly rule in or out a diagnosis of NF. The criteria are not all-inclusive, and many of the clinical features are age-dependent. Also, the requirement that at least two features be present is somewhat arbitrary. This requirement avoids mislabeling some people who have only a single

Table 2-1. Diagnosis of Neurofibromatosis Type 1

Six or more café au laut macules over 5 mm in greatest diameter in prepubertal individuals and over 15 mm in greatest diameter in postpubertal individuals
Two or more neurofibromas of any type or one plexiform neurofibroma
Freckling in the axillary or inguinal regions
Optic glioma
Two or more Lisch nodules (iris harmartomas)
A distinctive osseous lesion such as sphenoid dysplasia or thinning of long bone cortex with or without pseudoarthrosis
A first-degree relative (parent, sibling, or offspring) with NF1 by the above criteria

The diagnostic criteria are met in an individual if two or more of the features listed are present.

feature, such as café au lait spots, although in fact some of these people do have NF. An individual who fulfills the diagnostic criteria can confidently be said to be affected, but in someone who has only one of the listed features, the diagnosis cannot be considered either established or ruled out. It should also be noted that no single feature is pathognomonic for NF1, and therefore at least two features from the list must be present to make a diagnosis.

The diagnosis of NF1 is most commonly suggested by cutaneous features (4,13). Café au lait spots (Fig. 2–1) may be present at birth, but often are not noticed until after the first few months of life. There is no relationship between their location and the occurrence of other NF-related lesions, or between their number and the severity of NF. It is not uncommon to see up to six café au lait spots in people without NF (4,14,15) and even six or more have been reported in some people who apparently are not affected (16). Freckling within skin folds appears to be highly specific for NF1 (17). It appears in later childhood, and is best seen under the arms or in the groins (Fig. 2–2). Occasionally there is a diffuse freckling and "bronzing" of the skin in adults with NF1.

Neurofibromas are most often first seen on the skin, where they usually appear as small raised nodules (Fig. 2–3), which are soft to the touch and have

Table 2-2. Diagnosis of Neurofibromatosis Type 2

1. Bilateral masses of the eighth cranial nerve seen with appropriate imaging techniques (e.g., CT or MRI)
   or
2. A first-degree with NF2 and either:
   a. Unilaterial mass of the eighth cranial nerve, or
   b. Two of the following:
      Neurofibroma
      Meningioma
      Glioma
      Schwannoma
      Juvenile posterior subcapsular lenticular opacity

The criteria are met by an individual who satisfies condition 1 or 2.

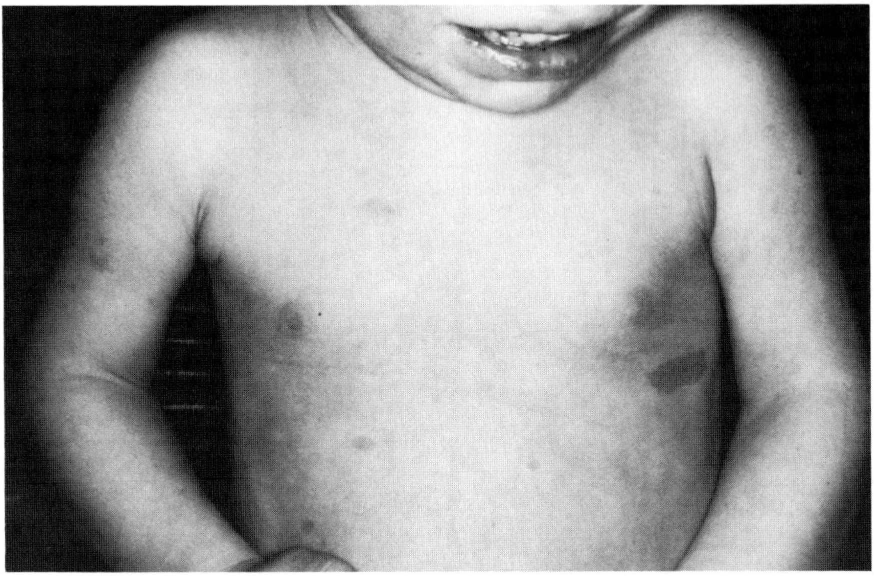

Figure 2–1. Café au lait spots on the chest of a child with NF1. A large spot is seen under the left nipple, and several smaller spots are seen elsewhere on the chest.

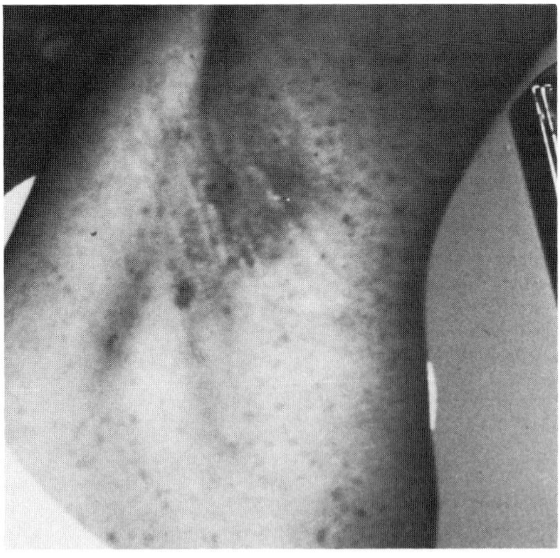

Figure 2–2. Freckling under the arm of an adult with NF1.

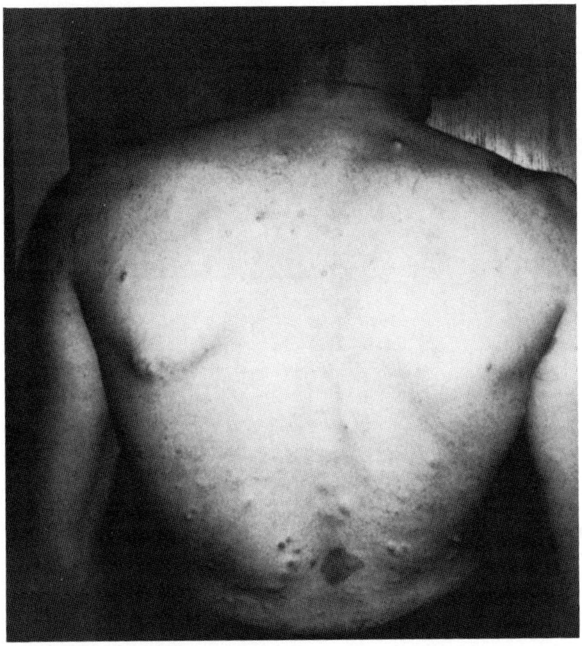

Figure 2–3. Multiple cutaneous neurofibromas on the back of an adult with NF1. Several café au lait spots are also visible.

a pink or purple hue. They can appear at any time in life, but most commonly not until late childhood or adolescence. Plexiform neurofibromas, in which multiple fascicles of a large bundle of nerves are diffusely thickened with neurofibroma-like growth, are often congenital. They appear as a soft-tissue mass under the skin, often following the course of a peripheral nerve. There may be hypertrophy or deformity of an involved part of the body and diffuse hyperpigmentation of the overlying skin (Fig. 2–4) (16). The occurrence of a single neurofibroma is well documented in people with no other stigmata of NF, which is why two neurofibromas are required as a diagnostic feature. The plexiform neurofibroma is more distinctive and only one is required to fulfill this criterion.

Lisch nodules (Fig. 2–5) are clumps of pigment cells that occur on the iris of the eye in many people with NF1 (18–21). They usually appear in late childhood, and require the use of a slit lamp to be detected and distinguished from iris nevi. The latter occur on many people and are not indicative of NF. Lisch nodules do not interfere with vision. Their detection often provides the basis for confirming a diagnosis in an individual suspected of having NF1 because of multiple café au lait spots.

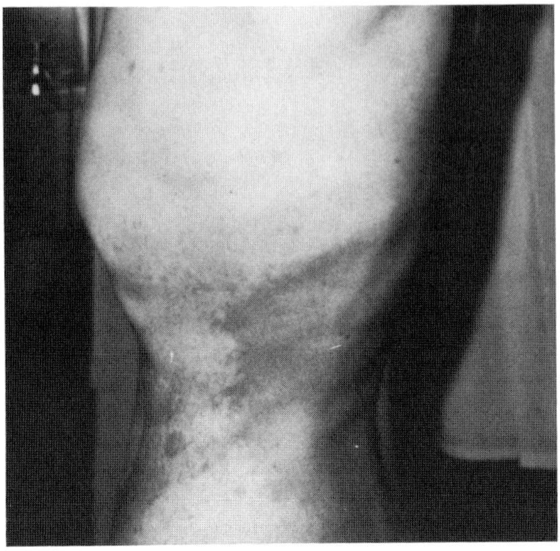

Figure 2–4. Hyperpigmentation associated with underlying plexiform neurofibroma.

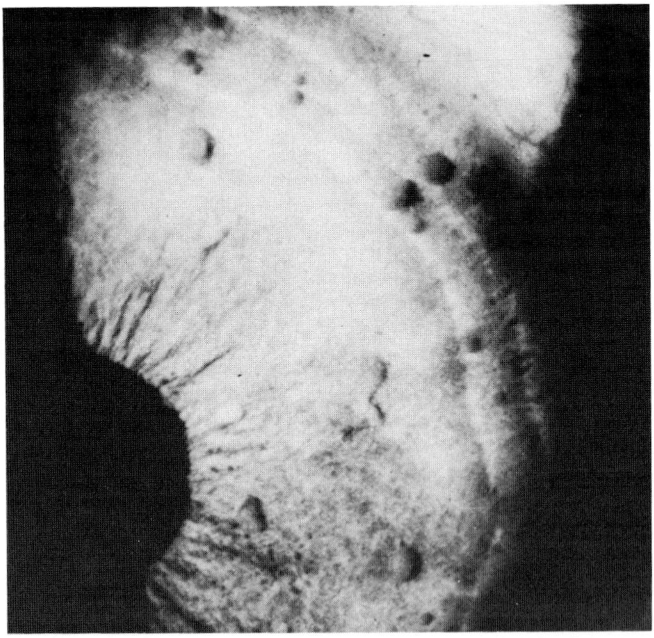

Figure 2–5. Iris Lisch nodules photographed through a slit lamp. (Photograph courtesy of Dr. Jane Kivlin, and reprinted from Postgraduate Medicine, 83:79–85, 1988, with permission of the publisher.)

Optic glioma and distinctive osseous lesions are listed as diagnostic criteria because their occurrence should suggest the possible diagnosis of NF1. People with optic glioma have thickening of the optic nerve due to the presence of excessive abnormal glial tissue (22) (Fig. 2–6). In some instances these gliomas cause interference with vision or neurological problems, but most often they cause no trouble at all. Optic glioma can occur without NF, but thickening of the optic nerve, usually without symptoms, is common in NF1 (23). Computed tomography (CT) or magnetic resonance imaging (MRI) scanning is useful in establishing the presence of optic glioma in an individual with clinical evidence of such a lesion.

Likewise, bony abnormalities (Fig. 2–7) such as dysplasia of a long bone or the sphenoid wing can be useful diagnostic clues if they are clinically evident (24). These skeletal abnormalities are fairly distinctive in NF, but have been seen in people without the disorder in rare instances.

The occurrence of a first-degree relative affected with NF fulfills one diagnostic criterion. It is important, therefore, to examine these relatives (parents, sibs, offspring) as part of the evaluation of any individual for NF. Obviously, the affected relative must fulfill at least two clinical criteria other than positive family history. It is not unusual to identify subtle signs of NF1 in a family member who was hitherto unaware that they were affected with the disorder (25).

In summary, a diagnostic evaluation for NF1 includes a careful history and examination for café au lait spots, skin freckling, neurofibromas, Lisch nodules, bony deformities, and ocular or neurological problems. Laboratory tests or x-rays are used only if clinical findings raise suspicion that a specific lesion is present. Occasionally it may be useful to biopsy a skin lesion suspected of being a neurofibroma, to confirm this by histological examination. Biopsy of

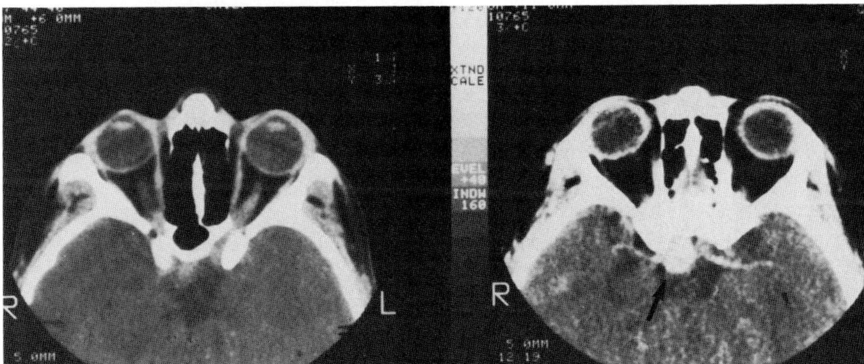

Figure 2–6. CT scans from individual with NF1 and optic glioma. Both optic nerves are thickened, and there is lucency and increased uptake of contrast in the chiasm (arrow).

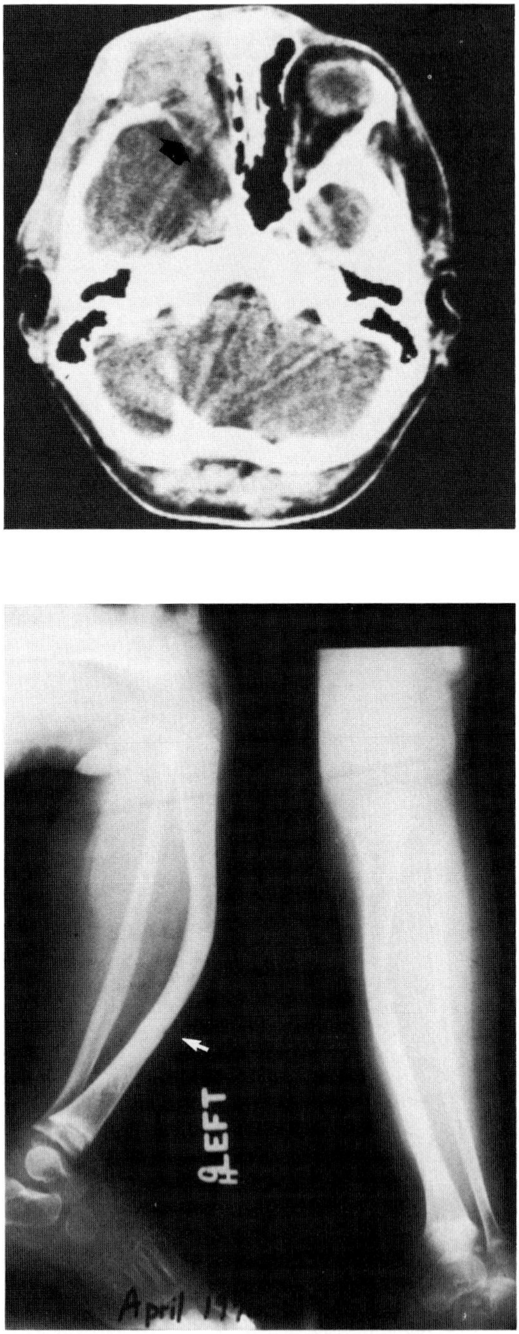

A

B

Figure 2–7. (A) Absence of the sphenoid wing (arrow) in patient with NF1. (B) Bowing of the tibia (lateral and frontal view) with fracture (arrow).

café au lait spots does reveal distinctive features (26), but these have not been established as a reliable means of identifying café au lait spots as being caused by NF.

The diagnosis of NF2 is established in any individual with bilateral masses of the eighth cranial nerve (Table 2–2). These, however, may not be evident until well after the first decade, and even later in many. The diagnosis may be made earlier in people with an affected first-degree relative who also have one of the features listed in Table 2–2. A distinctive cataract occurring in the first two decades of life has recently been reported in many people with NF2 (27) and may aid in making the diagnosis.

MEDICAL CARE OF PEOPLE WITH NEUROFIBROMATOSIS

There is no single "correct" approach to providing care to persons with NF. The cardinal principles are to help the individual adjust to living with the condition and to offer the best available medical treatment for specific complications. The task begins with accurate diagnosis, and open communications both between health-care providers and affected individuals and among health-care providers themselves. The burden of NF is made greater when care providers lack familiarity with the disorder or do not coordinate their efforts.

Severity of Neurofibromatosis

When the diagnosis of NF is first suggested, many people panic on learning of the potential for severe, even life-threatening complications. To some extent their reaction is influenced by any prior experience with the disorder in other family members, and the severity of the manifestations at the time of diagnosis. In general, people with NF should be reassured with a number of facts. First, the majority of affected individuals have few or no medical problems related to their condition. Subtly affected people generally do not come to medical attention as having NF (13,25), and therefore do not get included in medical statistics on rates of complications. Such statistics invariably overestimate the rate of specific problems, especially the more severe ones. For every person who comes to the doctor with signs of NF, there are many who have only minor skin stigmata and are never diagnosed.

Second, many of the severe complications of NF, particularly those leading to major deformities, are congenital. Therefore, a child or adult in whom the diagnosis is made will not suddenly develop such a deformity if it is not already present. This is not to say that cosmetically objectionable neurofibromas might not someday develop, but significant bony deformities are unlikely to occur if examination fails to reveal some evidence for deformity already.

Finally, although there are many possible complications of NF, virtually no individual suffers from all of them. The physician must place the potential for developing medical problems into perspective, helping to provide care without leading the individual into a state of excessive dependency on the one hand or denial on the other. This is generally best achieved by an honest description of the clinical spectrum of NF-related problems, and a program of regular medical follow-up.

Principles of Medical Surveillance

There is some controversy among physicians regarding the most appropriate way to provide surveillance for NF-related problems. In many instances the uncertainty relates to the use of laboratory tests, and particularly imaging systems such as x-rays or MRI scans. Some advocate their use as screening tests because of a relatively high yield of abnormal findings (28,29), whereas others believe that such tests should only be used to investigate specific clinical signs or symptoms (1).

No general answer is possible to this question since the physician's approach must be individualized to the specific needs of each patient. This takes into account the medical facts as well as more subjective issues such as the needs of the patient for reassurance or the reliability of the history and examination in a particular case.

For people with NF2, there is clear benefit to early detection of acoustic neuromas. This is based on the possibility of preserving hearing if surgery is performed when tumors are small. Close monitoring of eighth nerve function by audiometry and brainstem auditory evoked response (BAER) testing is therefore recommended for these individuals, including first-degree relatives at risk for the disorder (1).

The Value of "NF Programs"

In recent years a number of "NF Programs" have been established at major medical centers. Although the specific formats differ, these commonly offer multidisciplinary assessment and medical follow-up to patients and family members. Typically included are medical services such as genetics, neurology, orthopedics, ophthalmology, hearing, psychology, and social services. Generally these programs do not substitute for an individual's primary physician, but serve as consultants for dealing with problems related to NF.

NF Programs can be helpful in providing coordination of care for people with NF, and are a source of expertise in dealing with a relatively rare condition. They also provide an important resource for clinical research. Yet participation in an NF Program should not be considered an absolute necessity in obtaining care for NF. There are no services provided by an NF Program which cannot also be obtained from a qualified health-care provider who is familiar with NF. As long as conscientious medical follow-up is provided, an individual may be very well served by their regular family physician. Both physicians and patients should be aware of the resource of NF Programs, however, which can be helpful for consultation on specific problems. A list of

NF Programs associated with the National Neurofibromatosis Foundation is provided in the Appendix.

Recommendations for Care

Recommendations for care in NF1 and NF2, as suggested by the NIH Consensus Development Conference (1), are presented in Tables 2–3 and 2–4. These are proposed as general guidelines, with specific approaches depending on the clinical situation.

A common question concerns the appropriate follow-up for an individual in whom a diagnosis of NF is suspected but not proved. This arises especially often in children who have multiple café au lait spots. The presence of multiple café au lait spots fulfills one diagnostic criterion for NF1, but is not alone sufficient to establish the diagnosis. Therefore, if no other clinical features are found, including no affected first-degree relatives (both parents must be examined), the diagnosis of NF1 cannot be established. Yet many of the clinical features, such as skin-fold freckling, cutaneous neurofibromas, and Lisch nodules are age-dependent, and so the diagnosis also cannot be ruled out. In such an instance it is wise to provide regular medical follow-up on the assumption that the child is affected. This will ensure that potentially serious problems, such as symptomatic optic glioma, will not go undetected. Insofar as the suggested program of medical follow-up does not involve potentially dangerous or expensive testing, this approach is not harmful. Most of these children will develop other signs of NF1, confirming the diagnosis, over the years.

LIVING WITH NEUROFIBROMATOSIS

NF is a disorder, not a disease, and most people who are affected are healthy. Yet in spite of this, many affected individuals cannot escape a greater-

Table 2–3. Recommendation for Care of Individuals with Neurofibromatosis Type 1

History	Cognitive or psychomotor deficits, pain, vision problems, progressive neurological deficit, constipation
Examination	Hypertension, scoliosis, skeletal anomalies, macrocephaly, focal neurological deficits, developmental disabilities, proptosis, Lisch nodules, short stature, abnormal puberty, café au lait macules, neurofibromas
Tests	Dictated by findings on clinical evaluation
Counseling	Prognosis, genetics, psychosocial adjustment, family history, resources for support and information
Follow-up	Annual visits (more often if indicated) with a clinician familiar with the disorder.

Adapted from statement by NIH Consensus Development Conference on Neurofibromatosis, July 1987.

Table 2-4. Recommendation for Care of Individuals with Neurofibromatosis Type 2

History	Hearing loss, tinnitus, dizziness, loss of balance, pain, headache, seizures
Examination	Neurofibromas, café au lait macules, cranial nerves, balance, coordination
Tests	Audiogram and brainstem auditory evoked responses: MRI scan by puberty; tests of vestibular function; other tests dictated by clinical evaluation
Counseling	Prognosis, genetics, psychosocial adjustment, resources for support and information
Follow-up	Annual visits (more if indicated) with a clinician familiar with the disorder.

Adapted from statement by NIH Consensus Development Conference, July 1987.

than-average awareness of the fragility of life. Living with NF calls for inner strength, support from family and friends, as well as alert medical care.

Life Expectancy in Neurofibromatosis

Most people affected with NF die with their disorder rather than from it. Life-threatening complications do occur in people with NF, but fortunately this is the exception rather than the rule. Because of this, studies of life expectancy in people with NF who were not diagnosed because of some already existing medical problem have revealed a slightly decreased average life expectancy (30). This is mostly accounted for by the premature death of a minority of people at a young age due to rare NF-related problems. Most people with NF have a near-normal life expectancy, and should plan on living a full and reasonably healthy life.

Hope through Research

Research provides the major source of hope for many people with NF. The ultimate goal of this research is to provide means of preventing or treating the problems due to the disorder, as well as means of more accurate diagnosis. Recently, great progress has been made through the application of tools of molecular genetics, which permit study of the genetic basis of human disorders (see Chapter 16). The genes for NF1 and NF2 have been mapped, and efforts are now underway to identify the genes themselves.

To individuals afflicted with NF the pace of research cannot be fast enough. Indeed, at times it may seem that exciting findings are described too cautiously, and that the clinical application of these findings is too slow. It must be recognized, however, that the premature clinical use of unconfirmed data can at times be disastrous. The medical research community has evolved a mechanism for validating research results and testing new methods of treatment and diagnosis before allowing their use in people. The lay press is often not a reliable source of information about new advances in medicine. Questions about new approaches in NF are best addressed to one's health-care provider. The National Neurofibromatosis Foundation, through its Clinical Care Advisory Board, closely monitors current medical practice, and can also be a source of information.

CONCLUSION

NF has been known to medicine for over 100 years, yet our approach to the disorder still is largely empirical. Good medical care of people with NF consists essentially of the practice of good medicine, with particular alertness to the possibility of NF-related problems. In the coming years it is likely that research advances will significantly change our methods of diagnosing and treating the disorder, but our goal—helping affected individuals to adjust and live healthy and productive lives—will be the same.

REFERENCES

1. D.A. Stumpf, J.F. Alksne, J.F. Annegers, et al. Neurofibromatosis. Arch Neurol 1988;45:575–578.
2. V.M. Riccardi and J.E. Eichner. Neurofibromatosis: Phenotype, natural history, and pathogenesis. Baltimore, Johns Hopkins University Press, 1986.
3. V.M. Riccardi. Neurofibromatosis: Clinical heterogeneity. Curr Probl Cancer 1982;7:1–34.
4. F.W. Crowe, W.J. Schull, and J.V. Neel. A clinical, pathological, and genetic study of multiple neurofibromatosis. Springfield, IL, Charles C Thomas, 1956.
5. R.M. Miller and R.S. Sparkes. Segmental neurofibromatosis. Arch Dermatol 1977;113:837–838.
6. R.R. Roth, R. Martines, and W.D. James. Segmental neurofibromatosis. Arch Dermatol 1987;123:917–920.
7. C.E. Rawlings, III, R.H. Wilkins, W.A. Cook, and P.C. Burger. Segmental neurofibromatosis. Neurosurgery 1987;20:946–949.
8. J.M. Opitz and D.D. Weaver. The neurofibromatosis-Noonan syndrome. Am J Med Genet 1985;21:477–490.
9. H.M.M. Mendez, The neurofibromatosis-Noonan syndrome. Am J Med Genet 1985;21:471–476.
10. R.A. Saul. Noonan syndrome in a patient with hyperplasia of the myenteric plexuses and neurofibromatosis. Am J Med Genet 1985;21:491–492.
11. J.E. Allanson, J.G. Hall, and M.I. Van Allen. Noonan phenotype associated with neurofibromatosis. Am J Med Genet 1985;21:457–462.
12. A. Shuper, M. Mukamel, M. Mimouni, and R. Steinherz. Noonan's syndrome and neurofibromatosis. Arch Dis Child 1987;62:196–198.
13. S.M. Huson, P.S. Harper, and D.A.S. Compston. Von Recklinghausen neurofibromatosis. A clinical and population study in south-east Wales. Brain 1988;111:1355–1381.
14. R.G. Burwell, N.J. James, and D.I. Johnston. Café-au-lait spots in schoolchildren. Arch Dis Child 1982;57:631–632.

15. D. Whitehouse. Diagnostic value of the cafe-au-lait spot in children. Arch Dis Child 1966;41:316–319.
16. V.M. Riccardi. Pathophysiology of neurofibromatosis. V. Dermatologic insights into heterogeneity and pathogenesis. J Am Acad Dermatol 1980;3:157–166.
17. R.W. Crowe. Axillary freckling as a diagnostic aid in neurofibromatosis. Ann Intern Med 1964;61:1142–1143.
18. K. Lisch. Ueber Beteiligung der Augen, insbesondere das Vorkommen von Irisknotchen bei der Neurofibromatose (Recklinghausen). Z Augenheil 1937;93:137–143.
19. R.A. Lewis and V.M. Riccardi. Von Recklinghausen neurofibromatosis: Incidence of iris hamartomas. Ophthalmologica 1981;88:348–354.
20. C. Zehavi, A. Romano, and R.M. Goodman. Iris (Lisch) nodules in neurofibromatosis. Clin Genet 1986;29:51–55.
21. U. Flueler, E. Boltshauser, and A. Kilchhofer. Iris hamartomata as diagnostic criterion in neurofibromatosis. Neuropediatrics 1986;17:183–185.
22. P.K. Duffner and M.E. Cohen. Isolated optic nerve gliomas in children with and without neurofibromatosis. Neurofibromatosis 1988;1:201–211.
23. R.A. Lewis, L.P. Gerson, K.A. Axelson, et al. Von Recklinghausen neurofibromatosis II. Incidence of optic gliomata. Ophthalmologica 1984;91:929–935.
24. J.F. Holt. Neurofibromatosis in children. AJR 1978;130:615–639.
25. J.C. Carey, J.M. Laub, and B.D. Hall. Penetrance and variability in neurofibromatosis: A genetic study of 60 families. Birth Defects 1979; Original Article Series 15, No. 5B:271–281.
26. R.L. Martuza, I. Philippe, T.B. Fitzpatrick, et al. Melanin macroglobules as a cellular marker of neurofibromatosis: A quantitative study. J Invest Dermatol 1985;85:347–350.
27. M.A. Pearson-Webb, M.I. Kaiser-Kupfer, and R. Eldridge. Eye findings in bilateral acoustic (central) neurofibromatosis: Association with presenile lens opacities and cataracts but absence of Lisch nodules. N Engl J Med 1986;315:1553–1554.
28. V.M. Riccardi. Routine cranial neuroimaging of patients with or at risk for neurofibromatosis. Neurofibromatosis 1988;1:65–68.
29. J.R. Bognanno, M.K. Edwards, T.A. Lee, et al. Cranial MR imaging in neurofibromatosis. AJNR 1988;151:381–388.
30. S.A. Sorensen, J.J. Mulvihill, and A. Nielsen. Long-term follow-up of von Recklinghausen neurofibromatosis. N Engl J Med 1986;314:1010–1014.

3

Neurofibromatosis Type 2

Roswell Eldridge, M.D.

It is now recognized that there are several distinct forms of neurofibromatosis (NF) (1). The most common form is NF1, or von Recklinghausen NF, which was previously referred to as "peripheral" NF because the skin, or "periphery" of the body, is marked by light brown spots (café au lait spots) and lumps (neurofibromas). Another form of NF, NF2, has as its hallmark the development of tumors on both acoustic nerves, or the two nerves of hearing (Fig. 3–1); hence the name bilateral acoustic NF (2–5). This condition was previously called "central" NF because of the characteristic involvement of the central nervous system. It accounts for about 5 to 10% of all NF cases.

It is important to distinguish NF-2 from NF-1, because its clinical features, management, and genetic basis are distinct. It is also important to distinguish NF-2 from a single acoustic nerve tumor. The solitary acoustic nerve tumor, or unilateral acoustic neuroma, tends to develop later in life, is not inherited, and raises far fewer management issues.

Although it is not possible to cure or prevent NF-2, we do know its cause in a general sense. Family studies indicate that a single mutant, or altered, gene is responsible, and that the gene is on chromosome 22 (6,7). In time, we should be able to characterize the abnormal product of this gene and determine its precise location. With this information, it may be possible to prevent or even correct the disorder.

History

Isolated cases of bilateral acoustic neuromas were reported over 100 years ago. In reporting such a case in 1917, the famous neurosurgeon Harvey Cushing considered the condition a form of NF because the pathological changes were similar to those seen in von Recklinghausen NF (8).

In 1930, Gardner and Frazier (9) reported a large family from Pennsylvania in which at least 38 members were affected. Forty years later, Young et al. (10) restudied the family, this time documenting bilateral acoustic NF in more than 100 members. Because most of those affected had other evidence of NF, such as

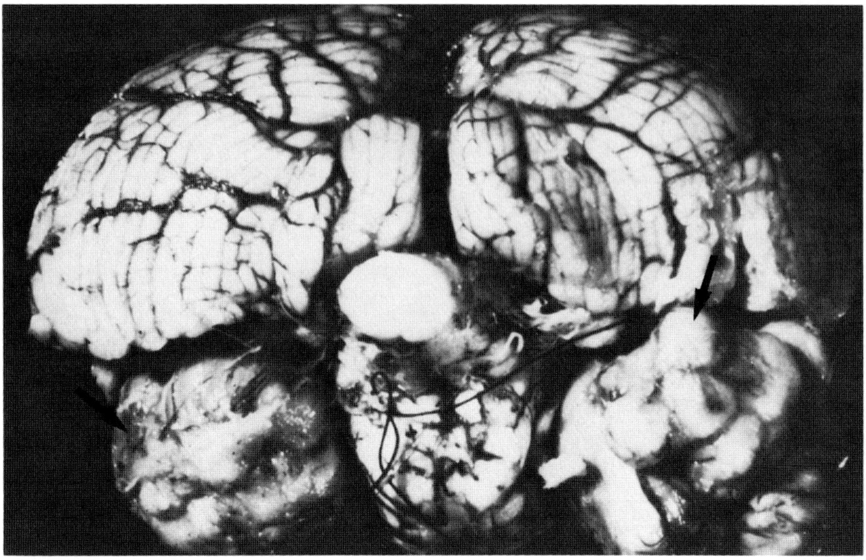

Figure 3–1. Bilateral acoustic neuromas (arrows) in patient with NF2.

one or more neurofibromas or several café au lait spots, they also considered the condition a distinct form of NF.

CLINICAL FEATURES

The patient usually is first aware of symptoms at about 20 years of age, but the symptoms may begin before 15 years of age or not until 30 years of age or later. The initial symptoms may involve one or both ears. When one ear is first affected, 10 or more years may elapse before the other ear becomes involved (2,7).

The patient's first complaint related to acoustic neuroma is usually loss of hearing in one or both ears. Careful questioning may reveal that the hearing loss was preceded by an intermittent ringing or roaring in one or both ears, or some unsteadiness, especially while walking at night on uneven ground. Other complaints may include facial weakness, headache, and change in vision. The earliest telltale sign in some patients, however, may be a lump or swelling under the skin caused by the development of a neurofibroma. Findings on routine physical and neurological examinations in the early stages of the disorder may be entirely normal with respect to the eighth cranial nerve complex. In a family member at risk for NF-2, the diagnosis should be suspected if mild signs of NF are found elsewhere, such as one or two café au lait spots or a small lump under the scalp or skin. Occasionally, related tumors of the spinal cord may produce a weakness of one or more limbs.

Slit lamp examination of the eyes with a beam of specially focused light does not reveal Lisch nodules, the slightly raised spots on the iris or pigmented membrane about the pupil, which are noted in NF-1. What have been found by careful examination of the eyes in about half of the individuals with NF-2 are changes indicating that cataracts are developing toward the rear of the lens (11) (Fig. 3–2). Sometimes the cataracts have interfered enough with vision that they require removal.

Other tumors of the brain occur with increased frequency in NF-2. These are often schwannomas, tumors originating from the cell forming the sheath about each of the cranial nerves, or meningiomas, tumors originating from the meninges, or protective membranes of the brain.

NATURAL HISTORY

An important but disturbing feature of NF-2 is its unpredictability. During or following puberty, the growth of one or both acoustic tumors may commence

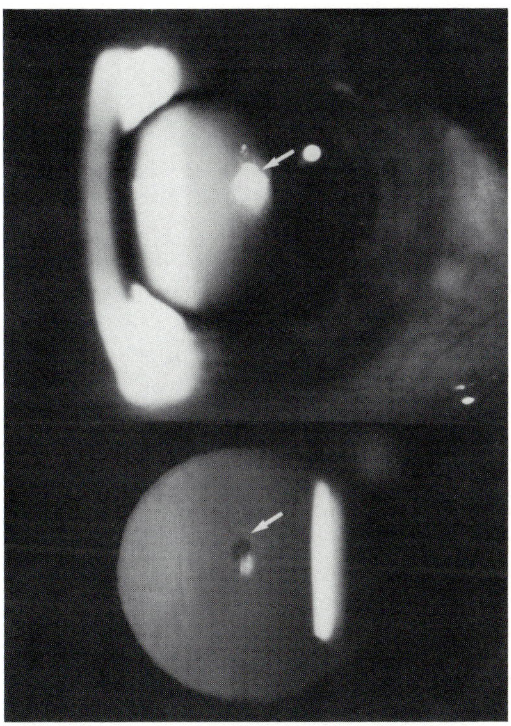

Figure 3–2. Posterior subcapsular cataract (arrow) in patient with NF2 seen on dilated biomicroscopy of the right lens. (Photograph provided by Dr. Muriel I. Kaiser-Kupfer, National Eye Institute, National Institutes of Health, Bethesda, MD.)

and progress relentlessly, leading to deafness, severe gait disturbance, chronic headache, or visual impairment. Eventually, death can result from the consequences of pressure and displacement of the brainstem. Alternatively, there may be only minimal growth for many years, so that the individual has few if any limitations. Typically, the course lies somewhere between these extremes. Although there may be other tumors of the brain, spinal cord, or peripheral nerves, it is generally possible to treat them surgically if their size or location warrants.

Unlike NF-1, NF-2 is not associated with bone changes or malignant transformation of the tumors. Also, some intellectual impairment is said to be common in NF-1, but this does not seem to be the case in NF-2.

Diagnosis

It is important to note that in NF-2 no single feature of the clinical evaluation or specific laboratory study may be diagnostic (12). The evaluation must be comprehensive and should be repeated after an interval of some months if the results are borderline.

In taking the history, emphasis should be placed on age at onset of the disease, initial symptoms, presence of symptoms directly referable to the eighth cranial nerve complex, and rate of disease progression. In addition to careful neurological assessment of cranial nerve and spinal cord status, the skin should be examined meticulously for café au lait spots or lumps suggestive of neurofibromas; the latter are frequently found beneath the scalp. The eyes should be examined by an eye specialist with particular attention given to the iris and the lens. Cataracts have been seen in an unusual number of patients with NF-2, but the presence of iris nodules would be highly unusual in this form of NF.

Audiological and vestibular assessment together with "imaging" of the eighth cranial nerve complex forms the critical laboratory studies. Auditory evoked response (Fig. 3–3) may be the most sensitive of the procedures but is not positive in all cases, especially when acoustic neuroma is small (13). Abnormality of vestibular nerve function may predate any other changes by a matter of months or years so that its assessment is essential when this condition is suspected (14).

Imaging of an acoustic neuroma can be performed using x-rays or magnetic waves. Computed tomography (CT) scan involves the integration of "slices" of the brain obtained by x-ray by means of a computer. If there is a question of a small tumor, it may be necessary to inject a contrast solution into a vein to obtain better definition of the tumor, as the solution is concentrated by tumor tissue. This technique has detected acoustic neuromas that are pea-sized or smaller (15,16).

It is now possible to obtain images by use of magnetic waves instead of x-rays. In the presence of a magnetic field, or pulse, subatomic elements within

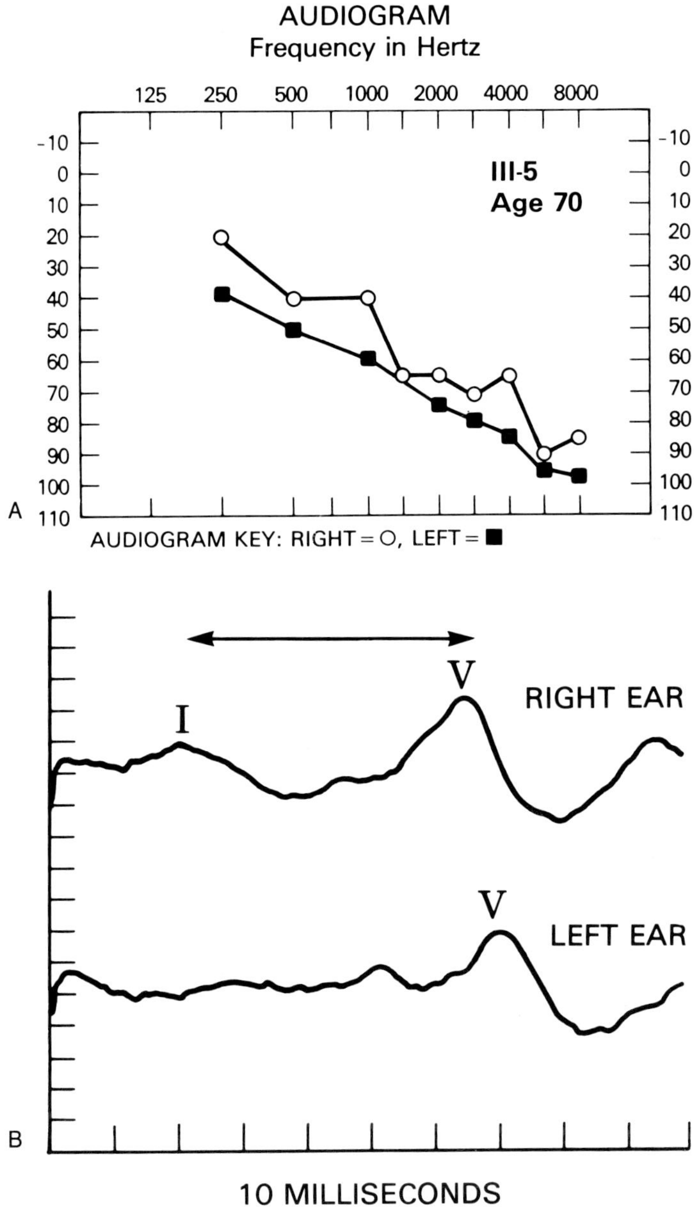

Figure 3–3. (A) Audiogram from patient with bilateral acoustic neuromas, showing 20 to 40 dB sensorineural hearing loss at 250 Hz, increasing to 80 to 100 dB at 8000 Hz. The left side is worse than the right. (B) Auditory evoked potential tracing from patient with NF2. Right wave I to V interpeak interval of 4.47 msec is more than 2.5 standard deviations beyond the clinic norm of 3.95 msec. Left I to V interpeak interval could not be measured. (Illustrations provided by Mrs. Anita Pikus, National Institute of Deafness and Other Communication Disorders, National Institutes of Health, Bethesda, MD.)

cells are "tipped" in one direction. The energy release when the magnetic force is removed can generate a detailed anatomical image. In theory, this technique, called magnetic resonance imaging (MRI), should permit detection of even smaller acoustic tumors and without the risk involved with x-ray (Fig. 3–4) (17–21).

Several other studies are used by some medical scientists, and there undoubtedly will be new and more precise diagnostic procedures developed soon.

Absolute confirmation of the diagnosis of an acoustic neuroma requires study of tissue from the tumor by a pathologist. This step requires surgical removal of the tumor. In familial cases, there is often sufficient evidence from the imaging studies to permit management and counseling decisions without tissue confirmation.

DIFFERENTIAL DIAGNOSIS

NF-2 must be clearly distinguished from NF-1 and from a unilateral acoustic neuroma occurring in one ear only. Acoustic neuromas have been reported to

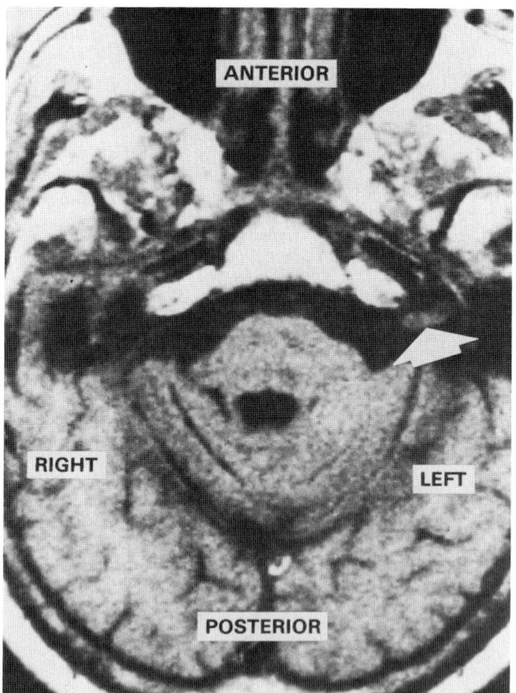

Figure 3–4. MRI scan of brain, showing acoustic neuromas within the left internal auditory canal (arrow). The right canal was not sufficiently well visualized to diagnose tumor. (Photograph provided by Dr. John L. Sherman, Magnetic Imaging of Washington, Chevy Chase, MD.)

occur in NF-1, but based on our experience at the National Institutes of Health, the occurrence must be rare. We have evaluated more than 100 families with NF-1 and have not encountered anyone with an acoustic neuroma. However, we have also evaluated more than 50 members of families affected by NF-2 and none have had the extensive skin changes or Lisch nodules of NF-1.

Unilateral acoustic neuromas generally occur in older individuals, with no other family member affected (22). They are more common in the general population than are neuromas due to NF-2. Although both unilateral and bilateral acoustic neuromas arise from the superior vestibular nerve of the eighth cranial nerve complex and both appear similar microscopically, they are generally different morphologically and require different surgical considerations. Unilateral tumors arise as a single mass and compress the eighth nerve complex but do not, as a rule, crowd into neighboring nerves. Bilateral tumors consist of several lobes, which suggests that the tumors arise at several sites along the sheath of the vestibular nerve and are more likely to invade, or interdigitate, with fibers of adjoining nerves within the internal auditory canal.

Several examples of familial unilateral acoustic neuroma have been reported, but in each instance onset was relatively early and the presence of bilateral tumors in the affected adults was not definitely excluded. Since management implications are quite different for unilateral versus bilateral tumors, it is important for those caring for such patients to be aware of the two kinds of acoustic neuromas.

MANAGEMENT

Diagnosis of NF-2 in an individual brings with it the immediate question of what, if anything, to do about the tumors (23–26). If the patient is having rapid progression of the symptoms or other evidence of tumor growth, or if symptoms are interfering with work or daily routine, then intervention is in order. If the tumor is small and the patient is asymptomatic or only minimally troubled, a dilemma is posed. With very small tumors, it is sometimes possible to operate and to save useful hearing, as well as preserve facial nerve function so that facial expression is near normal (27,28). This is not the case with larger tumors. Even with small tumors, however, there is often significant damage to the eighth cranial nerve complex. Another problem is that a tumor seeming small by a standard imaging procedure can prove to be larger when it is actually visualized by the surgeon. Also, the acoustic tumors in NF-2 seem to be more invasive than a single, isolated acoustic tumor, so that even small tumors may grow into the auditory nerves and make preservation of the nerves impossible.

Balanced against these disquieting features of NF-2 is the fact that tumor growth may be slow or even nonprogressive for years. It is possible for individuals with known tumors to live with them for years or decades, pursuing useful lives meanwhile.

There are several surgical approaches to an acoustic neuroma, depending in part on the size of the tumor and the specialty of the surgeon. In addition, considerable experience has been accumulated by at least one group that employs highly focused radiation instead of surgery.

The decision as to whether to intervene, and if so, when and in just what manner, must be made by individuals familiar with the natural history of NF-2 and the consequences of the intervention process itself. An effort should be made to determine the specific experience of the management team with bilateral acoustic tumors. Although these considerations apply when an initial acoustic neuroma develops in NF-2, it is when the second acoustic neuroma has been demonstrated that they become critical. This is especially true if hearing impairment or hearing loss in one ear resulted from the first tumor.

Once a diagnosis of NF-2 has been made, either by the demonstration of an acoustic neuroma or through the presence of neurofibroma elsewhere, certain measures are in order. The patient, immediate family members, and friends should all be encouraged to learn nonverbal means of communication such as sign language (the third most common language in the United States). If there is troubling hearing loss, amplification of sound may be helpful.

Because the vestibular portion of the eighth nerve complex may be involved early but go unrecognized until the individual requires precise balance or sense of direction, special care must be taken of those at risk and under age 30 in such situations as swimming, diving, or climbing heights, as on a ladder. Swimming alone underwater should be avoided entirely.

Family members at risk for NF-2, that is, first-degree relatives under the age of 35 who are asymptomatic, should have a CT or MRI scan and baseline audiological assessment, including auditory evoked response (1). About 5% of those affected do not have symptoms until the age of 35 or later. Genetic counseling for such important personal considerations as career choice and family planning should be conducted by a practitioner familiar with clinical and genetic aspects of NF-2. The counselor should be able to determine the probability of carrying the NF-2 gene at various ages in a person who has no signs or symptoms of the disease.

ETIOLOGY: GENETICS AND ENVIRONMENT

NF-2 is caused by a single mutant, or altered, gene located on chromosome 22 (6,7). The resulting trait behaves in an autosomal dominant manner; that is, approximately half of the offspring of an affected parent will be affected. Unknown, however, is how this mutant gene exerts its deleterious effect. In tumors, it has been found that the normal copy of the region of chromosome 22 where the NF2 gene resides is deleted (29). Theories about how this contributes to tumor formation are reviewed in Chapter 16. Knowledge in this area is advancing rapidly and soon should allow improved management or even prevention of the disorder.

The gene is highly "penetrant"; that is, when someone carries the gene, the acoustic neuromas almost always develop. Only a few examples exist of an individual who has no evidence of tumors yet must carry the gene because both a parent and a child have the tumors. None of these individuals has been thoroughly examined to be sure there is no medical evidence of the trait.

The gene is usually uniform in its expression. Bilateral acoustic neuromas develop in over 90% of those with the gene. Other nervous system tumors are reported to occur in about half of those affected, but the percentage is undoubtedly higher, particularly for spinal cord tumors. The presence of other tumors is a function of the patient's age and sex, with females apparently more prone.

The gene for NF-2 is apparently distributed throughout the world, but most of the families reported have been from the United States. Four large kindreds are all of English ancestry, suggesting that each family may have had the same common ancestor many generations ago.

Several observations suggest that hormones or growth factors may play a role in the initiation and subsequent growth pattern of acoustic neuromas. The first signs often occur in relation to puberty. Pregnancy is often associated with the onset of symptoms or worsening of existing symptoms (30), and women are thought to have more problems in general, as well as larger and more vascular tumors. When the gene is transmitted by the mother, the onset of the disease tends to be earlier. Tumors that develop in the central nervous system invariably involve the sensory nerves, which are known to have a high concentration of receptors, or attachment sites, for the female hormone estrogen (31). In contrast, motor nerves, which are seldom involved, have more male hormone receptors.

So far it has not been possible to document a specific role for estrogen or other hormones. A recent study suggests that a glial nerve growth factor is present in unusual concentration in tumors of family members affected by NF-2 (32), but this observation requires confirmation. Very likely, specific hormones or other factors regulating tumor cell growth are involved, but they themselves may not be abnormal.

CONCLUSION

NF-2 (bilateral acoustic NF) is a distinct but not well-known form of NF. The acoustic tumors are amenable to specific management, especially in their early stages, and relatives who are at risk of contracting the disease can be screened to permit early diagnosis. This disorder has much to teach us regarding the function of the eighth cranial nerve complex and about tumor formation.

REFERENCES

1. D.A. Stumpf, J.F. Alksne, J.F. Annegers, et al. Neurofibromatosis. Arch Neurol 1988;45:575–578.
2. R. Eldridge. Central neurofibromatosis with bilateral acoustic neuroma. Adv Neurol 1981;29:57–65.
3. R.L. Martuza and R. Eldridge. Neurofibromatosis 2. N Engl J Med 1988;318:684–688.
4. W.R. Kanter, R. Eldridge, R. Fabricant, et al. Central neurofibromatosis with bilateral acoustic neuroma: Genetic, clinical and biochemical distinctions from peripheral neurofibromatosis. Neurology 1988;30:851–859.
5. S.M. Huson and D.C. Thrush. Central neurofibromatosis. Q J Med 1985;55:213–224.
6. G.A. Rouleau, W. Wertelecki, J.L. Haines, et al. Genetic linkage of bilateral acoustic neurofibromatosis to a DNA marker on chromosome 22. Nature 1987;329:246–248.
7. W. Wertelecki, G.A. Rouleau, D.W. Superneau, et al. Neurofibromatosis 2: Clinical and DNA linkage studies of a large kindred. N Engl J Med 1988;319:278–283.
8. H. Cushing. Tumors of the nervus acusticus. Philadelphia, W.B. Saunders, 1917.
9. W.J. Gardner and C.H. Frazier. Bilateral acoustic neurofibromatosis: A clinical study and field survey of a family of five generations with bilateral deafness in thirty-eight members. Arch Neurol Psychiatry 1930;23:266–302.
10. D.F. Young, R. Eldridge, G.T. Nager, et al. Hereditary bilateral acoustic neuroma (central neurofibromatosis). Birth Defects 1971;7:73–86.
11. M.A. Pearson-Webb, M.I. Kaiser-Kupfer, and R. Eldridge. Eye findings in bilateral acoustic (central) neurofibromatosis: Association with presenile lens opacities and cataracts but absence of Lisch nodules. N Engl J Med 1986;315:1553–1554.
12. R.L. Martuza, S.W. Parker, J.B. Nadol, et al. Diagnosis of cerebellopontine angle tumors. Clin Neurosurg 1985;32:177–213.
13. A.D. Legatt, T.A. Pedley, R.G. Emerson, et al. Normal brain-stem auditory evoked potentials with abnormal latency-intensity studies in patients with acoustic neuromas. Arch Neurol 1988;45:1326–1330.
14. M. Bodard, P. Pialoux, G. Freyss, et al. Comparative values of unilateral and bilateral caloric bithermal vestibular tests in the diagnosis of acoustic neurinoma. Ann Otolaryngol Chir Cervicofac 1981;98:9–13.
15. D.W. Johnson. Air cisternography of the cerebellopontine angle using high-resolution computed tomography. Radiology 1984;151:401–403.
16. S.H. Lee, E. Lewis, J.H. Montoya, and J.F. Seelaus. Bilateral cerebellopontine angle air-CT cisternography. AJNR 1981;2:105–106.
17. D.L. Daniels, R. Herfkins, P.R. Koehler, et al. Magnetic resonance imaging of the internal auditory canal. Radiology 1984;151:105–108.
18. B.D. McGinnis, T.J. Brady, P.F. New, et al. Nuclear magnetic resonance (NMR) imaging of tumors in the posterior fossa. J Comput Assist Tomogr 1983;7:575–584.
19. C. Ochiai, K. Takakura, N. Basugi, et al. Visualization of cerebellopontine angle disease by nuclear magnetic resonance imaging. No To Shinkei 1983;35:1191–1198.
20. I.R. Young, G.M. Bydder, A.S. Hall, et al. The role of NMR imaging in the diagnosis and management of acoustic neuroma. AJNR 1983;4:223–224.
21. M.E. Glasscock, III, K.X. McKennan, and S.C. Levine. False negative MRI scan in an acoustic neuroma. Otolaryngology Head Neck Surg 1988;98:612–614.
22. M. Tos and J. Thomsen. Epidemiology of acoustic neuromas. J Laryngol Otol 1984;98:685–692.
23. G.B. Hughes, A. Sismanis, M.E. Glasscock, III, et al. Management of bilateral acoustic tumors. Laryngoscope 1982;92:1351–1359.
24. F.H. Linthicum, Jr., and D.E. Brackmann. Bilateral acoustic tumors. A diagnostic and surgical challenge. Arch Otolaryngol 1980;106:729–733.

25. R.L. Martuza and R.G. Ojemann. Bilateral acoustic neuromas: Clinical aspects, pathogenesis, and treatment. Neurosurgery 1982;10:1–12.
26. C.H. Tator. Acoustic neuromas: Management of 204 cases. Can J Neurol Sci 1985;12:353–357.
27. R.G. Ojemann, R.A. Levine, W.M. Montgomery, and P. McGaffin. Use of intraoperative auditory evoked potentials to preserve hearing in unilateral acoustic neuroma removal. J Neurosurg 1984;61:938–948.
28. P. Piffko and E. Pasztor. Operated bilateral acoustic neurinoma with preservation of hearing and facial nerve function. ORL J Otorhinolaryngol Relat Spec 1981;43:255–261.
29. B.R. Seizinger, G. Rouleau, L.J. Ozelius, et al. Common pathogenetic mechanism for three tumor types in bilateral acoustic neurofibromatosis. Science 1987;236:317–319.
30. J. Allen, R. Eldridge, and T. Koerber. Acoustic neuroma in the last months of pregnancy. Am J Obstet Gynecol 1974;119:516–520.
31. R.L. Martuza, D.T. Maclaughlin, and R.G. Ojemann. Specific estradiol binding in schwannomas, meningiomas, and neurofibromas. Neurosurgery 1981;9:665–671.
32. J.P. Brockes, X.O. Breakefield, and R.L. Martuza. Glial growth factor-like activity in Schwann cell tumors. Ann Neurol 1986;20:317–322.

4

Neurological Aspects of Neurofibromatosis

Allan E. Rubenstein, M.D., and Bruce R. Korf, M.D., Ph.D.

The two disorders that are now known as NF1 and NF2 primarily involve the nervous system. Indeed, von Recklinghausen's name is associated with NF1 because he was the first to recognize that neurofibromas arise from nerves. NF1 is associated with two major forms of neurological problems: abnormalities of nervous system development and an increased risk of neural tumors. NF2 is associated only with neural tumors; no developmental problems are known to occur. NF2 is covered in a separate chapter (Chapter 3) and therefore only NF1 will be discussed here.

Abnormalities of Nervous System Development

Developmental abnormalities represent problems in the way the nervous system is formed. Therefore, for the most part, these are present from birth, and can be diagnosed early in life. Some of the more important types of developmental problems affecting the nervous system associated with NF1 are listed in Table 4–1.

Megalencephaly

Megalencephaly is one of the more common neurological features of neurofibromatosis (NF). Head circumference is generally measured around the widest portion of the top of the head and is compared with normal values on standard growth curves. Head growth occurs particularly rapidly in all children in the first year of life. Yet many children with NF1 have head sizes that are well above average for age, often exceeding the 98th percentile. In general, head growth for these children tends to follow a curve that is parallel to normal growth rate, but well above normal. In most instances this appears to be completely harmless. There are no associated neurological problems, and no correlation with learning disabilities. If a computed tomography (CT) or magnetic resonance imaging (MRI) scan is done, it usually shows a general

Table 4–1. Some Major Developmental Anomalies of the Nervous System Associated with Neurofibromatosis Type 1

Structural
Megalencephaly
Hydrocephalus
Abnormal neuronal migration or differentiation
Vascular occlusion
Dural ectasia
Absence of sphenoid wing
Lambdoidal suture defect
Function
Seizures
Learning disabilities
Mental retardation (rare)

increase in brain substance, without disproportionate increase in the size of the fluid-filled spaces, the ventricles (Fig. 4–1). Other than monitoring head growth by periodic measurement, to determine that growth rate is consistent, no special medical follow-up or evaluation is necessary.

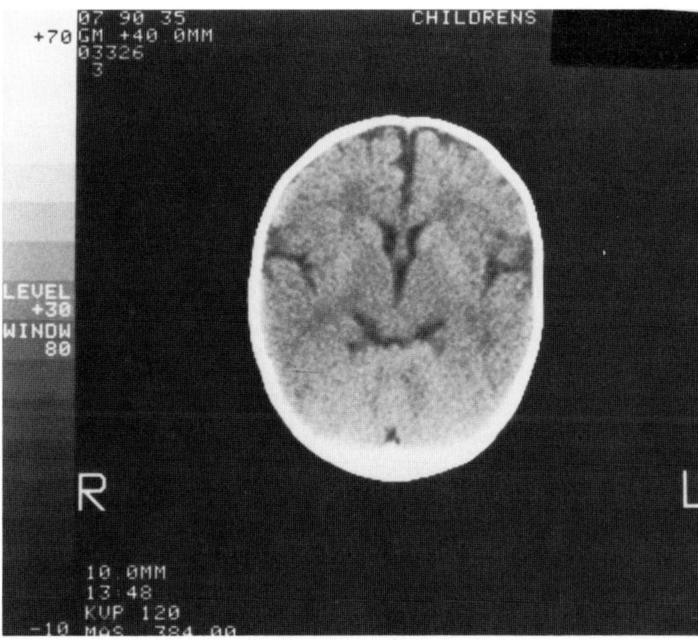

Figure 4–1. CT scan of child with NF and megalencephaly. The ventricles are slightly enlarged but otherwise the study is normal.

Hydrocephalus

Hydrocephalus represents the buildup of fluid pressure inside the ventricles. In young children, whose skull bones have not yet fused together, this usually causes a progressive increase in head size. Unlike simple megalencephaly, head growth in hydrocephalus is not parallel in rate to normal growth. If hydrocephalus occurs later in childhood or in adulthood, after fusion of the skull bones, head size does not change, but neurological signs and symptoms related to increased intracranial pressure occur. These may include headaches, vomiting, irritability, lethargy, double vision, and buildup of fluid around the optic nerve (papilledema). In general, hydrocephalus may be caused by a variety of problems that interfere with the normal circulation of cerebrospinal fluid in and around the brain. Although not commonly associated with NF, some people with NF1 having hydrocephalus due to aqueductal stenosis have been reported (1). Neurological signs or symptoms suggestive of hydrocephalus would be evaluated by CT or MRI scan of the brain. If a cause of spinal fluid obstruction, such as tumor, is found, it would be treated. Usually the hydrocephalus is treated by shunting the spinal fluid through a tube that drains into the abdomen. This is usually left in place permanently.

Functional Problems in the Nervous System

Aside from obvious structural anomalies of the nervous system, such as megalencephaly, some individuals with NF1 display signs of nervous system dysfunction, which apparently are not due to tumors. These problems include learning disabilities and seizures. Learning disabilities are discussed in detail in Chapter 5. It is worth noting here, however, that learning disabilities as a group include a wide spectrum of difficulties in cognitive function. Some degree of learning impairment, typically affecting some single skill such as language or mathematical ability, is common in individuals with NF (and in the general population, to a lesser degree). Most individuals with specific learning disabilities are generally intelligent, sometimes very intelligent, yet have an area of weakness that they must learn to live with. There are some with NF whose cognitive impairment is more severe and affects learning abilities more generally. Some of them might be labeled as mentally retarded, although there is no universal definition of mental retardation. Fortunately, such severe cognitive impairment is very rare in NF (2,3). Also, individuals with severe developmental disabilities are usually recognized as impaired early in life. Except in situations where brain tumors develop (see next section), it is very unusual to experience a significant loss of previously gained developmental function due to NF.

Seizures represent the abnormal discharge of electrical activity in the brain, and produce symptoms that vary according to the region of the brain involved. These may vary from brief episodes of staring and fidgeting of the hands, to major convulsions involving the entire body. Some include unusual symptoms such as the impression of an unpleasant taste or odor, or unusual behaviors. Overall, seizures are not very common among people with NF. When they do occur, it is necessary to evaluate the individual to determine the cause of the seizures. The evaluation usually includes recording of brain waves (the electroencephalogram, or EEG) as well as a CT or MRI scan of the brain. Seizures that emanate from a single region of the brain may signal the presence of a tumor, or of a region of abnormal development. In some cases the testing will reveal such a localized abnormality, which, depending on what it is, may be treated by surgery, radiation therapy, etc. In other cases, the abnormality may be missed by currently available techniques, perhaps because it is too small or subtle to be seen. Such instances would likely be treated with antiseizure medications (anticonvulsants) and repeated examinations by EEG and CT or MRI over the course of time. Seizures that are generalized might still originate in a single area due to a localized problem, but often truly occur in all regions simultaneously. In the latter case, the exact cause is unknown, but the seizure disorder would be viewed as a form of epilepsy, and treated with anticonvulsant medications.

The cause of learning disorders or seizures in people with NF who do not have evidence for tumors in the central nervous system is unknown. It is often assumed that, in these individuals, the formation of the brain has been disturbed in some way, so that the function of nerve cells is impaired. There is evidence that minor structural abnormalities of the brain, visible only with the microscope, do occur in some people with NF (4). How this correlates with learning problems or seizures has not been worked out, but it implies that the NF gene mutation can, in some cases, have subtle but important effects on brain development.

Developmental Anomalies of Peripheral Nervous System

The nervous system is not limited just to the brain and spinal cord, but includes a vast network of nerves that extend to all parts of the body. Dysfunction of a nerve due to compression by a tumor will be considered in the next section, but abnormal formation of nerves deserves mention as a developmental anomaly. One example which has been seen rarely in people with NF is abnormal formation of nerve cells in the wall of the bowel. These nerves are vital to normal bowel motility, and their absence produces problems such as severe constipation. In some cases the motility problem is so serious as to lead to a back-up of intestinal contents leading to expansion of a portion of the intestine. This problem, although rare, can represent a surgical emergency.

Skull Defects

Two forms of skull defect occur rarely in some people with NF, although neither involves the brain directly. One is absence of a portion of the sphenoid bone (see Chapter 2, Fig. 2–7A). This bone comprises part of the rear portion of the orbit. Its absence is usually associated with deformity of the orbit, and often plexiform neurofibroma within the orbit. The brain itself is usually normal. The other is a defect in the back of the skull, near the junction of the occipital and temporal bone (lambdoidal suture) (Fig. 4–2). For unknown reasons this most often occurs on the left side of the head (5). It results in a space between the bones which is soft, and bulges with coughing or other maneuvers that temporarily increase venous pressure. This gap may tend to enlarge through midchildhood. The cause of this defect is unknown, but it appears to be harmless. It is not associated with neurological abnormality.

Vascular Anomalies

NF1 may be associated with abnormalities of the structure of blood vessels anywhere in the body, including the nervous system. The abnormality usually takes the form of increased thickness of the vessel wall, and narrowing of the lumen. In the extreme, the vessel may be blocked entirely. When this occurs in the central nervous system, often there are no associated problems because collateral flow develops through alternative vascular pathways (Fig. 4–3). However, if blood flow is compromised, for example, by a transient decrease in blood pressure, the region supplied by the occluded vessel may not be supplied with sufficient blood. This can cause transient symptoms of neurological impairment, or even stroke. Serious vascular problems involving the

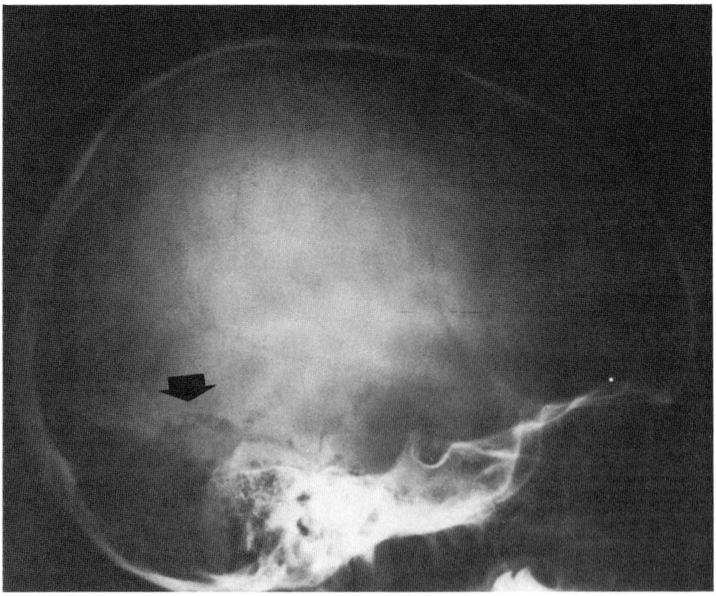

Figure 4–2. Skull x-ray illustrating defect in lambdoidal suture (arrow) in child with NF1.

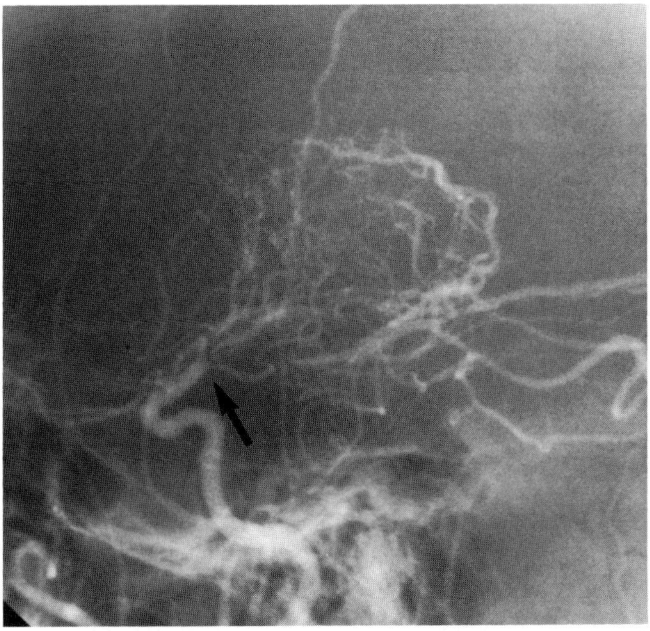

Figure 4–3. Angiogram demonstrating occlusion of the carotid artery (arrow) and collateral flow (moyamoya syndrome) which occurred in a child with NF1 who had received radiation therapy for optic glioma.

central nervous system are rare in NF1 (6). They may be more common in those who receive radiation therapy for brain tumors, however (7).

NEURAL TUMORS IN NEUROFIBROMATOSIS TYPE 1

Predisposition to tumor formation is one of the cardinal features of NF, and indeed is the feature that gives the disorder its name. Neural tumors associated with NF1 occur in both the central and the peripheral nervous system and together account for a substantial portion of the medical burden of NF.

Peripheral Nervous System

The neurofibroma is the most common tumor type associated with NF1. Neurofibromas arise from the proliferation of cells that surround and ensheathe nerves, rather than from the nerves themselves (Fig. 4–4) (8). They can occur along nerves anywhere in the body, and can occur at any time in life. The most common place to first notice neurofibromas is on the skin (3,9) (see Chapter 2, Fig. 2–3), where they first appear in most people in late childhood or during puberty. Initially they are small bumps, which may resemble mosquito

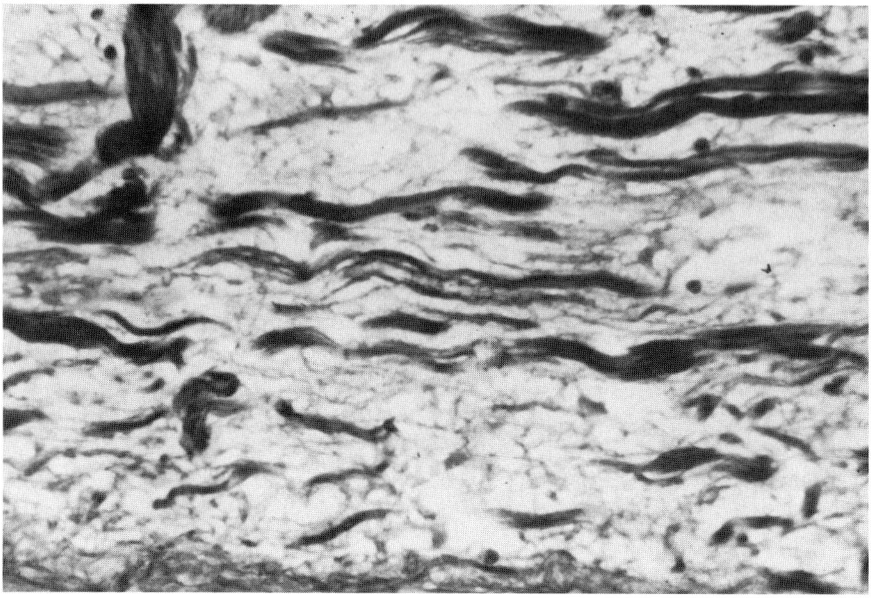

Figure 4–4. Photomicrograph of neurofibroma. There is a proliferation of spindle-shaped cells and a large amount of extracellular material.

bites, although they do not itch and do not go away. They are soft and fleshy to the touch, and often the overlying skin has a pink or purple hue. Most people with NF1 eventually get at least some dermal neurofibromas, but it is impossible to predict how many for any individual; some people have just a few, whereas others develop hundreds. Dermal neurofibromas rarely, if ever, impair nerve function. Their major impact is usually cosmetic. Surgical removal is possible, although regrowth sometimes occurs.

Neurofibromas also occur deeper inside the body along the course of peripheral nerves. Some may be palpated through the skin as discrete masses. These, too, usually do not have an effect on nerve function. If they do cause trouble, it may be because of their location. For example, if a neurofibroma grows to the point where it presses the nerve against a bone, the nerve may be damaged by the constant pressure. This nerve damage typically presents with pain, weakness, and numbness or tingling in the area of the body supplied by that nerve. If such symptoms occur, neurological evaluation should be sought. Physiological studies of nerve function such as nerve conduction velocity studies (NCV) and electromyography (EMG) may be ordered, and x-ray or MRI tests of the involved area may be necessary. If a neurofibroma is found to be compressing a nerve, surgery may be indicated.

Although most neurofibromas arise from a small portion of a nerve sheath and grow as discrete masses, some take a more diffuse form. This is the plexiform neurofibroma, which represents the involvement in neurofibroma-like growth of the sheath of a major nerve for considerable distance. Often a whole group of major nerves in a particular region of the body may be involved (Fig. 4–5). The nerves may be palpated as a network of cord-like masses under the skin in some cases, or may lie deeper inside the body. Occasionally plexiform neurofibromas may be associated with overgrowth of surrounding skin and bone, which can cause an enlargement of one side of the face, arm, hand, or leg (Fig. 4–6). If severe, this can cause significant disfigurement. Plexiform neurofibromas are often apparent at the time of birth, but may continue to grow during childhood, or later in life. Sometimes the growth is inexorable and disfiguring. In most cases this is not due to malignancy, and therefore treatments such as radiation or chemotherapy are ineffective. Surgical removal of at least a portion of the growth is the only available treatment, although it is usually impossible to completely remove a plexiform neurofibroma. This is because the tumor may be wrapped around many vital structures, including many nerve trunks. Limited surgical treatment to reduce the bulk and improve appearance is usually the best that can be done, and often repeated procedures are necessary.

In addition to neurofibromas, another tumor type that arises from the nerve sheath, the schwannoma, is associated with NF. Schwannomas are discrete

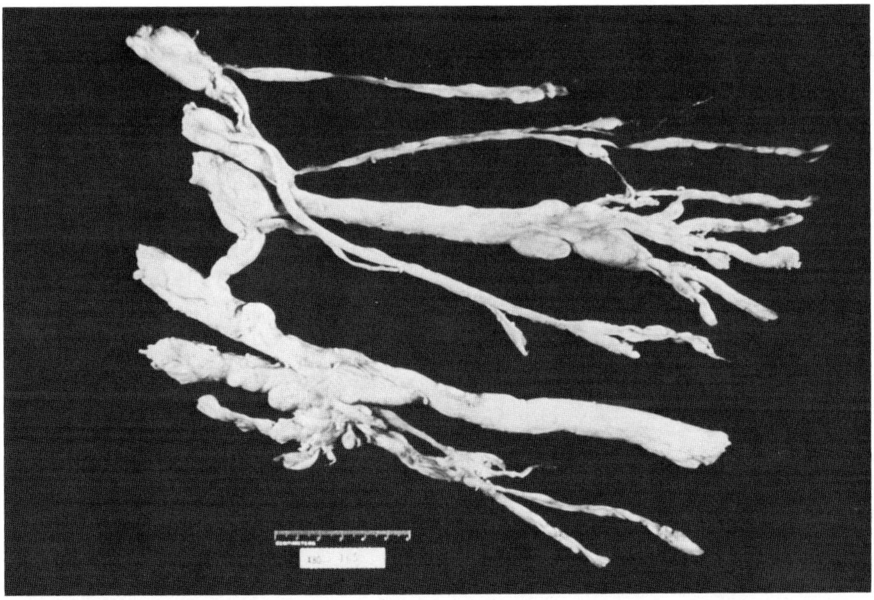

Figure 4–5. Plexiform neurofibroma of the lumbar plexus showing thickened nerve trunks and several masses of neurofibroma. (Photograph provided by Dr. Curt Dohan.)

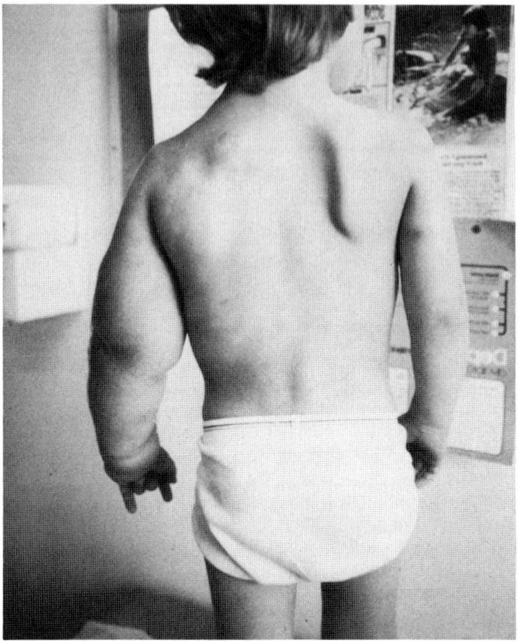

Figure 4–6. Enlargement of the arm due to plexiform neurofibroma in child with NF1.

masses of Schwann cells which have a different pattern of growth than neurofibromas. The former tend to push the nerve to one side, whereas in the latter, the nerves tend to course through the substance of the tumor. This difference is usually only appreciated on microscopic examination, and is not important from the clinical point of view.

As just noted, neurofibromas can appear and grow at any time. The stimuli responsible for this growth are unknown. Since growth commonly occurs in association with puberty and pregnancy, hormonal factors have been implicated. Yet no specific hormone that influences neurofibroma growth has been identified. Neurofibromas are generally benign growths, in the sense that they do not have the tendency to spread and invade tissues typical of a malignancy, or cancer. There is some risk of the development of malignancy within a neurofibroma, however. Overall, this risk is thought to be about 5% or less for an individual over their lifetime. Malignancy is virtually never seen in dermal neurofibromas, and appears to be limited to plexiform neurofibromas. The signs of malignancy are sudden growth of a portion of a tumor, or the sudden occurrence of pain. Such symptoms should be brought to medical attention promptly. Often biopsy of the portion that is growing or painful is necessary to determine if malignancy is present. Treatment would include surgical removal or radiation treatments, and often chemotherapy as well. For additional information about malignant schwannoma, see Chapter 10.

Central Nervous System

Tumors of the central nervous system are less common in NF1, but when they occur they have the potential of causing more severe problems. As for the peripheral nervous system, most of these tumors involve cells that surround nerves, rather than the nerve cells themselves. In the central nervous system these cells are referred to as glia, and the tumors as gliomas. Most of the glial tumors associated with NF arise from astroglia, and are referred to as astrocytomas.

The signs and symptoms associated with gliomas depend on the size and location of the tumors. Many have no detectable effects because they are too small, or are located in a region whose functional impairment may be quite subtle. Such tumors may be present for years without being noticed, and may even remain quiescent for a lifetime. In other cases, neurological problems, sometimes quite severe, can result. These include seizures, behavioral changes, lethargy or coma, weakness, sensory loss, headache, vomiting, visual disturbance, etc. Symptoms of headache and vomiting may signal increased intracranial pressure due to the presence of a tumor. It should be noted, however, that many people with NF get ordinary tension or migraine headaches, the latter commonly being accompanied by vomiting. Therefore, not every headache signals a brain tumor. On the other hand, recurrent headaches or other symptoms just listed should be brought to medical attention for further evaluation.

Medical evaluation of suspected brain tumor begins with a careful neurological examination. This is done specifically to look for evidence of impairment that can be localized to a particular region of the nervous system. Suspected brain or spinal cord tumors are usually investigated by contrast-enhanced CT scans or by MRI scans (Fig. 4–7) (10,11). In some cases, tumors identified by such tests need to be biopsied to determine their exact type and degree of malignancy. Treatment depends on the nature of the tumor and rate of progression. Small tumors that are not causing symptoms and do not appear to be growing may not be treated at all, but may be observed for future growth. This may entail repeated neurological examination and CT or MRI scan. The physician must weigh the risks of treatment against the risks of progression of a tumor in making this decision. Tumors that are clearly progressive or causing significant neurological impairment may be treated with a combination of surgery, radiation, and, in some cases, chemotherapy. The specific means of treatment depends on the location of the tumor, its degree of malignancy, and the general health of the patient. The outcome likewise depends on the specific situation, and the likely side effects vary with the treatment used. Additional discussion of these issues will be found in Chapter 7.

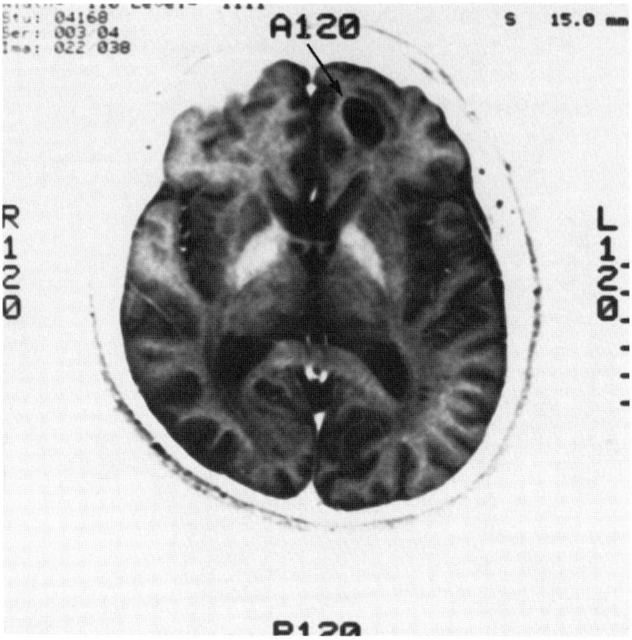

Figure 4–7. MRI scan demonstrating brain tumor (arrow) in individual with NF1.

One important type of glioma associated with NF1 which deserves special mention is the optic glioma. This tumor affects the optic nerves, which connect each eye to the brain (see Chapter 2, Fig. 2–6). Studies have shown that thickening of the optic nerve occurs commonly in individuals with NF1, perhaps as many as 15% (12–14). Most of these people have no signs or symptoms of visual or neurological impairment, and most never develop such problems (3). A few, however, do develop difficulties such as loss of vision in one or both eyes, pain in or behind the eye, or even generalized signs of neurological impairment due to spread of tumor from the optic nerve to the rest of the brain. Symptomatic optic gliomas associated with NF1 most commonly occur in children. They are often treated with radiation therapy, which may arrest further progression of the tumor. On the other hand, asymptomatic optic nerve thickening, which may not really be malignant tumor so much as abnormality of the structure of glial tissue in the optic nerve, does not require treatment.

Routine Neuroimaging

The relatively high frequency of tumors of the central nervous system in people with NF1 has led some to recommend routine CT or MRI scanning in these individuals (10). This is not universally done, however, because many of the lesions seen do not require treatment, and in fact, it would be very unusual to recommend treatment for a lesion that was not causing signs or symptoms of neurological impairment. The decision to do such screening is best left as an individual decision made by the physician on a case-by-case basis, taking into account the specific needs of a given patient.

MRI scanning is a powerful recent addition to the list of tools available to study the nervous system. As this technique has been applied to people with NF1, a number of people have been found to have unexplained abnormalities (10). These appear as prominent bright spots often symmetrically placed in regions such as the basal ganglia and cerebellum (Fig. 4–8). In most cases they have not been associated with neurological problems, and do not appear to be progressive. Sometimes it may be difficult to distinguish such findings from brain tumor, but their location, symmetry, and lack of associated neurological impairment in spite of a seemingly large extent of involved brain may be clues. Sometimes these are referred to as "unidentified bright objects," or UBOs. Their significance is unknown, and is currently a subject of study.

Other Central Nervous System Tumors

A variety of other central nervous system tumors may occur in individuals with NF, albeit less commonly. Acoustic neuromas, which are commonly seen in people with NF2 (see Chapter 3), have been reported in people with NF1.

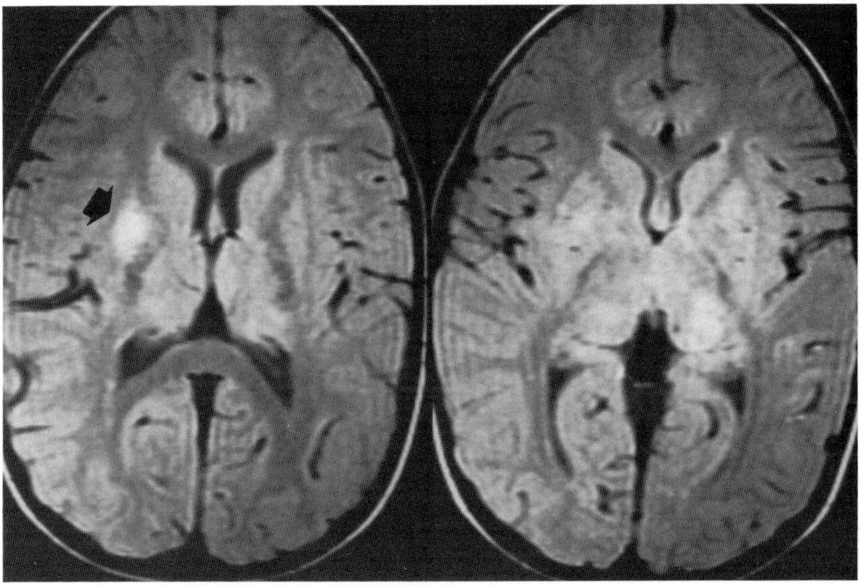

Figure 4–8. MRI scan in child with NF1 showing area of increased signal intensity with T2-weighted imaging in basal ganglia (arrow), corresponding with a UBO.

When they occur in NF1, they are usually unilateral, in contrast with bilateral tumors which occur in NF2. The acoustic neuroma is actually a schwannoma occurring along the vestibular portion of the eighth cranial nerve. Schwannomas may occur in association with other cranial nerves, such as the fifth, ninth, or tenth. These may present with impairment of function of the involved nerve as well as brainstem compression. Schwannomas may also occur along spinal

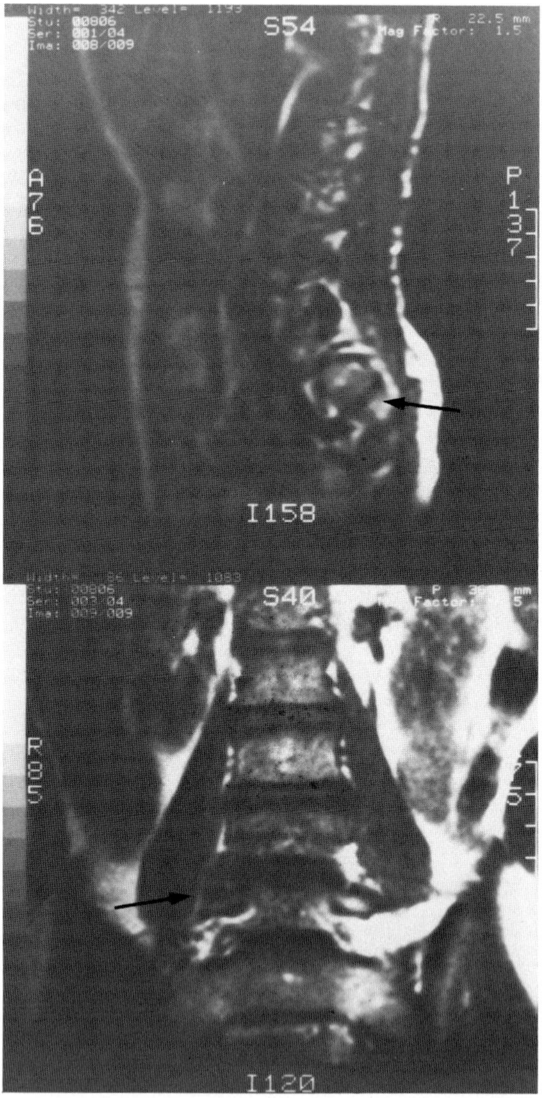

Figure 4–9. MRI scan of the spine, with a neurofibroma of the nerve root indicated by the arrows.

nerve roots. If these invade the neural foramen, they may not only compress the nerve root, but even compress the spinal cord itself. Symptoms of spinal cord compression (weakness and increased reflexes in muscle groups below the level of the tumor) are usually evaluated by spinal MRI scanning or myelography (Fig. 4–9). Treatment of these tumor types is mainly surgical.

SUMMARY

A wide variety of developmental problems involving the nervous system are seen more frequency in NF1 than in the general population. In addition, people with NF have an increased risk for certain types of neural tumors. Learning disabilities, megalencephaly, and dermal neurofibromas are the most common neurological complications seen. All other neurological problems are relatively uncommon. There is considerable variability in the spectrum of involvement of the nervous system in NF1. Most affected individuals have relatively minor problems, whereas some have multiple severe neurological complications. In addition to the deficits resulting from a neural tumor, the surgical removal of a tumor can result in additional motor or sensory deficits. The variability of neurological manifestations in NF1 extends to affected families. There is no known predictive value to the level of involvement of an individual as it relates to an affected sibling or child. The management of NF1 requires, from a neurologist's point of view, lifelong surveillance for the development of neural tumors, which includes periodic examination and in some cases imaging of the brain or spinal cord. Management in the childhood years involves screening and possible diagnostic testing for the wide range of developmental problems described in this chapter.

REFERENCES

1. A. Horwich, V.M. Riccardi, and U. Franke. Aqueductal stenosis leading to hydrocephalus: An unusual manifestation of neurofibromatosis. Am J Med Genet 1983;14:577–581.
2. J.C. Carey, J.M. Laub, and B.D. Hall. Penetrance and variability in neurofibromatosis: A genetic study of 60 families. Birth Defects 1979; Original Article Series 15, No. 5B:271–281.
3. S.M. Huson, P.S. Harper, and D.A.S. Compston. Von Recklinghausen neurofibromatosis. A clinical and population study in south-east Wales. Brain 1988;111:1355–1381.
4. N.P. Rosman and J. Pearce. The brain in multiple neurofibromatosis (von Recklinghausen's disease): A suggested neuropathological basis for the associated mental defect. Brain 1967;90:829–838.
5. J. Handa, T. Koyama, Y. Shimizu, and S. Yoneda. Skull defect involving the lambdoid suture in neurofibromatosis. Surg Neurol 1975;3:119–121.
6. T.A. Tomsick, R.R. Lukin, A.A. Chambers, and C. Benton. Neurofibromatosis and intracranial arterial occlusive disease. Neuroradiology 1976;11:229–234.

7. R.A. Beyer, P. Paden, D.F. Sobel, and F.G. Flynn. Moyamoya pattern of vascular occlusion after radiotherapy for glioma of the optic chiasm. Neurology 1986;36:1173–1178.
8. L. Rubenstein. The malformative central nervous system lesions in the central and peripheral forms of neurofibromatosis: A neuropathological study of 22 cases. Ann NY Acad Sci 1986;486:14–29.
9. F.W. Crowe, W.J. Schull, and J.V. Neel. A clinical, pathological, and genetic study of multiple neurofibromatosis. Springfield, IL, Charles C Thomas, 1956.
10. J.R. Bognanno, M.K. Edwards, T.A. Lee, et al. Cranial MR imaging in neurofibromatosis. AJNR 1988;151:381–388.
11. J. Gray and K.F. Swaiman. Brain tumors in children with neurofibromatosis: Computed tomography and magnetic resonance imaging. Pediatr Neurol 1987;3:335–341.
12. R.A. Lewis, L.P. Gerson, K.A. Axelson, et al. Von Recklinghausen neurofibromatosis II. Incidence of optic gliomata. Ophthalmology 1984;91:929–935.
13. P.K. Duffner and M.E. Cohen. Isolated optic nerve gliomas in children with and without neurofibromatosis. Neurofibromatosis 1988;1:201–211.
14. R.J. Packer, L.T. Bilaniuk, B.H. Cohen, et al. Intracranial visual pathway gliomas in children with neurofibromatosis. Neurofibromatosis 1988;1:212–222.

5

Learning Disabilities in Neurofibromatosis

Alan M. Aron, M.D., Allan E. Rubenstein, M.D.,
Sibylle A. Wallace, M.D., and Jane C. Halperin, M.S.

Parents frequently ask, "What is the relationship between neurofibromatosis and learning disability?" It is important to state honestly that the exact relationship is yet to be defined. We have been impressed that there is a significantly greater incidence of learning disability (LD) in children with NF1 than in the general pediatric population. It is estimated that between 6 and 9% of school-age children harbor some form of LD and males are more often affected than females. The ratio of affected males to females approximates 6:1. In the neurofibromatosis (NF) clinic of the Mt. Sinai Hospital in New York, we have found that between 40 and 50% of children with NF1 have a LD, approximately five to six times what would be expected. There is no increase in the frequency of LD in people with NF2.

Definition of Learning Disability

What do we mean when we say "learning disability"? We are talking about a child who shows unexpected school failure but has a normal intellectual potential. This, therefore, excludes cases of mental retardation. It is essential to emphasize that the IQ range in people with LD is extremely variable. It is possible to have LD with superior intellect; a large proportion of children with LD have IQs in the average or low-average range.

There are three common presentations in children with LD. The first may reflect a specific learning problem. This difficulty can be confined to reading, writing, calculating, or some combination of these skills. The second involves a lack of coordination of varying degree. Most frequently this involves fine-motor incoordination manifest by awkwardness in handling a pencil and performing activities like buttoning, zippering, or tying shoelaces. A third common presentation involves hyperactivity, distractibility, and variable attention span. This may be found in 50 to 70% of children with LD. There are substantial numbers of children who have LD but do not have hyperactivity. A child does not have to have all three of these problems. Any one of these can lead to difficulties which impair language reception, memory, attention, and motor agility. In addition, emotional factors frequently supervene because children perceive themselves as different from their peers.

In a recent study, Eliason (1) compared children ages 6 through 14 with NF1 with children without NF but with developmental LD. The groups were matched for age, sex, and full scale IQ. The children with NF were distinguished by a high frequency of visual-spatial problems (56% in the NF group vs. 6% in the non-NF LD group). Sixty percent of the children with LD without NF presented with primarily language disabilities. Thirty percent of the NF group also had language or verbal memory deficits.

Learning involves a complex sequence of reactions. A child reacts to a stimulus that produces a sensation. In order to obtain an impression of the object, kinesthetic (motion), cutaneous (touch), visual, auditory, and other information are integrated to produce a thought, which is then stored in memory. The child with LD may falter at any point in this sequence. While it is common for children with LD to have normal growth and developmental milestones, there is an increased incidence of both delayed speech development and articulatory difficulties, as well.

Diagnosis of Learning Disability

Many parents are unaware that their child has a LD. Frequently, it is a nursery or preschool teacher who singles out the youngster as being "different." The child is recognized because he calls attention to himself by disruptive behavior or by being awkward in gross-motor activities such as running or jumping. Such children manifest fine-motor problems by their inability to manipulate scissors or to color within boundaries. They are awkward in managing a pencil and have difficulty in learning to grip properly. It is not uncommon for the nursery school teacher to contact the family and report these observations.

It is important to screen the child with NF1 for ability in reading and writing. For the preschool child, tests of copying simple geometric shapes should be carried out. For the older child, reproduction of Bender Gestalt figures is important. For the school-age child, a sample of writing from spontaneous dictation can frequently be helpful. The examiner should also complete tests of fine- and gross-motor coordination and sensory deficits (vision and hearing). Attention must be paid to language development with the examination of articulation, grammatical usage (syntax), and vocabulary.

The workup for the child with LD and NF1 should include a detailed neurological examination. It is essential to document that vision and hearing are normal. Ophthalmological consultation should be carried out when indicated. Audiometric testing and brainstem auditory evoked responses

(BAER) are indicated for the speech-delayed child with NF1. Differences of opinion continue concerning the most effective imaging study of the brain. Consideration should be given to performing a computed tomography (CT) scan of the brain or a magnetic resonance imaging (MRI) study (2,3). An electroencephalogram (EEG) can be helpful in ruling out subtle subclinical seizure phenomena that could be contributing to learning difficulty and impaired attention. A complete psychometric battery should be performed by a psychologist skilled in dealing with LD children and adolescents. A battery of psych-educational tests should be administered to screen for the specific basis of a learning difficulty. It is of the utmost importance to attempt to specifically define the basis for a learning difficulty. It is only with such knowledge that an appropriate program of rehabilitation and educational therapy can be individually developed for the child.

TREATMENT OF LEARNING DISABILITY

Treatment is available once the diagnosis of LD has been made. The treatment of such a child involves a multifaceted, team approach. The single most important factor is specific remediation for the defined area of deficiency. This is why it is essential for a psychologist to assist a special educator in pinpointing the areas of deficiency in the learning schema of the child. It is important to determine whether the problem is an auditory difficulty or a visual problem or a combination of each. Special school placement is frequently a valuable help to the child. It assures a smaller student-to-teacher ratio. It provides a structured class setting where the child with a behavior problem and/or attentional distractibility is in an environment more conducive to learning.

Psychological counseling is often beneficial for it provides support for the child and his family. The youngster with a LD and with NF1 reacts to "being different." It is common for such children to harbor a poor self-image and poor peer relationships. This results in inevitable conflict with siblings and parents. A common first response of parents with children who have LD is to deny the problem. The next response is frequently one of parental anger and frustration. Such parental reactions can be dealt with through counseling to enlist active parental support in the total rehabilitative process.

The use of medications has been restricted to helping improve attention span in children with hyperactivity. Hyperactivity and distractibility interfere with the learning process and create social problems. Medication may enhance the child's ability to attend, thereby allowing the child an improved opportunity to learn. With maturation, there seems to be a spontaneous improvement in hyperactivity.

The medications that have been used to decrease distractibility and enhance attention can be classified into three categories: (1) stimulants, such as methylphenidate and amphetamines; (2) antihistamines, such as diphenhydramine hydrochloride, which are frequently less effective; and (3) psychotrophic agents typified by phenothiazines, which are indicated for more severe behavioral problems characterized by aggressivity and poor impulse control. All of these medications represent acceptable modes of therapy in specific instances. Treatments should be individualized according to specific traits of each child.

Controversial therapies that have not been shown to have a beneficial role in improving LD include patterning, optometric exercises, orthomolecular approaches, and biofeedback. The elimination of specific artificial coloring and food additives and the elimination of sugars, as emphasized in the Feingold diet, have not been demonstrated in any controlled study to have a positive effect.

SUMMARY

In summary, the specifics of the anatomical basis and the pathophysiology that lead to LD have yet to be defined. How LD relates to NF1 is also unknown. Present clinical research must address this relationship. We are unfortunately left with more questions than those for which we can provide answers. The association between LD and NF1 deserves further study. This relationship should be recognized by parents, by educators, and by physicians. The child with NF1 deserves careful screening for LD so that he or she may be able to utilize his or her fullest potential to learn.

REFERENCES

1. M.J. Eliason. Neuropsychological patterns: Neurofibromatosis compared to developmental learning disorders. Neurofibromatosis 1988;1:17–25.
2. J. Gray and K.F. Swaiman. Brain tumors in children with neurofibromatosis: Computed tomography and magnetic resonance imaging. Pediatr Neurol 1987;3:335–341.
3. J.R. Bognanno, M.K. Edwards, T.A. Lee, et al. Cranial MR imaging in neurofibromatosis. AJNR 1988;151:381–388.

6

Communication Disorders in Children with Neurofibromatosis Type 1

Cynthia B. Solot, M.A., Elaine H. Zackai, M.D., Ph.D., Angela C. Obringer, Ph.D., Dan F. Konkle, Ph.D., Steven Handler, M.D., and Anna T. Meadows, M.D.

Communication disorders of hearing, speech, and language are often cited as complications associated with neurofibromatosis (NF) in children (1). The incidence and nature of communication disorders in children with NF1, however, are unknown because most published reports that describe communication problems associated with NF1 are either anecdotal or based on data from severely affected or hospitalized children. Moreover, data on overall developmental and intellectual functioning of children with NF1 are inconclusive. Past reports have indicated that mental retardation occurs frequently in NF1; however, a more recent report suggests that learning disorders may be more characteristic of NF1 than is mental retardation (2).

In an effort to more clearly understand the prevalence and nature of specific communication disorders in NF1, a pilot study was undertaken at The Children's Hospital of Philadelphia (CHOP). Thus far, a total of 33 children diagnosed with NF1 were studied with 10 normal sibling controls. Subjects are drawn from the established NF1 clinic in which approximately 200 children have been followed in a comprehensive, multidisciplinary program.

Evaluations of hearing, speech, language, and voice are conducted by a speech-language pathologist and audiologist. In the NF1 clinic, children are evaluated by a geneticist and an oncologist and then referred as necessary to radiology, otolaryngology, neurology, ophthalmology, orthopedics, and surgery (see Chapter 14).

Preliminary findings from this ongoing investigation suggest that many children who are even mildly affected with NF1 experience some degree of speech and language problems, but do not appear to suffer hearing loss to an extent greater than children without NF1. Abnormalities have been identified in the areas of voice, speech, and language (see Table 6–1). These findings,

Table 6-1. Incidence of Speech-Language Disorders in 23 Children with Neurofibromatosis Type 1 and Their Siblings

	PROBANDS (N = 23)	SIBLING CONTROLS (N = 10)
Articulation disorders	11	2
Language disorders (n = 22)		
Mental retardation	3	0
Language learning disorders	9	1
Voice disorders		
Hypernasality	5	0
Hoarseness	5	0
Vocal nodules	2	0
Hearing impairment	0	0

coupled with the observation that learning problems can have an overall adverse influence on intellectual and sensorimotor functions, suggest that all children with NF1 be considered at risk for speech and language disorders.

The purpose of this chapter is to discuss the nature of speech and language problems that may exist in children with NF1. As an introduction to these concepts, this chapter is organized to present: first, a brief overview of terminology; second, a description of speech and language disorders commonly encountered in children with NF1; third, an overview of strategies used in speech-language evaluation; and fourth, a brief outline of therapies that can be used when speech and language disorders are identified.

TERMINOLOGY

Speech refers to the articulation, or formation, of sounds using the muscles and structures of the tongue, lips, palate, jaw, and teeth. These structures work in concert with the muscles of respiration to produce a stream of air and the structures of the larynx which vibrate the air stream to produce a voice. Speech is a physical process that requires anatomical integrity and adequate hearing acuity and perception.

It is important to distinguish between speech and *language*, which is an interactive, symbolic code by which infinite verbal and nonverbal messages are produced and understood. Language is comprised of the content of ideas, the form or structure into which ideas are organized, and the intent or reason for language use. Language is possible without speech, as in (severe) cerebral palsy where neuromuscular dysfunction may preclude speech because of impaired motor abilities. Meaningful speech, however, cannot occur without at least a rudimentary level of language.

Another important aspect of speaking is *voice*. Voice is the vehicle on which messages are carried. Technically, it is a vibrated stream of air that is produced by the muscles of respiration and phonation. The air stream is altered into various shapes and sizes to form the many sounds of speech. Without the carrying power of the voice, there may be significant distortion of the speech signal, and speech intelligibility may be severely reduced as occurs following a laryngectomy.

Normal development of speech and language processes depends upon adequate *auditory functions*. Sensory stimulation in the form of auditory input provides the basis for language development and the expression of linguistic concepts via speech. If auditory reception is impaired because of hearing loss, it follows that language development will be delayed, abnormal, or absent. Even mild forms of hearing loss have been associated with delays in language and in subsequent educational and psychosocial development (3).

Speech, language, audition, and voice are interrelated components of the communicative system. Disorders of one or more of these components may have potentially adverse influences on the overall development of children. However, disorders can vary widely in severity, and there is not always a direct relationship between severity of the disorder and any associated handicap. Generally, when communicative disorders are identified early and intervention strategies are initiated promptly, the effect of the handicap can be minimized.

Speech

Structural Anomalies

As speech production depends on a complex interaction of the structures of respiration and phonation, the growth of a neurofibroma on one of these structures can cause a reduction or alteration in the way the affected structure moves. The size, type, and location of a neurofibroma determines whether there will be interference in the speech process. Subcutaneous tumors were found to cause impairment in several children's speech. In one case, a child presented with a large plexiform neurofibroma under the left collar bone which extended into the neck. Speech and vocal quality were impaired and the voice was hypernasal. Speech rate was slowed. Because of difficulty sustaining phonation, phrases were short. Another child presented with a relatively small plexiform neurofibroma under the tongue. There was only very mild, inconsistent articulatory distortion. In a third child, a very large mass on the left side of the neck did not interfere with the production of speech. Thus, the position of the neurofibroma relative to speaking structures is a critical determinant of its effect on speech.

Similar tumors in the oral cavity or larynx or within the respiratory mechanism can also adversely affect speaking ability. In some cases, surgical removal of the neurofibromas is effective in eliminating the speech disorder.

Conversely, surgical excision of the tumor may itself cause speech disturbance. Therefore, there must be careful consideration of overall medical/ communication needs.

Of the speech disorders seen in children with NF1, structural anomalies account for only a small percentage of speech problems found.

Motor Speech Disorders

Motor speech disorders may present as weakness, paralysis, or incoordination of the speech musculature. Motor disorders result from damage within the central or peripheral nervous system. These problems can be present at birth or acquired with the growth of neurofibromas along neural pathways or within the brain. General symptoms observed with motor speech problems include excessive slowness or distortion in execution of speech movements, reduced range or strength of articulatory movements, weak or impaired vocal intensity, resonance or quality, and/or impaired speech breathing. Speech and non-speech functions may be affected. There may also be impairment in the prosodic features of speech, which include rate, rhythm, intonation, and stress. The term used to describe these types of speech disorders is dysarthria.

Another category of motor dysfunction is dyspraxia. In dyspraxia, muscle strength and range movement are intact. Oral motor performance of non-speech functions may be unimpaired. However, the neurological circuitry governing the planning or programming of coordinated speech movements and movement sequences is impaired. In this case, an individual has difficulty executing intended motor movements. Speech sound errors are made in the form of sound substitutions, omissions or distortions.

The data derived at CHOP suggest that motor speech disorders represent one of the most prevalent groups of speech disorders found in the NF1 children studied thus far. Many of the children mispronounced speech sounds or had difficulty sequencing sounds. Sometimes, sounds in words were produced out of order or sounds were entirely omitted. Syllables of polysyllabic words were also often transposed or omitted. In addition to errors forming speech sounds and sound sequences, it was common for NF1 children to demonstrate slight differences in their use of rhythm and speech rate. Typically, there was less variation in these prosodic features than is generally observed in ongoing speech. In very young children there may be a history of past or present disturbances in motor skills for feeding as well.

None of the unaffected siblings demonstrated this type of speech disturbance. Observed delay in speech development in the unaffected siblings was present to the same degree as in the general pediatric population.

Phonological Processing Disorders

Learning to speak requires the ability to perceive accurately the sounds of speech spoken by others. This process includes learning to differentiate speech from nonspeech sounds, to discriminate one sound from another, and, later, to ascribe meaning to groups of sounds. This process begins in infancy and depends upon normal hearing, adequate cognitive abilities, and language skills.

Every language has rules governing the use of sounds and sound sequences. Thus, after mastering the perceptual nature of sounds, it is necessary to learn how sounds are typically organized. Children must then learn to reproduce these patterns in their own speech, pairing what they have learned with motor patterns and vocabulary.

Disorders in the perception of sounds or sound patterns are almost always considered to be part of the larger category of language learning disabilities. Since learning disabilities are discussed in detail elsewhere in this volume, they are only briefly considered here.

When perception is impaired there may be a prolonged period of production of immature speech patterns in conjunction with errors of auditory-listening and discrimination. Problems in sound-symbol association and phonics, characteristic in this group, can lead to difficulties learning to read.

Cognitive Deficit

In mental retardation, there is subnormal functioning in all areas, including the development of language and speech. Strictly speaking, children with mental retardation develop language and speech following the usual sequences of development, but at a slower rate consistent with the degree of retardation. Therefore, for example, an 8-year-old child with mild retardation may have speech patterns similar to a normal 5-year-old, with the characteristic immaturities or patterns seen in children of that age. This is not considered a speech disorder, but rather a delay in the acquisition of speech milestones. With maturation, speech should continue to develop within the competencies of the individual.

Often, however, mentally retarded individuals have other developmental problems, such as motor dysfunctions and perceptual impairments, so that maturation alone may not necessarily produce optimum speech development. Therefore, it is important to evaluate speech to determine if it is commensurate with an individual's intellectual capacity or fails to meet developmental expectations.

In the group seen at CHOP, few children presented with mental retardation. Of those children, several presented additional speech disorders, distinct from the retardation.

Sensory Deficits

Speech disorders can also result from hearing impairment. Young children who were born with sensory defects do not hear speech sounds or hear them in a distorted way. They have difficulty learning the meaning of spoken language.

Congenital hearing impairment occurs infrequently in NF1. More commonly, in NF2, hearing loss may develop in adolescence and adulthood. While these individuals are already highly skilled users of speech and language, speech quality is likely to deteriorate without the tactile-kinesthetic and auditory feedback provided by hearing senses. Even when amplification is provided, speech therapy may be necessary to help maintain optimum speech performance.

In the sample of children at CHOP, there were no cases of congenital hearing loss.

LANGUAGE

The term language is often confused with the term speech. As noted, language refers to a symbolic process that incorporates elements of meaning, concepts, grammar, and memory. Language reflects a fund of information and vocabulary and an ability to think and reason with words, to interpret and assign semantic significance to spoken words, to select and retrieve words which express thoughts and feelings, and to organize words into sequences under the direction of a rule-governed grammatical code. The process of oral language can be subdivided into the following component processes: auditory reception and processing, cognitive and semantic language processing, verbal memory, organization and fluency, and pragmatic or social use of language. Each of these processes has receptive and expressive aspects. The abilities to read and write are secondary language systems learned after oral language mastery.

Language is the means by which we communicate with each other. It is how information is transmitted to children in school. Thus, language is essential to normal social, emotional, and intellectual development.

Language development may be delayed for a variety of reasons, including mental retardation, learning disabilities, hearing impairment, neurological disorders, and social-emotional problems. In the sample of children at CHOP, there were no instances of delayed language on the basis of emotional, sensory, or hearing deficit.

LEARNING DISABILITIES

Language learning disabilities are defined in the 1975 Education for All Handicapped Children Act as: "disorders of one or more of the basic psychological processes involved in comprehending or using language, either spoken or written, which result in difficulty listening, thinking, speaking, reading, writing, or doing mathematical calculations" (4). The definition excludes individuals with subnormal intelligence, sensory deficits, or emotional/behavioral disturbances, although it is now generally accepted that these conditions may coexist with language disabilities. Within the broad category of learning disabilities, there may be other impaired processes that adversely affect learning, such as visual-perceptual abilities, visual-motor skills, and gross- and fine-motor skills. In a recent study, 56% of a sample of NF children studied demonstrated disabilities in visual perceptual skills. Of those children with visual perceptual problems, 30% also presented with language problems (5). In contrast, surveys of disabilities in the general population indicate 40 to 60% are language based (6).

In Chapter 5 Aron et al. state that 40 to 50% of NF1 children have learning disabilities, a significantly greater proportion than found among school-age children in the general population where estimates range from 5 to 20% (7). The preliminary data in our study are consistent with this report and suggest a majority of NF1 children with learning disorders have language problems.

In our sample, children with NF1 scored lower than the sibling control group on several standardized measures. The most significant difficulties observed in the NF group were with vocabulary acquisition and various aspects of written language. In addition, many children exhibited difficulties at the syntactic, phonological, and semantic levels. All of the NF1 children with language learning disabilities were reporting problems in school. In our data, there was no apparent association between clinical severity of NF1 and language findings. In fact, in our sample, the two most clinically affected children were average to bright intellectually and showed no learning problems. The distribution of language learning problems also differs from the general population, where learning disabilities occur with a ratio of four males to one female. In our NF1 sample, there was equal sex distribution.

Mental retardation occurs with only a slightly increased frequency in NF1 in comparison to the general population (2,8). Our data support this assertion. As described earlier, mentally retarded individuals show a generalized slowness in all areas of development, including language. The level of language performance may be consistent with the magnitude of retardation. However, language problems may be more severe than the developmental deficiencies of the individual lead one to expect. When this occurs, a child is considered to have both a cognitive deficiency as well as a learning disorder.

VOICE DISORDERS

In order to produce a normal voice, the following prerequisites must be present: a source of air to vibrate, coordination of the respiratory and phonatory systems, intact structural mechanisms, and normal capacity for laryngeal movements.

In general, voice disorders can occur as a result of organic problems, such as congenital or acquired structural anomalies; trauma; neurological or motor impairments; or allergies. Nonorganic factors, such as vocal misuse of abuse, and psychological factors, may also cause vocal dysfunction.

Voice disorders in NF1 can be the result of neurofibromas that appear on structures associated with the production of sound. These include the muscles and structures of respiration as well as those of phonation.

The most common voice dysfunction in school-age children in the general population is vocal abuse/misuse often leading to vocal nodules (9). The most common symptom associated with vocal nodules is hoarseness, which occurred frequently in our clinical population. Two of the children with hoarseness were subsequently found to have vocal nodules. None of the sibling controls showed any degree of hoarseness.

Additional vocal difficulties often seen in children with NF1 are disorders of resonance, particularly hypernasality. In our sample, several children were hypernasal in comparison to none of the sibling controls. While the reason for this increased occurrence is unknown, impairment of motor control of the velopharynx is suspected. In one published report, observation of several NF1 children studied for hypernasal speech revealed a variety of velopharyngeal disorders (10).

EVALUATION

A comprehensive diagnostic assessment of speech and language is comprised of many elements. Prior to the speech-language assessment, however, it is important to obtain an audiological evaluation to determine overall hearing status. While the incidence of hearing loss in children with NF1 is essentially the same as that of the general population, it can be projected that some children will have transient hearing loss associated with middle ear infections. A few will have varying degrees of sensorineural involvement. However, since NF1 children are at risk for speech and language disorders, physicians, parents, and other professionals must be alert to the importance of monitoring hearing function through auditory assessment.

Assessment

In language and speech assessment a comprehensive history should be taken, including time of emergence of developmental milestones; patterns of development; history of school performance; family history of associated speech, language, and school problems; history of otolaryngological conditions; and pertinent medical background.

In general, the speech-language evaluation should include an examination of the different aspects of communication:

The size and shape of the oral structures are evaluated in addition to associated findings such as the presence, size, and symmetry of tonsils or neurofibromas; the strength, range, and functional mobility of structures; and coordination for speech and nonspeech movements.

Pitch, quality, and resonance characteristics of the voice should be evaluated in words, sentences, and spontaneous speech. Presence or absence of associated characteristics, such as hoarseness or pitch breaks, should be observed. Loudness level and respiratory control are noted. If vocal pathology is suspected, referral for laryngoscopic evaluation by an otolaryngologist is indicated.

Articulation is evaluated by listening to speech in several contexts and comparing performance to developmental norms. There are several good standardized tests that evaluate all of the speech sounds of the language in their respective places in words, for instance, initial (*s*ee), medial (pen*c*il), and final (hou*s*e). Production should also be assessed in sentences and in more spontaneous contexts, such as stories and conversation, to determine how well sound and motor patterns are mastered.

Language assessment should include a battery of standardized measures that comprehensively evaluate abilities in the various language domains. Test scores are compared to normative data and integrated in light of general intellectual capacities of the individual. The quality of performance (that is, the style or manner of performance, the relative ease or difficulty needed to complete tasks, associated behavioral/attentional factors, and the degree of examiner report required) is also analyzed.

The predominant referral sources in the clinic at CHOP are physicians, teachers, and parents. However, referrals may be made by anyone concerned about a child's development, including social workers, psychologists, and occupational and physical therapists. Because children with NF1 may have many medical needs, attention to communication may be delayed or overlooked.

THERAPY

When communication problems are identified, speech and language therapy can be helpful in remediating problems and in stimulating development. It is not sufficient merely to identify problems. When indicated, early intervention can make a critical difference in the outcome of a child's development.

The speech and language problems of NF1 children are amenable to traditional therapeutic methods. Therapy is a means by which communication problems can be hierarchically ordered and systematically treated. Therapy can change deficient behavior using specialized methods, or develop compensations to accommodate to a particular disability. Often, speech-language therapy is provided in school as part of a program of specialized education. However, speech-language therapy may be provided independently, in private offices, clinics, and hospitals.

With children, therapy is generally provided on an individual basis or in small, homogeneous groups. The approach can be direct or indirect in a context of play. With older children and adolescents, the therapy is often more direct. A warm, supportive relationship between therapist and child is a key factor in therapeutic effectiveness. Further, contact among parents, teachers, and the speech-language pathologist is important to reinforce therapeutic goals in different contexts of the child's life, and thereby to optimize learning.

Generally, articulation therapy proceeds systematically from one sound to another or from one sound group to another. Auditory, tactile, and kinesthetic cues are used to achieve sound production. The sounds are practiced using target sounds first in isolation, then words followed by phrases, sentences, stories, and spontaneous speech. Adaptations in the above procedures are made, depending on the etiology of the articulation problem (that is, motor, structural, cognitive, or phonetic). Motor speech problems generally take a longer time to correct than others. When problems are severe, compensating speech patterns or approximations of target speech sounds must be accepted. Motor speech problems require much practice with phonetic placement. Phonetic processing difficulties may require more auditory training than other types of articulation problems. With hearing loss, visual feedback devices give a visual representation of sound and assist the affected individual in matching sensorimotor patterns to desired acoustic signals.

Voice therapy should always be preceded by otolaryngological examination. The purpose of such an evaluation is to obtain a view of laryngeal structure and function and to determine the etiology of a voice disorder. Proper diagnosis is critical to correct treatment.

Through specifically designed exercises, voice therapy can change the way the vocal folds are used or alter speaking habits that are harmful to the larynx. Further, sluggish muscles can be strengthened or nasality and pitch characteristics altered. Often, respiration training is part of a voice therapy program since breath support provides the foundation for vocalization. Voice therapy is sometimes used on a trial basis before surgical interventions are made, to determine if pathological conditions can be corrected by changing vocal use.

Language therapy is highly complex and the methods of therapy are more variable. Therapy can be didactic or experiential, direct or indirect, structured or open. Specific verbal games or activities are used to correct specific aspects of language deficiencies. Activities isolate the problem for practice and then integrate the selected target into functional language use. Therapy can be effective in providing remediation and/or compensation to any or all of the areas of language processing/development, including comprehension, concepts, vocabulary, recall, organization, syntax, and pragmatics.

A certified speech-language pathologist can be found within most communities in the following places:

- Local hospitals or medical centers
- School district or intermediate units
- University speech and hearing clinics
- Community mental health/mental retardation centers

- Rehabilitation centers
- Private schools
- Private practice
- Otolaryngologist's or pediatrician's office

State or local speech and hearing associations, or the American Speech-Language-Hearing Association, provide listings of qualified professionals. The address of the American Speech-Language-Hearing Association is: 10801 Rockville Pike, Rockville, MD 20852.

SUMMARY AND CONCLUSIONS

Speech and language problems occur to a significant degree in children with NF1. In an ongoing research project of CHOP, the majority of NF1 children seen to date presented with speech and/or language disabilities. Speech disorders comprised the largest disability group. In this group of children, there were many etiological factors, including primarily motor speech disorders, phonological disorders, and, less commonly, cognitive deficits and structural anomalies. The majority of children with language problems demonstrated impairments associated with learning disabilities. Language problems related to mental retardation were also seen to a degree slightly higher than in the general population. In addition, minor voice problems were also heard.

Because communication disorders, including speech, language, and voice (and hearing in the central form of NF1) occur with such frequency in children with NF1, they may constitute one of the most serious conditions associated with NF1. Therefore, it is extremely important that communication skills be evaluated. All NF1 children, regardless of severity, should be seen for a speech-language evaluation as a routine part of comprehensive care. Assessment should be conducted shortly after the initial diagnosis of NF1. Initial evaluations can be used as a baseline by which to measure growth in subsequent evaluations and/or as a means of planning for educational or therapeutic needs. Moreover, evaluation of speech and language can be an excellent screening mechanism to detect more widespread developmental or physical problems. Once identified, children with communication problems can be offered appropriate remedial assistance. Early intervention is of the utmost importance in minimizing the negative impact of a communication disorder and maximizing a child's social, emotional, and developmental potential.

More information about specific characteristics and patterns of development of communication in NF1 is needed. Such information can assist the overall understanding and treatment of NF1 as well as, perhaps, shed light on the nature of developmental disabilities in general.

REFERENCES

1. V.M. Riccardi, and J.E. Eichner. Neurofibromatosis: Phenotype, natural history, and pathogenesis. Baltimore, Johns Hopkins University Press, 1986.
2. J.C. Carey, J.M. Laub, and B.D. Hall. Penetrance and variability in neurofibromatosis: A genetic study of 60 families. Birth Defects 1979; Original Article Series 15, No. 5B:271–281.
3. M. Downs, and J. Norther. Hearing in children. Baltimore, Williams and Wilkins, 1978.
4. Public Law 94-142. Education for all handicapped children act. Washington, D.C., Federal Register, 1975.
5. M.J. Eliason. Neurofibromatosis: Implications for learning and behavior. J Dev Behav Pediatr 1986;7:175–179.
6. M. Miettinen. Gastrointestinal stromal tumors: An immunohistochemical study of cellular differentiation. Am J Clin Pathol 1988;89:601–610.
7. J. Coplan. Evaluation of the child with delayed speech or language. Pediatr Ann 1985;14:3–7.
8. S.M. Huson, P.S. Harper, and D.A.S. Compston. Von Recklinghausen neurofibromatosis. A clinical and population study in south-east Wales. Brain 1988;111:1355–1381.
9. D.K. Wilson. Voice problems in children. Baltimore, Williams and Wilkins, 1979.
10. M. Pollack, and R. Sprintzen. Velopharyngeal insufficiency in neurofibromatosis. Int J Pediatr Otorhinolaryngol 1981;3:251–262.

7

NEUROSURGICAL ASPECTS OF NEUROFIBROMATOSIS

Robert L. Martuza, M.D.

Neurosurgical problems are among those most feared by the patient or family with neurofibromatosis (NF). Although these problems can be very serious, they should be kept in perspective since such serious complications are relatively uncommon (1,2), and are usually caused by benign tumors that can be surgically removed if detected early.

As noted in Chapter 1, there are two types of NF. These two forms present distinct challenges in neurosurgical care. Type 1 (NF1), or von Recklinghausen form, causes multiple café au lait spots and neurofibromas, but is also associated with central nervous system abnormalities such as spinal or nerve root neurofibromas, optic gliomas, or, less commonly, meningiomas or gliomas. Type 2 (NF2), or bilateral acoustic NF, on the other hand, is characterized by the development of bilateral acoustic neuromas. Other central nervous system tumors such as meningiomas and cranial or spinal neurofibromas are also common in this disorder, but skin manifestations are few.

In both NF1 and NF2 the mere presence of a brain or nerve tumor does not necessarily mean that it needs to be surgically removed. The decision for or against surgery is made on the basis of the type and location of the tumor, whether or not it is growing, and the age and medical condition of the patient.

TUMORS OF THE NERVE SHEATH (SCHWANN CELL TUMORS)

The neurofibroma is the most common tumor associated with NF1. It has already been described in Chapter 4. Neurofibromas may be plentiful on the skin, where they can be a major cosmetic problem but rarely cause serious symptoms. When such tumors occur on deeper nerves in the arm or leg, however, they can cause pain, numbness, or weakness. Physical examination or various radiological studies may reveal the tumor which is usually a *plexiform neurofibroma* (Fig. 7–1). If the symptoms are minimal or the lesion is not

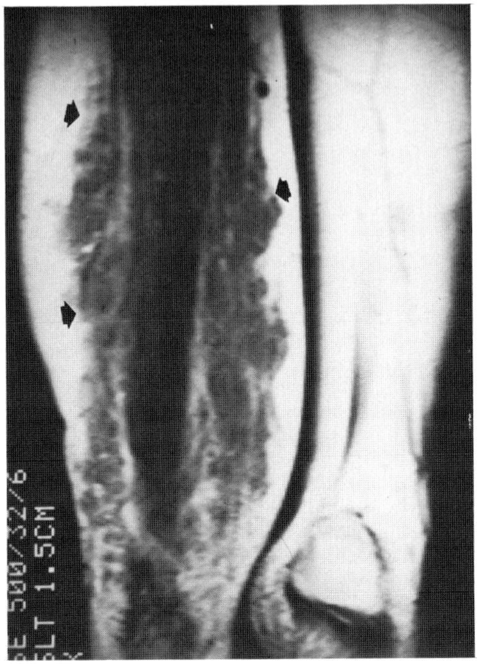

Figure 7–1. MRI of lower legs in a patient with NF1. This longitudinal section shows a leg enlarged by a plexiform neurofibroma (arrows).

growing, it is often decided not to operate. Such tumors may engulf many nerve fibers and the surgery itself can lead to numbness or weakness. However, if the symptoms are progressive, the risks are worth taking. If the tumor is not surrounded by many fibers, it can often be removed with little or no neurological deficit. In cases where an important nerve must be sacrificed, the surgeon may choose to remove only part of a benign tumor or to insert a nerve graft. Fortunately, most of these tumors are benign. However, some rapidly growing tumors may be found to be malignant. In such cases, more extensive surgery and postoperative radiation are usually needed (see Chapter 10).

The most difficult plexiform neurofibromas to treat are those in the brachial plexus (Fig. 7–2). The brachial plexus is an intricate web of nerves, between the neck and shoulder or upper arm, which connects the spinal cord with the arm and hand. Complete removal of a brachial plexus neurofibroma is often impossible because of the serious hand or arm difficulties that can be produced.

Modern surgical techniques utilize an operating microscope, electronic nerve stimulation and recording during surgery, and, in some cases, surgery under local anesthesia with the patient awake so that nerve function can be tested during surgery. With these methods, surgery of peripheral nerve tumors can be safely performed.

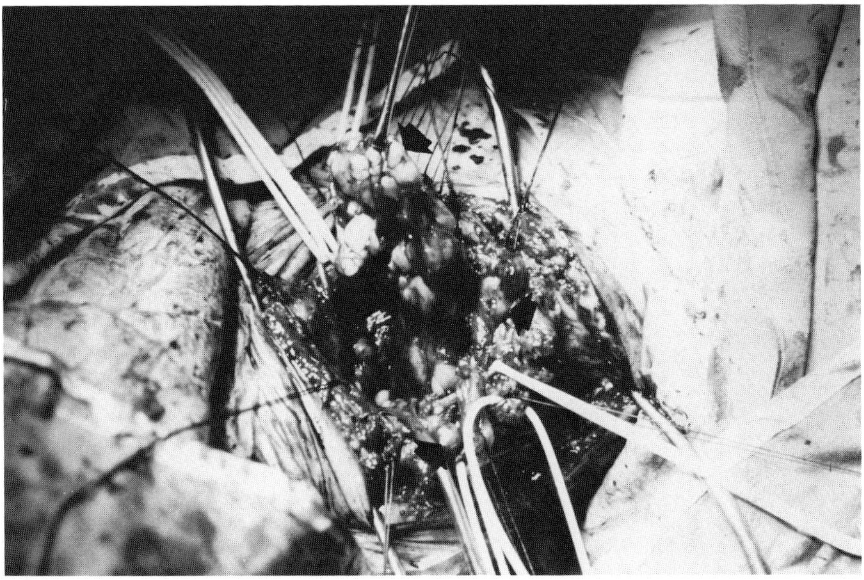

Figure 7–2. A patient with NF1 has multiple plexiform neurofibromas of the brachial plexus. At surgery tumors are found on many nerves (arrows).

Spinal neurofibromas are Schwann cell tumors that form at or near the point where nerves from the arms or legs join the spinal cord (3). Many patients have multiple spinal neurofibromas noted on a computed tomography (CT) scan, myelogram, or magnetic resonance imaging (MRI) (Fig. 7–3). Most do not grow or cause symptoms, and are best left alone. When symptoms occur, these often relate to compression of the nerve on which one of these tumors is growing and may include pain, numbness, or weakness in a specific area. With large tumors, the spinal cord may be compressed, causing bilateral symptoms, walking difficulty, or poor control of bowel or bladder function. Such symptoms should never be ignored. Evaluation with x-rays, CT scan or MRI, or myelography is usually urgently done and surgery is virtually always indicated. With the operating microscope and newer operating techniques such as the laser and the ultrasonographic aspirator, such tumors can usually be completely and safely removed.

Schwann cell tumors may form on any cranial nerve. These nerves join the brain to the eyes, face, ears, throat, or tongue. The most common cranial Schwann cell tumor is the *acoustic neuroma*. This is a tumor of the vestibular (balance) nerve. The earlier an acoustic neuroma is found, the better the result of surgery will be (4). Detailed testing of hearing with audiograms and brainsteam auditory evoked responses (BAER) is essential to early detection (5) (see Chapter 3). With very small tumors, complete removal can often be done while saving hearing and facial function (6). As the tumor enlarges, it

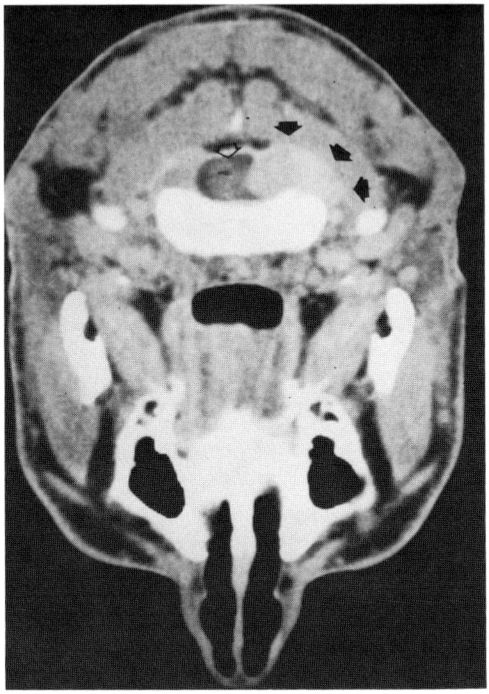

Figure 7–3. This CT scan demonstrated a spinal root neurofibroma (closed arrows) pressing on the spinal cord (open arrow).

becomes difficult or impossible to save hearing, and surgery may be associated with facial weakness.

In patients without NF or with NF1, if an acoustic neuroma develops, it likely will occur only on one side (Fig. 7–4). In this case, although hearing loss may be caused by the tumor or by surgery, useful hearing remains in the opposite ear. In contrast, patients with NF2 have acoustic neuromas on each side and face total deafness (7). In such patients, the indications for surgery and the type of surgery differ from the patient with one acoustic neuroma. In the NF2 patient, the goal is to preserve hearing for as long as possible. In some cases, this may require deferring surgery and following the size of the acoustic neuromas by CT scan or MRI. In other instances, the removal of a small tumor may be done with intraoperative monitoring (BAER) to preserve hearing. The surgeon may elect partial tumor removal to spare hearing in the only hearing ear. These decisions are complex and must be individualized to the needs, medical condition, and age of the patient.

Tumors of the Covering of the Brain and Spinal Cord

Meningiomas are benign tumors that arise from a protective layer (meninges) which covers the brain and spinal cord (Fig. 7–5) (8). Meningiomas may occur in both NF1 and NF2 but are more common in the latter. Although not an

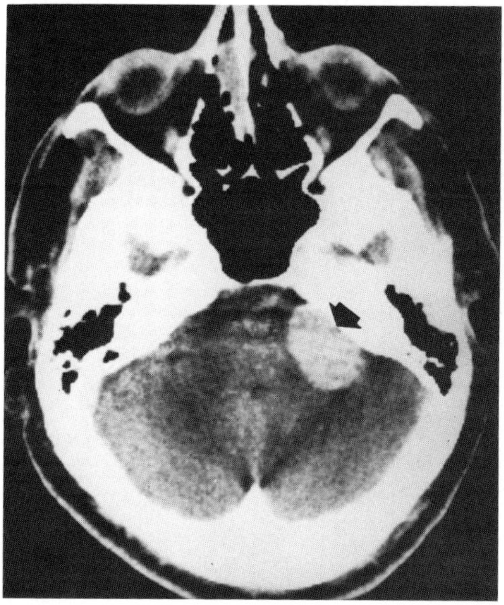

Figure 7–4. This contrast-enhanced CT scan shows a unilateral acoustic neuroma (arrow).

intrinsic part of the brain or spinal cord, meningiomas cause symptoms by pressing on these structures. Since they can occur over any part of the central nervous system, they can produce a wide variety of problems. On the brain, they can cause seizures, weakness, numbness, visual problems, memory disturbance, or personality changes. In the spinal area, they can lead to weakness, numbness, bowel or bladder trouble, or impotence. A CT scan or

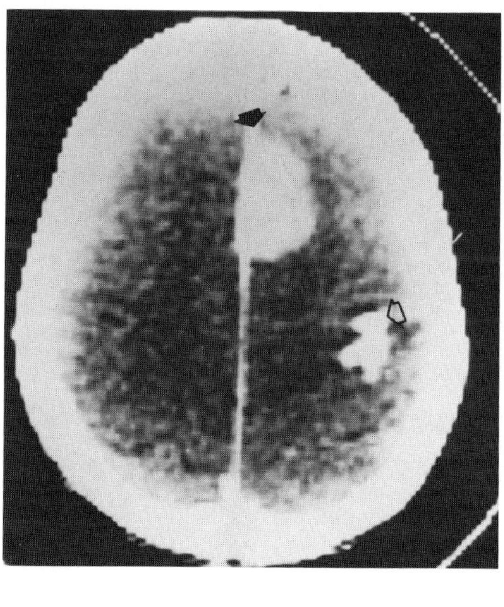

Figure 7–5. A meningioma (closed arrow) is noted in this CT scan from an NF2 patient. A second tumor of unknown type is also seen (open arrow).

contrast-enhanced MRI will usually detect the tumor. Often an angiogram is done to confirm that a tumor is a meningioma. Meningiomas are almost always benign, and, since they are usually located on the surface of the brain (just under the skull), they can be safely and completely removed in most instances. Postoperative radiotherapy is not necessary unless the tumor is malignant. In some patients, multiple meningiomas may be present. If they are easily approachable, they may be removed at the time of removal of the symptomatic tumor. In other instances, small lesions may simply be observed with sequential CT scans.

TUMORS WITHIN THE BRAIN OR SPINAL CORD

In both types of NF, a tumor may form within the substance of the brain or spinal cord. These do not arise from the nerves themselves but rather from the glial cells surrounding the nerves, and are called gliomas.

Optic gliomas form in the nerves of vision just behind the eye (Fig. 7–6). In some cases they are present from birth and cause few or no symptoms (9). In other patients, they may cause progressive visual loss or blindness (10). In the past, a biopsy was often recommended for diagnosis, but current radiological techniques (CT scan, MRI) eliminate the need for biopsy in most cases (11,12). Surgery is reserved for those tumors that are very localized in one nerve, for tumors that are rapidly enlarging and cause pressure on other brain structures, or for instances in which diagnosis is uncertain (13,14). Often it is unwise or

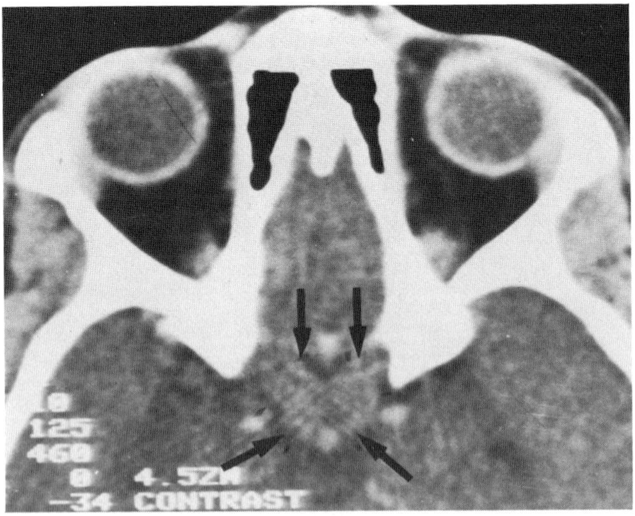

Figure 7–6. This CT scan demonstrates a glioma of the optic chiasm (arrows).

impossible to completely remove an optic glioma, and either sequential scanning to follow growth or radiotherapy to arrest growth may be necessary.

Gliomas within the brain or spinal cord (15–17) are the most difficult tumors of NF for the surgeon to treat. The symptoms relate to their location in the central nervous system and are as varied as those described for meningiomas. Some are benign or slowly growing and can be extensively removed. Others infiltrate deeply in the brain and can be removed only at great risk. Generally, complete removal is not possible and recurrence depends upon the rate of growth of the infiltrating cells left behind. Some gliomas are malignant and removal is followed by rapid recurrence (Fig. 7–7). Radiotherapy (and sometimes chemotherapy) is needed to slow the growth of these tumors but a cure has not been found for the malignant glioma. Fortunately, such tumors are very uncommon in both types of NF.

Cerebrospinal Fluid Flow Problems (Hydrocephalus)

The brain is constantly producing cerebrospinal fluid. It forms in cavities deep within the brain (ventricles) and flows through narrow passageways out of the brain. It then bathes the spinal cord and brain and finally flows to the top of the brain where it is absorbed and returned to the bloodstream. This complex

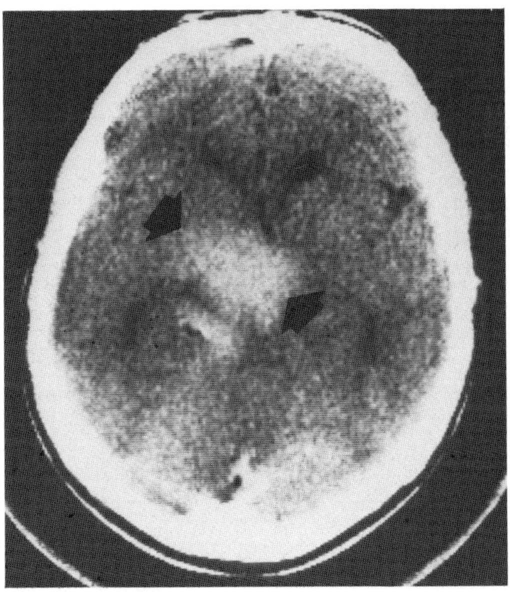

Figure 7–7. This CT scan demonstrates a malignant glioma (arrows) in a patient with NF1.

pattern of flow can be blocked at any number of locations by a tumor, scarring from hemorrhage, trauma, past surgery, or congenital narrowing of one of the passageways. When this happens, pressure builds up in the ventricles of the brain, causing headache, walking difficulty, or poor bladder control. In infants it can cause an abnormal increase in head size. When the blockage is more acute, it can cause blurred vision, blackouts, or even death. This condition is called hydrocephalus and is easily treated by an operation in which the surgeon places a soft tube containing a one-way valve (shunt) beneath the skin. The shunt drains cerebrospinal fluid from the ventricles of the brain to the bloodstream or to the abdomen. The operation is safe and the shunt is left permanently in place. Occasionally, the shunt valve may malfunction, the original symptoms recur, and a revision of the shunt system is necessary.

The diagnosis of hydrocephalus in a patient with NF (18) is complicated by the fact that the average head size of most NF patients is larger than that of the rest of the population (19,20). A CT scan may even show enlarged ventricles (ventriculomegaly). However, a larger than average head and ventriculomegaly do not mean that a shunt is necessary. A shunt is placed only when symptoms, signs, and radiological studies suggest progressive hydrocephalus.

SUMMARY

In this brief overview of the more common neurosurgical problems encountered by NF patients, it has been emphasized that the patient and family keep these problems in perspective. Most NF patients will never have a need to see a neurosurgeon. Others may have spinal neurofibromas or other tumors that remain quiescent and do not need surgery. However, some will have enlarging tumors. The development of symptoms described should lead to seeking attention, since the smaller the tumor is and the milder the symptoms are, the better the surgical prognosis will be. It is heartening to know that most of the tumors are benign and, in many cases, completely removable.

REFERENCES

1. J.C. Carey, J.M. Laub, and B.D. Hall. Penetrance and variability in neurofibromatosis: A genetic study of 60 families. Birth Defects 1979;Original Article Series 15, No. 5B:271–281.
2. S.M. Huson, P.S. Harper, and D.A.S. Compston. Von Recklinghausen neurofibromatosis. A clinical and population study in south-east Wales. Brain 1988;111:1355–1381.
3. W.J. Levy, J. Latchaw, J.F. Hahn, et al. Spinal neurofibromas: A report of 66 cases and a comparison with meningiomas. Neurosurgery 1986;18:331–334.
4. R.L. Martuza, and R.G. Ojemann. Bilateral acoustic neuromas: Clinical aspects, pathogenesis, and treatment. Neurosurgery 1982;10:1–12.

5. R.L. Martuza, S.W. Parker, J.B. Nadol, et al. Diagnosis of cerebellopontine angle tumors. Clin Neurosurg 1985;32:177–213.
6. R.G. Ojemann, R.A. Levine, W.M. Montgomery, and P. McGaffin. Use of intraoperative auditory evoked potentials to preserve hearing in unilateral acoustic neuroma removal. J Neurosurg 1984;61:938–948.
7. R.L. Martuza, and R. Eldridge. Neurofibromatosis 2. N Engl J Med 1988;318:684–688.
8. D.F. Merten, C.A. Gooding, T.H. Newton, and N. Malamud. Meningiomas of childhood and adolescence. J Pediatr 1974;84:696–700.
9. R.A. Lewis, L.P. Gerson, K.A. Axelson, et al. Von Recklinghausen neurofibromatosis II. Incidence of optic gliomata. Ophthalmology 1984;91:929–935.
10. P.K. Duffner, and M.E. Cohen. Isolated optic nerve gliomas in children with and without neurofibromatosis. Neurofibromatosis 1988;1:201–211.
11. J. Gray, and K.F. Swaiman. Brain tumors in children with neurofibromatosis: Computed tomography and magnetic resonance imaging. Pediatr Neurol 1987; 3:335–341.
12. J.R. Bognanno, M.K. Edwards, T.A. Lee, et al. Cranial MR imaging in neurofibromatosis. AJNR 1988;151:381–388.
13. D.E. Spitzer, and J.T. Goodrich. Optic gliomas and neurofibromatosis: Neurosurgical management. Neurofibromatosis 1988;1:223–232.
14. J.D. Easley, L. Scharf, J.L. Chou, and V.M. Riccardi. Controversy in the management of optic pathway gliomas. Neurofibromatosis 1988;1:248–251.
15. H.A. Rodriguez, and M. Berthrong. Multiple primary intracranial tumors in von Recklinghausen's neurofibromatosis. Arch Neurol 1966;14:467–475.
16. A. Horie, U. Shigemi, T. Fukushima, and K. Tanaka. Neurofibromatosis complicated by intracranial tumors. Acta Pathol Jpn 1974;24:705–716.
17. E.B. Ilgren, L.M. Kinnier-Wilson, and C.A. Stiller. Gliomas in neurofibromatosis: A series of 89 cases with evidence for enhanced malignancy in associated cerebellar astrocytomas. Pathology Ann 1985;20:331–358.
18. A. Horwich, V.M. Riccardi, and U. Franke. Aqueductal stenosis leading to hydrocephalus: An unusual manifestation of neurofibromatosis. Am J Med Genet 1983;14:577–581.
19. J.F. Hall, and L.R. Kuhns. Macrocranium and macroencephaly in neurofibromatosis. Skel Radiol 1976;1:25–28.
20. K.A. Weichert, M.S. Dine, C. Benlon, and F.N. Silverman. Macrocranium and neurofibromatosis. Radiology 1973;107:163–166.

8

Ocular Features of Neurofibromatosis

Richard A. Lewis, M.D.

Both major forms of neurofibromatosis (NF) can have important effects on the visual system. Ocular manifestations often provide important signs of the disorder that may be valuable in establishing a diagnosis. Visual disturbance may also constitute a serious potential complication of the disorder. The chief ocular manifestation of NF2 is posterior subcapsular cataract (1). This is a helpful diagnostic clue, but rarely causes visual loss or requires cataract surgery. Moreover, this lesion has already been described in Chapter 3. This chapter will therefore concentrate on involvement of the eye in NF1.

Neurofibromas Involving the Eye

Neurofibromas, the characteristic tumors of NF1, may occur anywhere in the body, including the face and eye. Here they range in size from less than 3 mm, thus forming dot-like elevations often of the eyelid or eyelid borders (and are thus called punctiform neurofibromas), or they may be larger and form lumps or nodules of 6 to 3 mm in diameter (nodular neurofibromas) and be distributed over the face and lids. About 20% of adult patients with NF1 have punctiform neurofibromas of the lids, often near or within the eyelash borders. In addition to being dome-shaped and elevated under the skin, these tumors rarely may have a stalk and be pedunculated. Diffuse neurofibromas with exuberant overgrowth of thickened, ropy nerves involving the face, the eyelids, and the tissue in the orbit occur occasionally, but fortunately in only 1 or 2% of all individuals with NF1.

The most frequent and disfiguring facial neurofibroma is a plexiform (meaning "net-like") neurofibroma involving the outer one-third of the upper lid (2). This lesion causes a thickening and redundancy of the lid tissue and a deformity that gives the appearance of a lazy S (Fig. 8–1). This is highly characteristic of NF1 when it occurs, although fewer than 5% of all individuals with NF1 have this type of neurofibroma of the lid.

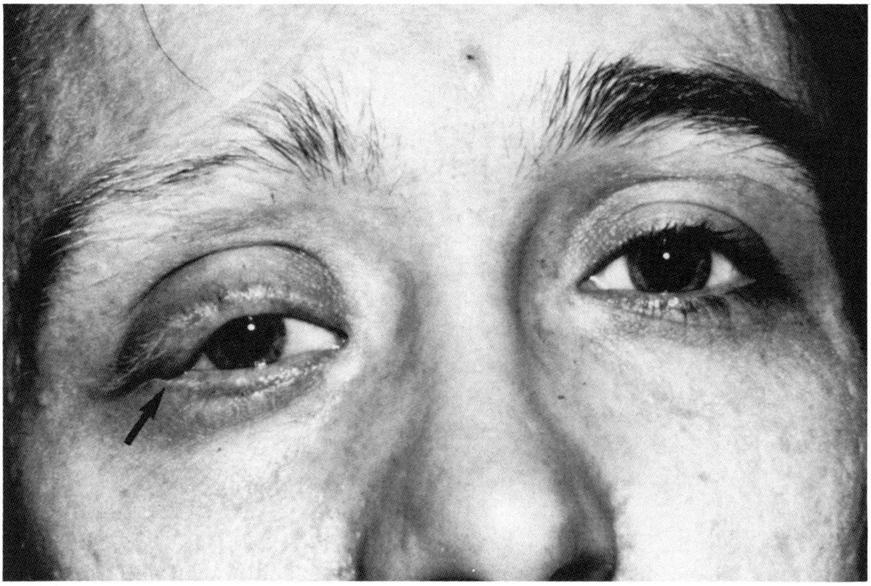

Figure 8–1. Plexiform neurofibroma of the right orbit, causing deformity of the eyelid on that side (arrow).

It has long been taught that there is a risk of congenital glaucoma, almost always in one eye only, in patients who have diffuse plexiform neurofibroma involving tissues of both lids and the orbit. The frequency of this diffuse involvement of all these tissues at the same time is quite low, probably less than 2% of all subjects with NF1. However, any infant or child who is born with or who develops massive thickening of the eyelid and orbital tissues should be examined carefully for the possibility that the eyeball is also malformed and that there is an increase in pressure inside the eye. Unfortunately, the developmental abnormalities of the nerves and other structures in the eye are sometimes so severe that control of ocular pressure by either medicines or surgery is almost impossible. Maintenance of good vision in an eye with congenital glaucoma in an orbit with a diffuse plexiform neurofibroma can seldom be achieved and often the patient and family must be content to preserve the eye intact, even if it does not have useful sight.

Crossed eyes or other abnormalities of movement of the eyes have been thought by some investigators to be more common in children and young adults with NF1 than in the rest of the population. However, in a survey of over 500 subjects with NF (R.A. Lewis, unpublished observations), the frequency of crossed eyes (either turned in or turned out) appears to be no different than that for the population in the United States without NF.

The cornea is the transparent covering of the front surface of the eye, through which must pass all light that enters the eye. When an ophthalmologist examines the cornea under high magnification with a microscope or slit lamp, occasionally thickening or prominence of the nerves that normally pass through the cornea is noted (3). This thickening or hypertrophy occurs in approximately 10 to 20% of individuals with NF, but tumors of these nerves are never seen in the cornea. Thus, although prominence of corneal nerve fibers is probably more frequent in NF than in the normal population, this observation is not a useful diagnostic sign for NF1 and it has no effect or vision even when it does occur.

LISCH NODULES

In 1937, Karl Lisch, an Austrian ophthalmologist, noticed some small tan bumps on the surface of the iris of three adult patients with NF1 (4). These bumps have subsequently been called Lisch nodules, out of respect for his observation, even though they were seen as early as 1930 by two American physicians. Lisch nodules are tan to glassy, smooth-bordered, dome-shaped elevations that contain no blood vessels and that may occur anywhere along the iris surface, from its margin at the pupil into the angle where the iris joins the inside of the cornea (Fig. 8–2). Lisch nodules are almost never present at birth but tend to appear at about the age of 5 years. Before the age of 6 years, Lisch nodules occur on average in one or both irises of some 15 to 20% of all children with NF1 (5).

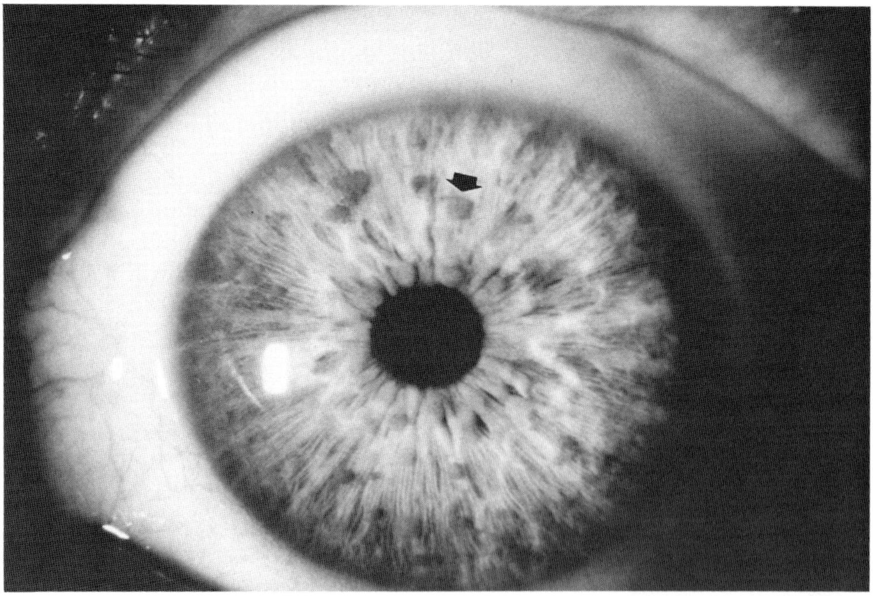

Figure 8–2. Multiple iris Lisch nodules (arrow).

Numerous other conditions may cause bumps and discolorations on the surface of the iris and usually they are either too tiny or too transparent to be seen with the naked eye. Therefore only an experienced ophthalmologist can distinguish the structure and appearance of Lisch nodules from a number of other hereditary, congenital, and acquired variations of the iris surface. In addition, the ophthalmologist must use an illuminated microscope called a slit lamp to examine the iris to find Lisch nodules as part of a complete medical eye examination. Most pediatricians, internists, neurologists, and geneticists do not have the skills and experience to identify Lisch nodules.

After age 6 years, some 95% of individuals with NF1 develop Lisch nodules of the iris (3,5–7). Lisch nodules occur just as commonly among people who have inherited NF1 as they do when the affected person is the first person in the family to have the disorder. It makes no difference whether the NF was inherited from the patient's father or mother; the number of Lisch nodules, their distribution on the iris surface, and their appearance are not related to the parent who transmitted the gene. Lisch nodules appear to be the most frequent ocular feature of NF and are nearly diagnostic of the disease when they appear, particularly when associated with café au lait spots and neurofibromas of the skin. However, Lisch nodules are not correlated with the severity of the disease, the number of café au lait spots, the number of neurofibromas of the skin, other tumors of the eye and central nervous system, mental retardation, or head circumference in patients with NF. Because of the distinctive nature of these nodules, a careful and complete medical eye examination in a person who is suspected of having NF is the second best test for this diagnosis after a thorough skin examination, especially if the person is old enough to have Lisch nodules.

STRUCTURES INSIDE THE EYE

After the ophthalmologist has examined the face, eyelids, eye muscle movements, and the front parts of the eye with the slit lamp microscope, drops will be used to dilate (enlarge) the pupil, to allow examination of the inside of the eye, most especially the retina, the choroid, and the optic nerve. The retina is a thin sheet of nerve tissue that lines the inside of the back two-thirds of the eye and serves like the film in a camera to capture images. Electrical images from the retina are carried up to the brain through the optic nerve, which functions like a large telephone cable to connect the retina to the brain. The choroid is a thick spongy blood vessel coat that lines the inside of the eye behind the retina.

The choroid gives an overall reddish-brown hue to the inside of the eye, darker in blacks and Hispanics than in most whites, and darker in brunettes than in blonds. When the ophthalmologist examines the inside of the eye, most properly with a bright light called an indirect ophthalmoscope, occasionally tan, flat discolorations in the back half of the eye are seen, and in some cases resemble the tan café au lait spots seen in the skin of patients with NF (3). These "freckles" are best seen after the teen years, have no affect on eyesight, and have extremely low potential for malignancy. In the past, it was said that there is a higher risk for melanomas inside the eyes of people with NF1. However, there is no evidence to substantiate this old idea. It is almost impossible to see these tan freckles inside the eyes of Hispanics or blacks, because of the dark natural coloring of the lining of their eyes. Presumably the freckles are actually there but they cannot be seen.

Optic Glioma

Another concern for people with NF1 is a tumor called an optic glioma. Gliomas are tumors (or swellings) made up of the supportive cells, called glial cells, which nourish and maintain the integrity of the optic nerve. Optic gliomas may occur at any point in the visual pathway (8). In some instances the tumor is confined to the portion of the optic nerve within the orbit. In other cases the tumor may include or be confined to the optic chiasm, where the optic nerves from the two eyes meet. This structure is adjacent to the hypothalamus, a part of the brain involved in control of hormone secretion, among other things. Involvement of the nerve fibers extending from the chiasm to the brain is also found, although rarely.

In a study of several hundred individuals with NF1, in which everyone underwent detailed, high-resolution, thin-section computed tomography (CT) scans of the brain, orbit, and optic nerves, 15% of subjects were found to have tumors of one or both optic nerves or the chiasm (9). Gliomas of the optic nerve are rarely malignant. Unfortunately, there is very little space in the optic nerve for normal tissue, let alone the slow growth of the nearly normal cells that form the glioma. Therefore, these tumors may damage the vision from the eye because of where they are rather than what they are. Actually, fewer than 5% of patients with NF1 develop any problems or damage to sight from this type of tumor (10). The remaining tumors are silent and can be detected only by careful use of sophisticated CT or magnetic resonance imaging (MRI) scans (11). Unfortunately, the natural history and progression of these tumors which are found on routine scanning are unknown.

Gliomas of the brain or optic nerve(s) occur equally often in both males and females with NF and equally often in whites, blacks, and Hispanics. In addition, there is no greater risk of having a glioma among people who have inherited NF from a parent than those who represent a new genetic mutation or are the first instance of NF in their families.

Because of the excellent detail obtainable from present-day CT or MRI scans, the diagnosis of optic glioma by a radiologist using these imaging machines is usually not difficult (Fig. 8–3) (12). However, standard skull x-rays and x-rays of bony tunnels through which the optic nerves travel from the orbit into the

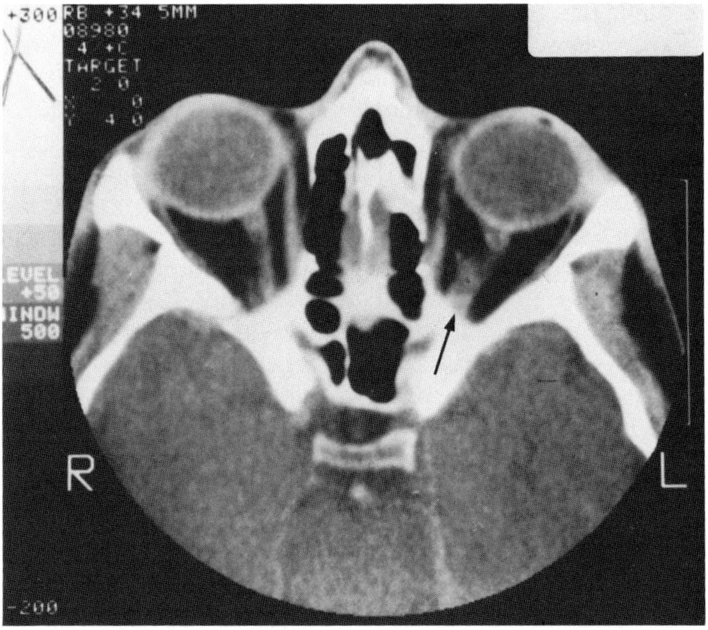

Figure 8–3. Optic glioma involving the left optic nerve (arrow).

brain are not helpful in detecting optic gliomas, especially those that do not involve those canals themselves. Visual evoked potentials (recording of electrical activity in the brain resulting from presenting flashes of light or a changing pattern in front of the eyes) can also be of use in establishing a diagnosis of optic glioma (13,14). Loss of vision or atrophy (loss of color and substance) of the optic nerve when the inside of the eye is examined by an ophthalmologist strongly suggests the presence of an optic glioma in a patient with NF. Most importantly, however, the obverse is not true: a normal eye examination does *not* eliminate the possibility of an optic glioma in NF, since at least two-thirds of the time patients with this tumor have completely normal vision, normal visual fields, and normal findings on eye examinations. Although there is not universal agreement on this point, I believe strongly that all patients with NF1 should have at least one CT or MRI scan with views of both orbits and both optic nerves. Why do I make such a recommendation? First, of course, the natural history of these optic gliomas is unknown. Where do they come from? Which ones will cause problems? Unless a detailed examination is done, physicians will not be able to make informed judgments about who should be studied more carefully, or even who should have a biopsy of the tumor to identify whether it is malignant or benign. The second reason for knowing whether optic gliomas are present is to alert physicians to carefully follow those asymptomatic individuals with tumors, who have completely normal results on eye examinations. Infants and children, for example, may not complain of problems caused by slowly growing tumors; their care must be supervised by informed parents and scrupulously attentive physicians who know about the presence of a potential problem. Lastly, by studying everyone with this disease, we will develop a better understanding of the risks of these tumors, who is likely to have them, and who is likely to develop complications.

Unfortunately, the treatment of optic glioma remains controversial (15,16). No good medical study has evaluated the natural history of untreated tumors over a long period of time. Therefore, any recommendations for treatment may only be general guidelines and may not be applicable to any one particular patient or any one particular tumor. To some degree, differences in behavior of the tumor and its potential damage to sight depend on whether the tumor involves the optic nerve within the orbit, within the bony canal in the skull, or inside the brain. Patients who develop symptoms (including changes in peripheral vision or eyesight) may have more severe complications from their tumor(s) than those who go for several decades totally unaware of the tumor's existence except by radiological detection. Most physicians believe, however, that anterior optic gliomas (involving the tumors in the orbit) should be observed and followed when the patient is asymptomatic (8,17,18). When the tumor causes problems with vision or damages the appearance of the optic nerve, some physicians may recommend that the optic nerve should be removed surgically. Unfortunately, removal of the (entire) optic nerve irreversibly blinds that eye.

In posterior optic gliomas, especially those that involve the base of the brain and other structures inside the skull, most physicians think that asymptomatic tumors should be observed. Occasionally, the tumor might be biopsied to firmly establish an exact diagnosis, lest some other confusing tumor be missed. However, if a posterior optic glioma creates damage to vision, then it should be explored and biopsied to find out if it may respond to radiation therapy or even extensive surgical removal (17). However, the role of radiation therapy in posterior optic gliomas also is a matter of considerable controversy among radiation therapists, neurosurgeons, neurologists, and ophthalmologists (16,19). Complications of radiation therapy include loss of ability to make pituitary hormones such as growth hormone, and occlusion of major blood vessels, sometimes leading to stroke (20). As we gain more experience with the natural (untreated) evolution of some of these tumors, and compare the progress to groups of tumors that have been treated with surgery or x-rays, we may learn better guidelines for recommendations in the future.

SUMMARY

In summary, the complete medical eye examination is the next most important way to diagnose NF1 after the skin exam. The eye and its adjacent structures show many different features of this disease as well as several of its most important complications. The ophthalmologist plays a key role in the team of physicians and specialists in the diagnosis and management of NF.

REFERENCES

1. M.A. Pearson-Webb, M.I. Kaiser-Kupfer, and R. Eldridge. Eye findings in bilateral acoustic (central) neurofibromatosis: Association with presenile lens opacities and cataracts but absence of Lisch nodules. N Engl J Med 1986;315:1553–1554.
2. J. van der Meulen. Orbital neurofibromatosis. Clin Plast Surg 1987;14:123–135.
3. S.M. Huson, D. Jones, and L. Beck. Ophthalmic manifestations of neurofibromatosis. Br J Ophthalmol 1987;71:235–238.
4. K. Lisch. Ueber Beteiligung der Augen, insbesondere das Vorkommen von Irisknotchen bei der Neurofibromatose (Recklinghausen). Z Augenheil 1937;93:137–143.
5. R.A. Lewis, and V.M. Riccardi. Von Recklinghausen neurofibromatosis: Incidence of iris hamartomas. Ophthalmology 1981;88:348–354.
6. C. Zehavi, A. Romano, and R.M. Goodman. Iris (Lisch) nodules in neurofibromatosis. Clin Genet 1986;29:51–55.
7. U. Flueler, E. Boltshauser, and A. Kilchhofer. Iris hamartomata as diagnostic criterion in neurofibromatosis. Neuropediatrics 1986;17:183–185.
8. W.F. Hoyt and S.A. Baghdassarian. Optic glioma of childhood. Br J Ophthalmol 1969;53:793–798.
9. R.A. Lewis, L.P. Gerson, K.A. Axelson, et al. Von Recklinghausen neurofibromatosis II. Incidence of optic gliomata. Ophthalmology 1984;91:929–935.
10. S.M. Huson, P.S. Harper, and D.A.S. Compston. Von Recklinghausen neurofibromatosis. A clinical and population study in south-east Wales. Brain 1988;111:1355–1381.
11. J.R. Bognanno, M.K. Edwards, T.A. Lee, et al. Cranial MR imaging in neurofibromatosis. AJNR 1988;151:381–388.
12. P.K. Duffner, and M.E. Cohen. Isolated optic nerve gliomas in children with and without neurofibromatosis. Neurofibromatosis 1988;1:201–211.
13. B. Jabbari, C.G. Maitland, L.M. Morris, et al. The value of visual evoked potential as a screening test in neurofibromatosis. Arch Neurol 1985;42:1072–1074.
14. M.E. Cohen, and P.K. Duffner. Visual evoked responses in children with optic gliomas, with and without neurofibromatosis. Child's Brain 1983;10:99–111.
15. E.C. Alvord, Jr., and S. Lofton. Gliomas of the optic nerve or chiasm. J Neurosurg 1988;68:85–98.
16. J.D. Easley, L. Scharf, J.L. Chou, and V.M. Riccardi. Controversy in the management of optic pathway gliomas. Neurofibromatosis 1988;1:248–251.
17. D.E. Spitzer, and J.T. Goodrich. Optic gliomas and neurofibromatosis: Neurosurgical management. Neurofibromatosis 1988;1:223–232.
18. S.M. Chung, and J.A. McCrary, III. Management of pregeniculate anterior visual pathway gliomas. Neurofibromatosis 1988;1:240–247.
19. W.A. Fletcher, R.K. Imes, and W.F. Hoyt. Chiasmal gliomas: Appearance and long-term changes demonstrated by computerized tomography. J Neurosurg 1986;65:154–159.
20. R.A. Beyer, P. Paden, D.F. Sobel, and F.G. Flynn. Moyamoya pattern of vascular occlusion after radiotherapy for glioma of the optic chiasm. Neurology 1986;36:1173–1178.

9

The Skin in Neurofibromatosis

Arthur K.F. Tong, M.B., B.S., and
Thomas B. Fitzpatrick, M.D., Ph.D.

Neurofibromatosis (NF) is a relatively common inherited disorder of the neuroectoderm, characterized by the presence of a variety of tumors of neural crest-derived cells and other systemic disorders, such as macrocephaly, mental retardation, seizures, bone cysts, and short stature. The original descriptions of the disease by Smith (1849) (1) von Recklinghausen (1882) (2) did not include macular pigmentary changes. The addition of pigmentary changes to the complex is credited to Marie and Bernard (1896) (3) and to Chauffard (1896) (4). These changes are melanic in origin and consist of the café au lait macules and the hyperpigmented macules associated with an underlying plexiform neurofibroma. Crowe (5) subsequently added axillary freckling as a diagnostic marker of NF.

There are two forms of NF: (1) the classic von Recklinghausen NF (NF1) and (2) the central type, characterized by bilateral acoustic neuromas (NF2). NF2 is genetically distinct from NF1. Both types may have café au lait macules and neurofibromas. NF1 may rarely have unilateral acoustic neuroma, but only NF2 has bilateral acoustic neuroma. The following discussion will emphasize NF1, especially the cutaneous findings.

Clinical Features

Café au Lait Macules

Café au lait macules (Fig. 9–1) are pigmented macules of melanic origin. They are so-called because of their characteristic color—that of coffee with milk.

The café au lait macule has a homogeneous "very clear" brown color. In white persons with light constitutive skin color (skin type I and II), the hue is light tan and may only be visible with the aid of Wood lamp examination. The Wood lamp emits short-wavelength blue light, in which the contrast of pigmented skin lesions is enhanced, especially in fair-skinned individuals. In brown and black persons, the hue is dark brown or virtually black. On close

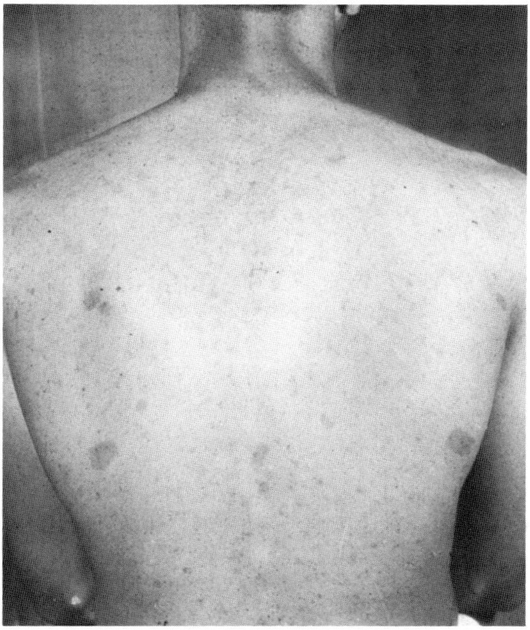

Figure 9–1. Von Recklinghausen NF (NF1). Many varying-sized café au lait macules in a 40-year-old male with brown constitutive skin color. The hue of the macule is quite dark brown.

examination with magnification of 10× or more and with the aid of mineral oil, there is an absence of a reticulated network of melanocytes as is regularly seen in melanocytic nevi. Café au lait macules in NF1 are indistinguishable from the brown macules in McCune-Albright polyostotic fibrous dysplasia (Fig. 9–2) (6). See Table 9–1 for a comparison of the melanotic macules of McCune-Albright syndrome and of NF1. Table 9–2 lists the various types of brown macules.

Café au lait macules are variable in size, configuration, and number. They may be located on any part of the body surface, but have a predilection for areas not exposed to sun. They are asymptomatic and are not known to undergo malignant change.

The incidence of café au lait macules that are larger than 1.5 cm in the widest diameter was determined to be about 10% in the normal adult population (7). About 90% of patients with proven NF by other criteria have at least one café au lait macule larger than 1.5 cm. Of NF patients, 68.3% were found with six or more café au lait macules while no adult found with six or more did not have NF. Thus Crowe and Schull (7) suggested that any person with more than six macules that are greater than 1.5 cm in diameter must be considered to have NF. If a person with no family history has fewer than six café au lait macules,

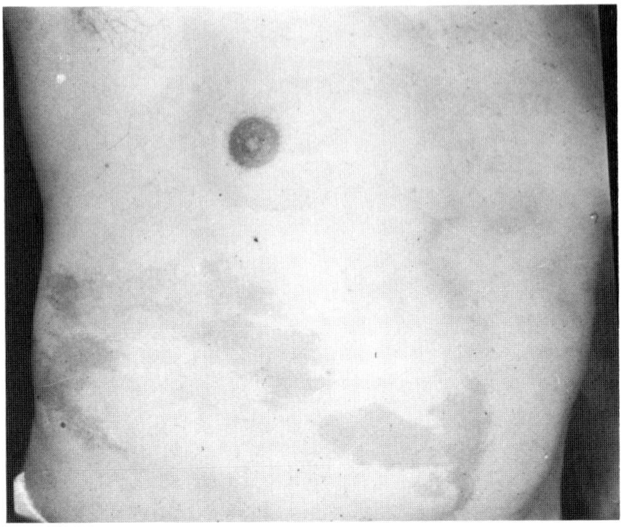

Figure 9–2. McCune-Albright syndrome. Note large café au lait macules occurring in a 6-year-old male with bone cysts. There was no precocious puberty.

then the probability of the person having NF is directly related to the number of café au lait macules on that person.

Whitehouse (8) studied 365 children under the age of 5 and noted that two or less café au lait macules are common in children, but more than two

Table 9-1. Clinical Features of Melanotic Macules in McCune-Albright Syndrome and In Neurofibromatosis

	McCUNE-ALBRIGHT SYNDROME	NF1
Distribution pattern	Tend to remain on either side of the midline; tend to be unilateral in a given area, e.g., neck, buttocks, and thorax	Tend to be generalized and irregularly distributed; axillary freckle-like pigmentation is characteristic of NF
No. of lesions	Few	Many
Configuration	Borders tend to be jagged and irregular, "coast of Maine"	Borders are more often smooth
Color	In addition to hue of café au lait, medium to dark brown; in the scalp, the hair over the lesion may be more pigmented	Café au lait; in brown and black people can be dark brown
Size	From macules covering a few centimeters to macules covering large areas	May be generalized, freckle-like macules in addition to the café au lait spots

Comparison of some of the clinical features of hypermelanotic macules in McCune-Albright syndrome and in NF. These features by themselves are not enough to make a definitive clinical differentiation between the hypermelanotic macules in McCune-Albright syndome and those in NF, nor is it possible to make a clinical diagnosis of either McCune-Albright syndrome or NF on the basis of a single pigmented macule. In most instances, however, it is possible to make a clinical diagnosis of NF, especially if, in addition to the café au lait macules, there is also diffuse freckle-like pigmentation of the axilla. We have not yet seen this in McCune-Albright syndrome.

Table 9-2. Brown Spots (Macules)

CAFE AU LAIT TYPE	MELASMA (FACIAL)*
Normal persons (10-15%)	Pregnancy
NF1	Oral contraceptives
Bilateral acoustic NF (NF2)	Normal males
McCune-Albright syndrome	Phenytoin (?)
Juvenile xanthogranuloma	
Silver-Russell syndrome	
Nevus spilus	
Cowden disease (multiple hamartoma)	
Ataxia-telangiectasia	
Xeroderma pigmentosa	
Generalized melanosis secondary to malignant melanoma	
X-linked ocular albinism	
Multiple lentigines syndrome	
Nojmegan syndrome	

*Rarely on the forearms.

macules occur in only 0.75% of normal children. He therefore suggested that five macules of greater than 0.5 cm be considered diagnostic until proven otherwise.

Normal children of pigmented (brown and black) persons have an increased incidence of café au lait macules compared to the normal white population. However, Bloch (9) in his study of NF1 in Indian and black South African children still found the criteria set by Crowe and Schull to be valid.

Axillary Freckling

There are small pigmented macules found in the areas of the skin not exposed to sun (i.e., axillae and other intertriginous areas) (Fig. 9–3). They are 2 to 3 mm in diameter and have been suggested by Crowe (5) to be a pathognomonic of NF. They are, however, seen in progeria and in leopard syndrome.

Hyperpigmented Macules in Association with Underlying Plexiform Neuroma

Hyperpigmented macules are darker in color than the typical café au lait macule. The borders of the hyperpigmented macules are concordant with the borders of the underlying plexiform neurofibroma. Those extending to the midline often suggest involvement of the spinal cord by the tumor (10).

Neurofibromas

Neurofibromas on the skin present as small, pink to skin-colored, dome-shaped papules. They may appear on any part of the body, but have a predilection for the areola in females. They are soft to the touch and give the

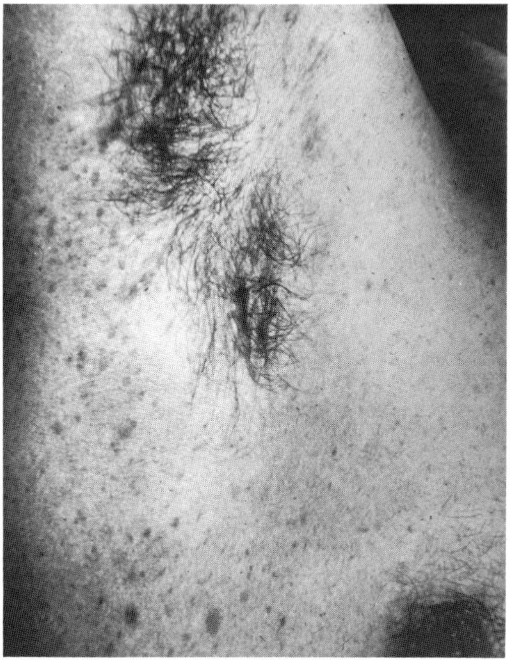

Figure 9–3. Axillary freckles. These are tiny versions of café au lait macules and are dissimilar from the common sun-induced ephelides (freckles).

feeling that the finger is herniating through the dermis on palpation (the "button hole" sign). With time, they become larger and pedunculated (Fig. 9–4). They may involve deeper peripheral nerves, nerve roots, and nerves of the autonomic nervous system.

The plexiform neuroma is a diffuse fibroma along the course of a nerve with a distinctive histology. They appear clinically as soft, drooping, and doughy masses. Elephantiasis neuromatosa is a diffuse NF of the nerve trunk associated with overgrowth of the subcutaneous tissue and of the skin, causing gross disfigurement.

Pregnancy and puberty may lead to an increase in the number and size of neurofibromas in any location. Rapid growth of a plexiform neuroma may suggest transformation to neurofibrosarcoma.

Blue-Red Macules and Pseudoatrophic Macules

Blue-red macules are located on the skin, mainly on the trunk. They average 3 cm in size and disappear on diascopy, indicating their vascular nature. These lesions may become slightly raised or even dome-shaped with time. Pseudoatrophic macules are oval-shaped, 5 to 10 cm in diameter, slightly depressed areas distributed mainly on the trunk. These areas are of normal

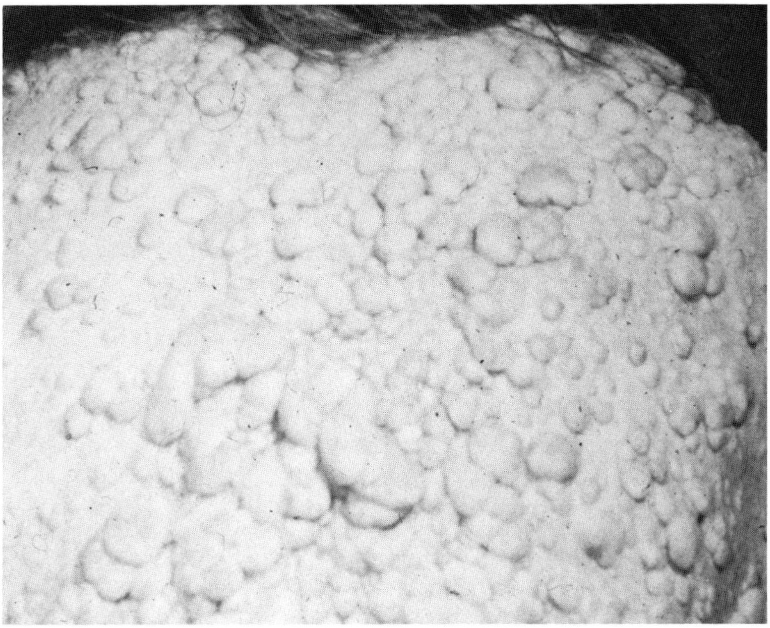

Figure 9–4. This 35-year-old female with NF1 has a grotesque appearance because of myriads of unsightly pendulous neurofibromas on the trunk and face.

skin color. The depression may be the result of a decrease of collagen bundles in the dermis of these areas. Both findings are claimed by Westerhof and Konrad (11) to be early indicators of the disease. However, the incidence of these findings and their specificity need to be further evaluated.

PATHOLOGY

Neurofibroma

The histology of neurofibroma in NF1 is identical to that of a solitary neurofibroma. On hematoxylin and eosin–stained sections, they appear as well circumscribed but nonencapsulated spindle cell tumors (Fig. 9–5). They are mostly in the dermis but may extend into the subcutaneous fat. The nuclei of the spindle cells are characteristically curved or S-shaped (Fig. 9–6). There is an increase in the number of mast cells within the tumor, which may account for up to 5% of the cells. A Giemsa stain would help to demonstrate these cells. Elastic fibers are absent in neurofibromas. A Bodian stain for nerves will demonstrate thin nerve fibers in most but not all tumors. The faintly eosinophilic, wavy fibers seen within the tumor stain positive with reticulin stain.

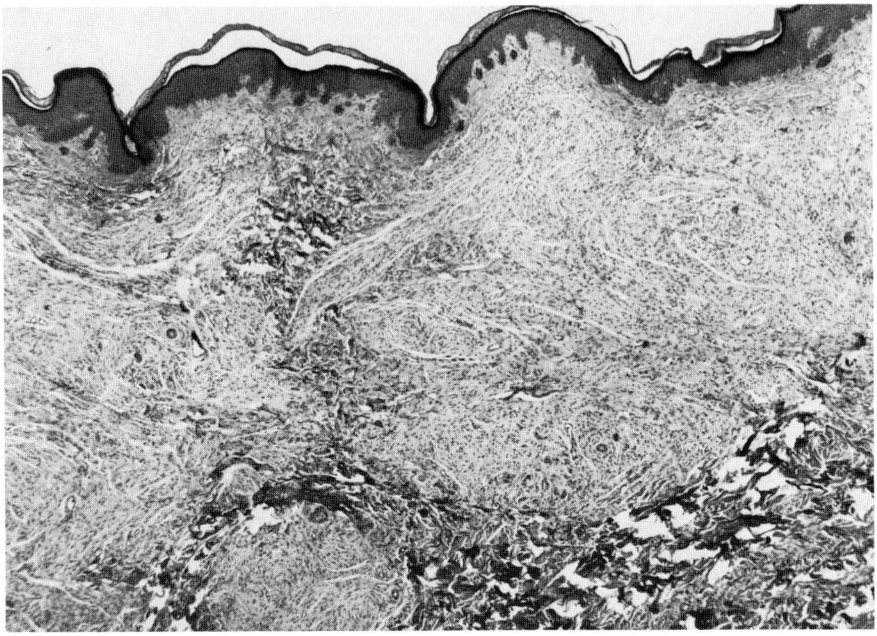

Figure 9–5. Neurofibroma, hematoxylin and eosin–stained section. Low-power view showing nonencapsulated, but well-circumscribed spindle-cell tumor in the dermis. (Original magnification = 45×.)

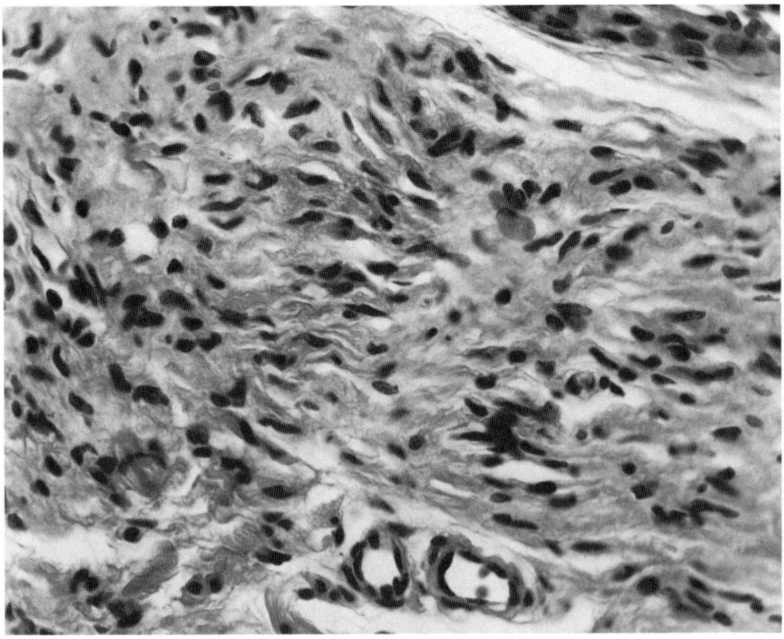

Figure 9–6. Neurofibroma, hematoxylin and eosin–stained section. A high-power view demonstrating the wavy nature of the cells and the curved or S-shaped nuclei. (Original magnification = 500×.)

Mucin may be found in the stroma. A cholinesterase stain is positive, further supporting a neural origin for these tumors.

Plexiform Neuromas

Plexiform neuromas are neurofibromas of large nerve tissues. Histologically they appear as globules of neural tissue (Fig. 9–7). The globules represent enlarged, tortuous plexi of Schwann cells and axons embedded in a mucinous stroma within a thickened perineurium.

Café au Lait Macules

The café au lait macules of NF1 patients contain more dopa-positive melanocytes per area than the surrounding skin. This is in contrast to café au lait macules on non-NF1 patients, which contain fewer dopa-positive melanocytes than the surrounding skin. Melanin macroglobules (MMG) are found in both hematoxylin and eosin–stained and dopa-stained sections. These appear on light microscopy as dark brown granules about 10 times the size of normal melanosomes. MMG can occur in a variety of disease conditions. However,

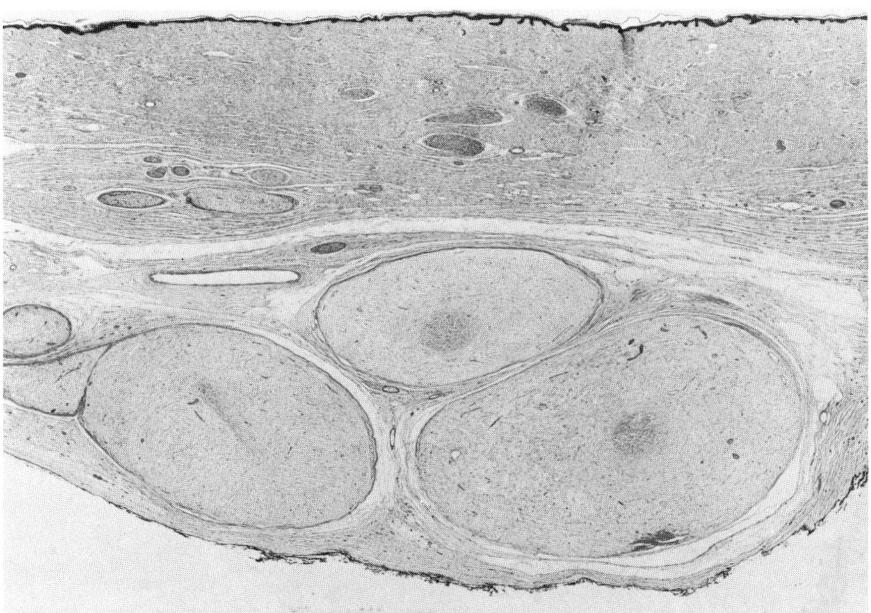

Figure 9–7. Plexiform neurofibroma, hematoxylin and eosin–stained section. This low-power view shows globules of enlarged nerves in the deep dermis and subcutaneous tissue. (Original magnification = 20×.)

Martuza et al. (12) found that whole mounts from café au lait macules that can be shown to contain more than 10 MMG per five high-power fields are present only in adult NF1 patients, compared to café au lait macules in normal persons, and in NF2 (see Table 9–3).

The ultrastructure of MMG has been studied by Nakagawa et al. (13) (Fig. 9–8). They do not represent true melanosomes. Instead, they are autolysosomes formed from the fusion of autophagosomes that contain variable numbers of melanosomes with primary and/or secondary lysosomes. The MMG are variable in size and internal structure, as would be expected if they represent various stages in the dynamic process of degradation of phagocytized melanosomes. The MMG may be retained within melanocytes or be transferred to keratinocytes, Langerhans cells, or dermal macrophages. After transfer, the MMG may fuse with other heterolysosomes and increase in size.

Table 9–3. Melanin Macroglobule in Various Disorders

Human
Neoplastic
Dysplastic melanocytic nevus
Melanocytic nevi (junctional and compound)
Lentigo simplex
Lentigo maligna
Nevus spilus
Dermal melanosis associated with metastatic malignant melanoma
Vitiligo-like leukoderma associated with malignant melanoma
Melanocytoma of the optic disc and the uvea
Genetic
NF1 (in café au lait macules and "normal" skin)
X-linked ocular albinism
Hermansky-Pudlak syndrome (oculocutaneous albinism and hemorrhagic diathesis)
Multiple lentiginous syndrome (Moynahan syndrome)
Xeroderma pigmentosum
Chemical/drug
Lentigines following oral PUVA photochemotherapy
Developmental
Becker hairy nevus
Microbiological
Tinea versicolor
Normal skin
Animal
Normal
Mouse—pallid (hair)
Rat—scrotum
Bovine—tapetum lucidum
Experimental
Gerbil—DMBA-induced dermal hyperpigmentation and blue nevus-like tumors

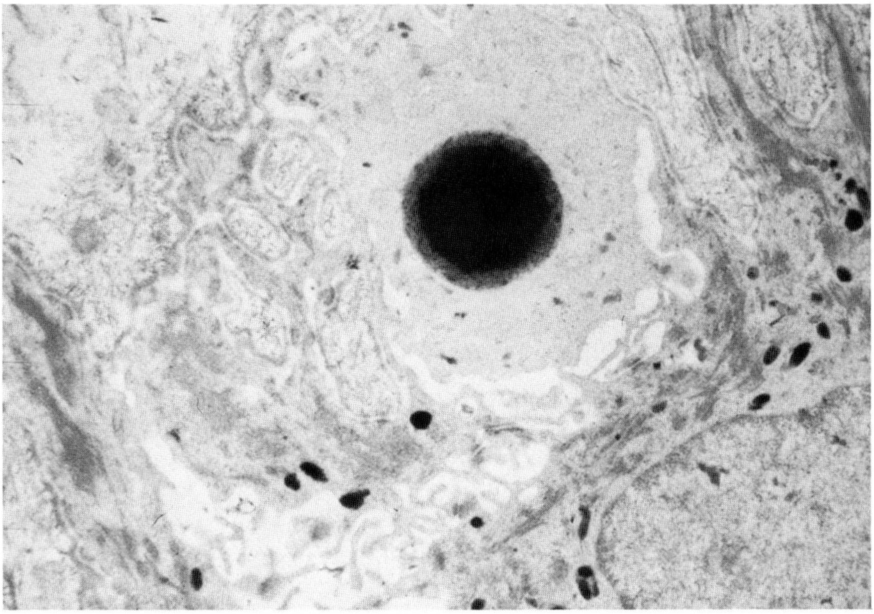

Figure 9–8. Melanin macroglobule. This very large intracellular organelle results from the merging of an autophagosome with a secondary lysosome. These are present in many and diverse diseases but only in large numbers in the café au lait macules that occur in NF1 vis-à-vis café au lait macules in normal skin or McCune-Albright syndrome. (Original magnification = 6900×.)

SUMMARY

Cutaneous features often are the first presenting signs of NF. The accurate recognition of these features can therefore be an important diagnostic aid. In addition, the skin is sometimes involved in disfiguring lesions, which can produce significant and difficult to manage problems.

REFERENCES

1. R.W. Smith. A treatise on the pathology, diagnosis and treatment of neuroma. In Atlas of illustrations of pathology. London, New Sydenham Society, 1898, p. 38.
2. F.D. von Recklinghausen. Ueber die multiplen Fibrome der Haut und ihre Beiehung zu den multiplen Neuromen. Berlin, Hirschwald, 1882.
3. P. Marie, and A. Bernard. Neurofibromatose generalisee. Soc Med Hop Paris 1896;13:200–209.

4. M.A. Chauffard. Dermato-fibromatose pigmentaire (ou neuro-fibromatose generalisee). Soc Med Hop Paris 1896;13:777–779.
5. F.W. Crowe, Axillary freckling as a diagnostic aid in neurofibromatosis. Ann Intern Med 1964;61:1142–1143.
6. P.H. Benedict, G. Szabo, T.B. Fitzpatrick, and S.J. Sinesi. Melanotic macules in Albright's syndrome and in neurofibromatosis. JAMA 1968;205:72–80.
7. F.W. Crowe, and W.J. Schull. Diagnostic importance of cafe-au-lait spot in neurofibromatosis. Arch Intern Med 1953;91:758–766.
8. D. Whitehouse. Diagnostic value of the cafe au lait spot in children. Arch Dis Child 1966;41:316–319.
9. C.A. Bloch. Cafe-au-lait spots in coloured and Indian children. S Afr Med J 1984;65:651–652.
10. V.M. Riccardi. Pathophysiology of neurofibromatosis. IV. Dermatologic insights into heterogeneity and pathogenesis. J Am Acad Dermatol 1980;3:157–166.
11. W. Westerhof, and K. Konrad. Blue-red macules and pseudoatrophic macules: Additional cutaneous sign in neurofibromatosis. Arch Dermatol 1982;118:577–581.
12. R.L. Martuza, I. Philippe, T.B. Fitzpatrick, et al. Melanin macroglobules as a cellular marker of neurofibromatosis: A quantitative study. J Invest Dermatol 1985;85:347–350.
13. H. Nakagawa, Y. Hori, S. Sato, et al. The nature and origin of the melanin macroglobule. J Invest Dermatol 1984;83:134–139.

10

Neurofibromatosis and Cancer: Incidence and Management

Ilene B. Lefkowitz, M.D., Angela C. Obringer, Ph.D., and Anna T. Meadows, M.D.

Neurofibromatosis (NF) is associated with an increased frequency of malignancy. Although this statement is indisputably true, the actual incidence and thus the relative risk of developing cancer in these individuals are not yet clearly known. The histological types of malignancy reported in NF are diverse but not random, and the evidence for some stated associations is much stronger than for others. The optimal treatment once cancer is diagnosed is also controversial due to concern about sensitivity to radiation and chemotherapy. This chapter will address these issues in an attempt to provide a comprehensive picture of cancer in NF. Most of these comments are directed at NF1, which is the most common type of NF.

Frequency of Cancer in Neurofibromatosis

Definition of Malignancy

A tumor is defined as any local accumulation of tissue producing a mass. Most of the tumors that occur in people with NF are neurofibromas, which are not malignant. Malignant tumors, or cancer, are characterized by their ability to invade surrounding tissues and spread from their point of origin to elsewhere in the body (metastasize). In this chapter all central nervous system tumors will be regarded as malignant regardless of histology.

Frequency of Malignancy

The ideal way to define the incidence of cancer in NF is to look for malignancy in a series of NF patients. Unfortunately, there have been few studies in which an unbiased population of NF individuals has been followed.

The two longest series, from Michigan and Denmark, included 395 and 201 families, respectively (1,2). The overall incidence of cancer in these groups was 8% (49 patients with 56 neoplasms), but neither study followed the patients or their families for any period of time. Thus the overall risk to an individual with NF of acquiring cancer during his or her lifetime cannot be established from this work. Recently, a 42-year follow-up study of the Danish patients has been published and will be discussed in detail below (3).

Despite the shortcomings of these studies, they present data that strongly suggest an increase in malignancy in NF and a shift of the age-specific incidence curve. The mean age at diagnosis of malignancy was 38 years (42 years in Denmark, 32 years in Michigan), compared to a mean age of 65 years in the general population of the United States (4). There was also an excess proportion of cancers in children. Pediatric malignancies make up approximately 1% of all cancers diagnosed each year in the United States (4); 20 to 25% of the NF patients with cancer in both studies were younger than 20 years.

Twelve percent of the NF patients in this group of 395 had more than one malignancy, an excess over the general population. Also the distribution of tumor types in this series is not typical of that seen in the general population, suggesting an increased propensity for specific malignancies. In particular, brain tumors (43% vs. 1.7% in the general population) and neurofibrosarcomas (14% vs. 0.04% in the general population) were overrepresented in the NF patients (1,2,4).

The long-term follow-up study of the original Danish cohort provides the most comprehensive information on the natural history of malignancy in NF (3). This study, published in 1986, reports 212 NF patients and their families followed over a 42-year period. Remarkably only 1% of the patients were lost to follow-up. The 76 probands in this study were all identified in hospital and therefore potentially had more severe disease. To diminish this bias, the analysis was performed separately for probands and affected relatives.

Overall, females had more malignant tumors than males and probands had more malignant tumors than relatives with NF. The observed-to-expected (O/E) ratio of cancer reached statistical significance in probands and female relatives only (4.0 and 1.9, respectively). The ratio for all affected relatives (1.5) was not significantly different from the population at large.

The observed disparity in cancer incidence between males and females with NF has also been reported by Bader et al. (5). In this questionnaire study mailed to member families of the National Neurofibromatosis Foundation, the O/E ratio for males was 3.43 and for females was 5.67. The increased rate of malignancy in men could be solely accounted for by the increase in neural tumors. When these tumors were omitted from analysis, the O/E ratio was not significantly different from 1. Females had an increased incidence of both neural and non-neural tumors. The average follow-up time in this report was 27 years for the 144 males and 28 years for the 168 females. This study had the advantage that many of its members were private-physician referred and therefore not necessarily identified from hospitalization. The study is marred by the low rate of compliance with approximately 50% of families responding to the questionnaire. It can be speculated that families with cancer were more prone to respond and therefore this report may represent an overestimation of cancer incidence. Other series in this literature also support the finding of female predominance in incidence of malignancy. The reasons for this are not yet understood.

The incidence of cancer does not appear to differ between sporadic and familial NF, although family history is not reported in several large series. There has been the suggestion of increased severity in maternally acquired NF, including malignancy (6). Of the patients with a positive family history (when available) in the Michigan and Denmark cohort studies, maternal inheritance was 1.5 times more common than paternal inheritance.

From the available literature it can be concluded that the frequency of cancer in NF is increased over the general population, and that more severely affected patients may be at greater risk. Incidentally diagnosed patients (relatives of probands) appear to have a lesser cancer risk.

Cancer in Children with Neurofibromatosis

Studies of malignancy in children with NF are plagued by the same general shortcomings just outlined. In addition, the relative lack of physical stigmata of NF in children makes case identification more difficult and therefore probably underreported. A review of the available literature reveals an overall frequency of cancer in hospitalized children with NF of 19% with a range of 8 to 35% (7–12). In a series of 4000 consecutive children (less than 15 years of age) throughout the United States and Europe with cancer, NF was the most frequent single gene defect noted (13). Thirty-eight NF patients were identified with this series for an incidence of 0.8%. Neural tumors, both central and peripheral, were by far the most common malignancy.

The Children's Hospital of Philadelphia (CHOP) has an established NF clinic and regional Tumor Registry that records cancer-prone conditions. Using both data sources, 69 children with NF and 76 malignant neoplasms have been identified (Table 10–1). The largest group consists of 25 patients with optic nerve gliomas. These occurred in 16 girls and nine boys at a median age of 4 years. It is especially interesting that eight of the 11 with inheritance of NF have fathers affected with the condition.

In the records of the CHOP other tumors of the brain occurred in 15 children at a median age of 12 years. Neurofibrosarcomas (nineteen), other soft-tissue sarcomas (five), leukemia (five acute lymphoblastic leukemia, two chronic myelogenous leukemia), Wilms tumor, ganglioneuroblastoma, non-Hodgkin lymphoma, and osteosarcoma were the remaining neoplasms. Five children were diagnosed with more than one malignant neoplasm; one of them developed four cancers. Two were neurofibrosarcomas; one of these was

Table 10–1. Neurofibromatosis and Childhood Cancer*

	NO.	INHERITED
Optic nerve glioma	25	11
Astrocytoma	8	4
Other glioma	5	2
Meningioma	2	0
Neurofibrosarcoma (3)	19	6
Rhabdomyosarcoma	5	1
Acute lymphocytic leukemia (1)	5	2
Chronic myelogenous leukemia	2	1
Wilms tumor	1	1
Non-Hodgkin lymphoma (1)	1	0
Osteosarcoma (1)	1	0
Ganglioneuroblastoma	1	0

*75 tumors in 69 children. In parentheses are the number of second neoplasms.

in the field of irradiation for a rhabdomyosarcoma, as was the third tumor, an osteosarcoma.

The Late Effects Study Group, an international consortium of 12 pediatric oncology centers, has the largest registry of children with second malignant neoplasms (14). All tumor types were seen in NF; some followed radiation therapy and some occurred spontaneously. A recent summary is presented in Table 10–2. The excess number of children with NF and second cancers (15 vs. 0.1 expected in 300 cases) attests to the increased cancer susceptibility in early life in NF patients.

Symptoms

In general, the signs and symptoms of cancer in patients with NF are the same as in the general population: easy bruising and anemia with leukemia, uncontrolled hypertension with pheochromocytoma, etc. More difficulty

Table 10–2. Neurofibromatosis and Multiple Cancers In Childhood

	SECOND				
	SOFT TISSUE	BRAIN	BONE	LEUKEMIA	SKIN
First					
Soft tissue	+/−	+/−	+		
Brain	+/−	+		+	+
Neuroblastoma	−				+
Leukemia/lymphoma		−		−	
Wilms tumor	+/+				−
Adrenocortical carcinoma			−		

+ Radiation associated; − No radiation.

arises in the evaluation of neural tumors. The presentation of intracranial tumors reflects the location of the mass lesion. Headaches, seizures, emesis are all nonspecific symptoms of an expanding intracranial mass. One-sided weakness, difficulty walking, and facial paralysis are all signs helpful in localizing a tumor. Computed tomography (CT) scans and especially magnetic resonance imaging (MRI) studies may show multiple intracranial abnormalities and only through serial evaluations can the growing lesion be identified (15).

Serial evaluations are particularly important in peripheral nerve tumors. Neurofibrosarcoma may arise de novo or within existing neurofibroma (16). Change in texture, change in size, pain, and attachment to surrounding tissues are all symptoms of "malignant degeneration" of existing benign neurofibromas. These changes may be subtle and slowly evolving and patients should be taught to evaluate palpable lesions regularly and to report changes promptly. As with any malignancy, therapy is more effective when the tumor is small and has not metastasized (spread to other parts of the body).

SPECIFIC TUMORS

The list of tumors reported to be associated with NF continues to grow. Although there is substantial evidence of an increased occurrence of certain malignancies (e.g., neurofibrosarcoma (17–19), leukemia (20–22), the data supporting other associations are questionable. Originally thought to be a disorder of only neural crest cells, there is substantial evidence that cancer arises with increased frequency in cells of diverse embryological origin.

Intracranial Tumors

As mentioned previously, the incidence of intracranial tumors is increased in NF in both children and adults. The frequency reported in the literature varies from 4 to 17%, with 5% of the patients in both the Denmark and the Michigan cohorts having brain tumors. The inclusion of bilateral acoustic neuromas (a separate entity from classic NF1) in some series serves to account for the wide range of reported incidence (16). Brain tumors appear to be more common in younger patients, with 62% developing before age 30 years versus 34% of non-neural tumors occurring before age 50 years in the Denmark study (3). This is largely due to optic glioma.

Central nervous system tumors may appear histologically benign but can be lethal by virtue of their location. The skull acts as a closed space, and therefore expanding intracranial masses can cause significant damage by invasion or increased pressure. Presenting signs and symptoms are as described already.

Histologically, the most common type of tumor encountered is the glioma, a neoplastic proliferation of glial cells. Optic nerve and chiasmatic gliomas are particularly frequent, generally occurring in young children. In an earlier series of 51 children with NF tumors, from the CHOP 13 of 22 central nervous system tumors were optic glioma (23). Other pediatric series support the predominance of optic nerve neoplasia (7–10). The diagnosis and treatment of optic gliomas is discussed further in Chapter 8.

Gliomas also tend to involve the brain parenchyma. Other central nervous system tumors described in the literature include ependymomas, giant cell astrocytomas, and hemangiomas, the latter tending to appear at an older age (24). The two cases in the Denmark cohort appeared when the patients were 56 and 72 years of age (3). When meningiomas are diagnosed in childhood, they are frequently associated with NF. In a series of 75 childhood meningiomas, 23% had associated NF1 (25). Meningiomas tend to be benign but can undergo malignant degeneration. They occur commonly in association with NF2 but rarely with NF1.

Medulloblastoma, the most common posterior fossa tumor of childhood, is surprisingly underrepresented in patients with NF. No cases of medulloblastoma were reported either in the Denmark series (3) or in 17 children with NF and brain tumors reported by Blatt et al. (12). One case of medulloblastoma in nine children with NF and brain tumors has been described as well as a case report of a child with multiple malignancies including medulloblastoma (26). The incidence of medulloblastoma may be similar to that in unaffected children and, therefore, may comprise a smaller proportion of central nervous system tumors in NF.

Peripheral Nerve Tumors

Benign neurofibromas are the hallmark of NF. Case reports exist on the literature of “malignant degeneration” of benign neurofibromas into neurofibrosarcomas (also called malignant schwannoma) and other sarcomas (17,18). These reports do not reveal the incidence of this phenomena and recent data from the Danish cohort suggest that transformation is uncommon (3). Of the six patients with peripheral nerve sarcomas, none could be confidently stated to arise from preexisting benign tumors. Estimates of frequency of “sarcomatous degeneration” in other series range from 2 to 29%, the highest value being reported from Memorial Hospital, which is biased toward malignant diseases (1,27,28). Another confounding factor is that some early series do not differentiate de novo nerve sarcomas from those arising in neurofibromas, thus making the literature impossible to interpret.

The incidence of de novo peripheral neurofibrosarcoma was 11% (6/51) in the Danish cohort with tumors or 2.8% of the total study population (3). In the series of 151 patients from the CHP, these values were 37% (19/51) and 11% (19/151), respectively. In the most recent analysis, neurofibrosarcomas comprised 25% of the neoplasms and were diagnosed in 9% of patients with NF. Although these tumors were thought to arise de novo, three of four were located in an area adjacent to benign plexiform neurofibromas. The higher incidence in this series can be accounted for by inclusion of patients referred due to malignancy.

Despite the uncertainty of tumor origin, peripheral nerve sarcomas occur with increased frequency in NF. In a recent series 52% of patients with neurofibrosarcoma had NF (29). Tumors were most common in the upper extremities followed by trunk and head and neck. As mentioned already, self-examination and reporting are important in early diagnosis and treatment.

Other Neural Crest Tumors

Neuroblastoma, a pediatric tumor of immature nerve cells, neuroblasts, has been reported in patients with NF, a frequency apparently no different from that in the general population. Recently Kushner et al. questioned the diagnosis in several of these reported cases (30). Although the occurrence of NF and neuroblastoma may be due to chance alone, the neural crest origin of both conditions suggests an association (31).

Pheochromocytoma, on the other hand, is strongly associated with NF, and reports of this association preceded von Recklinghausen's publication (32). This tumor arises from chromaffin cells of neural crest origin located in the adrenal medulla. Although initially reported in only one of 395 patients in the original population studies from Denmark and Michigan (1,2), the 42-year follow-up revealed three cases (1.4%) in 212 patients (3). The extreme rarity of the tumor in the general population makes this association unlikely to occur by chance alone. Whereas some cases of pheochromocytoma not associated with NF are familial (33), the epidemiological characteristics of pheochromocytoma in NF are more similar to the sporadic cases with an older age at diagnosis (mean, 38 years), lack of positive family history, and rare bilaterality (16). Significant hypertension, sweats, unexplained nervousness, or flushing may all be signs of pheochromocytoma and should prompt the physician to undertake a search for this tumor.

Medullary carcinoma of the thyroid, in theory, should be associated with NF. This tumor arises from a cell line derived from neural crest tissue and is associated with pheochromocytoma in the multiple endocrine neoplasia syndrome type III (Sipple syndrome). This syndrome has features in common with NF (multiple neuromas, café au lait spots, and scoliosis) and makes early case reports difficult to interpret. Although this theoretical association is interesting, there is currently no proof of a definite association (16).

Melanoma, another neural crest derivative affecting pigment cells in the skin (melanocytes), may be underrepresented in NF. Of the 22 cases in the literature there is a suggestion of increased frequency of the very rare uveal and leptomeningeal malignant melanoma, but reported cases of cutaneous melanoma are far below that expected in the general population. In fact, the large cohort studies (Michigan and Denmark) (1,2) contain no cases of melanoma and of 900 consecutive patients at a pigmented lesion clinic only one had NF (34).

Non-neural Crest Malignancies

Childhood leukemia is associated with NF. Although leukemia is the most common malignancy of childhood and many sporadically occurring cases would be expected in children with NF, the distribution of leukemia subtypes is so different from the general population that this association is very unlikely due to chance alone. In 1978 Bader and Miller reported 29 cases of leukemia in children with NF: nine patients had acute lymphoblastic leukemia (ALL) and 20 had nonlymphoblastic leukemia (NLL) (20), a distribution very different from that of leukemia in the general childhood population. Of the 20 patients with NLL, eight had acute myelomonocytic leukemia (AMML), eight had chronic myelogenous leukemia (CML), three had acute myelogenous leukemia (AML), and one had unspecified acute nonlymphoblastic leukemia.

The age distribution of these patients approximated the usual age of the various leukemia subtypes. Interestingly 70% (19/27) had a positive family history of NF and all patients with leukemia under age 2 had a positive family history. Looking more closely at the subtypes of leukemia, unusual associations can be seen. Eighty-three percent (15/18) with NLL had a positive family history of NF versus 44% with ALL. In sporadic cases of NF the ALL:NLL ratio of 5:3 is not very different from the 4:1 for this general pediatric population. Familial cases of NF showed a strikingly different ratio of ALL:NLL, 4:15, due to 13 cases of CML and AMML, which normally account for less than 10% of all cases of childhood leukemia. The overall ratio for patients with NF in this series is 9:20. Nineteen additional patients have been reported since Bader's series and these cases support the reversed ratio of leukemia subtypes, especially in familial cases. The underlying defect responsible for the increased susceptibility to unusual types of leukemia is unknown.

Rhabdomyosarcoma, a tumor arising from muscle, has also been reported to occur with increased frequency in NF. Of 84 patients with rhabdomyosarcoma seen at the CHOP and the National Cancer Institute, five had NF when only 0.03 were expected by chance (35). A total of 20 cases of rhabdomyosarcoma and NF have been reported with all but two occurring in familial NF. These tumors arose in the typical sites of sporadic rhabdomyosarcoma: genitourinary tract, extremities, orbit, paraspinal, chest, and nasopharynx.

Wilms tumor, and embryonic kidney tumor of childhood, has been linked to NF although the association is weak. Of 342 patients with Wilms tumor seen at one cancer center over 15 years, three cases were associated with NF, whereas only two cases with this association would be expected nationally (36). At the CHP we recently saw a child who developed ALL 6 years after her Wilms tumor had been treated with vincristine and actinomycin D alone. In the absence of carcinogenic therapy, this association suggests increased predisposition in NF to both types of tumors.

TREATMENT

The basic principle of cancer therapy is to kill tumor cells while minimizing toxic effects on normal cells in the body. No single mode of therapy is completely effective at achieving this goal. The specific therapy differs according to the particular tumor being treated, as well as other factors such as the age and state of general health of the patient, and the extent to which the tumor has invaded local tissue or spread through the body.

Surgery is the first-line treatment in many cases. Most tumors will at least be biopsied in order to firmly establish a diagnosis. In some instances a substantial bulk of tumor may be surgically removed. If examination of tumor tissue through the microscope reveals evidence of malignancy, or if the tumor has been found to have spread through the body, surgery alone will not be sufficient to prevent continued growth of the tumor.

In such cases, additional therapy is required. Typically, this consists of radiation and/or chemotherapy. Radiation therapy consists of aiming a beam of energy derived from a source of radioactivity at the tumor. All dividing cells, whether tumor or normal, within the path of the beam are killed. For the most part, selective killing of tumor cells depends on careful aiming of the radiation beam. Usually this procedure is performed in many sessions, so that the total dosage of radiation is given a little at a time. This tends to minimize side effects and increase the efficiency of killing tumor cells.

Chemotherapy consists of administering doses of chemical drugs, usually intravenously, which have the ability to kill tumor cells. There are a large number of such drugs, and the choice of which to use depends on the particular tumor being treated. Most side effects of chemotherapy relate to killing of nontumor cells that are also sensitive to the medications. These include the bone marrow, which results in transient susceptibility to infection, bleeding, and anemia, and the lining of the gastrointestinal tract, which results in diarrhea and vomiting. Usually these side effects are temporary, lasting until the normal cells are regenerated. One of the major causes of death from malignancy, however, is infection contracted during a time when the ability of the body to fight infection is impaired due to bone marrow suppression.

Early evidence had suggested that patients with NF were more susceptible than the normal population to carcinogenic/mutagenic effects of ionizing radiation (22). This led to reductions or avoidance of radiotherapy on the treatment of malignancies in patients with NF. Recently, this concept has received additional support from studies of chromosomal aberrations (37). It has been alternatively suggested that these patients are more resistant to the effects of radiation (38). Current recommendations are to treat the specific malignancy in the same manner as that for patients without NF (39). Thus, where indicated, surgery, chemotherapy, and radiation therapy should be used as aggressively as one would in non-NF patients.

The prognosis of treatment of cancer in patients with NF depends on the specific tumor being treated, the extent of disease, and on how soon after development of the tumor the treatment is begun. The means of treatment of specific tumors is beyond the scope of this book, and the treatments used are a rapidly evolving area. This is best discussed on a case-by-case basis with physicians familiar with the patient and currently available modes of treatment.

SUMMARY

Patients with NF do have an increased frequency of cancer. The types of malignancies encountered are different from the general population, although NF does not protect from common cancers. Tumors of the brain, peripheral nerves, muscle, and adrenal gland and also leukemia are more common than in the general population. The diverse embryological origin of the tissues that give rise to cancer in these patients questions the very nature of the defect in NF.

Recent data have revealed that certain patients with NF may be more prone to malignancy than others. In adults, but not children, more severely affected patients and females have a greater risk of developing a malignant tumor than others with NF. This information should be helpful to physicians who care for NF patients as well as to the patients themselves. Obviously more information is needed regarding incidence and tumor types. Research into the basic defect in NF is especially important as it may enhance our ability to understand the etiology of neoplasms in individuals with this condition, as well as in those with similar cancers, generally.

ACKNOWLEDGMENT —The authors wish to thank Jack L. Elias for his assistance in the preparation of this manuscript.

REFERENCES

1. F.W. Crowe, W.J. Schull, and J.V. Neel. A clinical, pathological and genetic study of multiple neurofibromatosis. Springfield, IL, Charles C Thomas, 1956.
2. A. Borberg. Clinical and genetic investigations into tuberous sclerosis and Recklinghausen's neurofibromatosis. Contributions to elucidation of interrelationship and eugenics of the syndromes. Acta Psychiatr Neurol Scand 1951; 71 (suppl):1–239.
3. S.A. Sorensen, J.J. Mulvihill, and A. Nielsen. Long-term follow-up of von Recklinghausen neurofibromatosis. N Engl J Med 1986;314:1010–1014.
4. S.J. Cutler, and J.L. Young, Jr. Third National Cancer Survey: Incidence data. Natl Cancer Inst Monogr 1975;41:1–454.
5. J.L. Bader, A.R. Kantor, A.E. Rubenstein, et al. Increased risk of cancer with neurofibromatosis (NF). Proc Am Soc Clin Oncol 1981;22:7.
6. M. Miller, and J.G. Hall. Possible maternal effect on severity of neurofibromatosis. Lancet 1978;2:1071–1073.
7. J.L. Fienman, and D.A. Yakovac. Neurofibromatosis in childhood. J Pediatr 1970;76:339–346.

8. W.G. Cole, and N.A. Meyers. Neurofibromatosis in childhood. Aust NZ J Surg 1978;48:360–365.
9. J.C. Adkins, and M.M. Ravitch. The operative management of von Recklinghausen's neurofibromatosis in children, with special reference to lesions of the head and neck. Surgery 1977;82:343–348.
10. A.H. Crawford. Neurofibromatosis in children. Acta Orthop Scand [Suppl] 1986;218:1–60.
11. R. Pollnitz. Neurofibromatosis in childhood: A review of 25 cases. Med J Aust 1976;2:49–52.
12. J. Blatt, R. Jaffe, M. Deutsch, and J.C. Adkins. Neurofibromatosis and childhood tumors. Cancer 1986;57:1225–1229.
13. J.L. Bader, A.T. Meadows, J. Lemerle, et al. Neurofibromatosis (NF) and other genetic diseases associated with childhood cancer. Am J Hum Genet 1980;32:97A.
14. A.T. Meadows, E. Baum, F. Fossati-Bellani, et al. Second malignant neoplasms in children: An update from the Late Effects Study Group. J Clin Oncol 1985;3:532–538.
15. J.R. Bognanno, M.K. Edwards, T.A. Lee, et al. Cranial MR imaging in neurofibromatosis. AJNR 1988;151:381–388.
16. D.G. Hope, and J.J. Mulvihill. Malignancy in neurofibromatosis. Adv Neurol 1981;29:33–56.
17. A.N. D'Agostino, E.H. Soule, and R.H. Miller. Sarcomas of the peripheral nerves and somatic soft tissues associated with multiple neurofibromatosis (von Recklinghausen's disease). Cancer 1963;16:1015–1021.
18. M.J. Sands, M.T. McDonough, A.M. Cohen, et al. Fatal malignant degeneration in multiple neurofibromatosis. JAMA 1975;233:1381–1382.
19. J.M. Friedman, P.J. Fialkow, C.L. Greene, and M.N. Weinberg. Probable clonal origin of neurofibrosarcoma in a patient with hereditary neurofibromatosis. J Natl Can Inst 1982;69:1289–1292.
20. J.L. Bader, and R.W. Miller. Neurofibromatosis and childhood leukemia. J Pediatr 1978;92:925–929.
21. R.D. Clark, and J.J. Hutter. Familial neurofibromatosis and juvenile chronic myelogenous leukemia. Hum Genet 1982;60:230–232.
22. S.D. Reich, and P.H. Wiernik. Von Recklinghausen's neurofibromatosis and acute leukemia. Am J Dis Child 1976;130:888–889.
23. M. Schneider, A.C. Obringer, E. Zackai, and A.T. Meadows. Childhood neurofibromatosis: Risk factors for malignant disease. Cancer Genet Cytogenet 1986;21:347–354.
24. J.V. Wander, and T.K. Das Gupta. Neurofibromatosis. Curr Prob Surg 1977;14:1–81.
25. D.F. Merten, C.A. Gooding, T.H. Newton, and N. Malamud. Meningiomas of childhood and adolescence. J Pediatr 1974;84:696–700.
26. A.G.L. Corkill, and C.F. Ross. A case of neurofibromatosis complicated by medulloblastoma, neurogenic sarcoma, and radiation-induced carcinoma of thyroid. J Neurol Neurosurg Psychiatry 1969;32:43–47.
27. E.S. Casselman, W.T. Miller, S.R. Lin, and G.A. Mandell. Von Recklinghausen's disease: Incidence of roentgenographic findings with a clinical review of the literature. CRC Crit Rev Diag Imaging 1977;9:387–419.
28. R. Brasfield, and T.K. Das Gupta. Von Recklinghausen's disease: A clinicopathological study. Ann Surg 1972;175:86–104.
29. B.S. Ducatman, B.W. Scheithauer, D.G. Peigras, et al. Malignant peripheral nerve sheath tumors. Cancer 1986;57:2006–2021.
30. B.H. Kushner, S.I. Hajdu, and L. Helson. Synchronous neuroblastoma and von Recklinghausen's disease: A review of the literature. J Clin Oncol 1985;3:117–120.
31. A.G. Knudson, Jr., and A.T. Meadows. Developmental genetics of neuroblastoma. J Natl Can Inst 1976;57:675–682.

32. M. Melicow. One hundred cases of pheochromocytoma (107 tumors) at the Columbia-Presbyterian Medical Center, 1926-1976: A clinicopathologic analysis. Cancer 1977;40:1987–2004.
33. E.G. Moorehead, II, M.J. Brennan, J.R. Caldwell, and W.C. Averill. Pheochromocytoma: A familial tumor. A study of eleven families. Henry Ford Hosp Med Bull 1965;13:467–477.
34. M.J. Mastrangelo, C.E. Goepp, Y.A. Patel, and W.H. Clark, Jr. Cutaneous melanoma in a patient with neurofibromatosis. Arch Dermatol 1979;115:846–865.
35. E.A. McKeen, J. Bodwitha, A.T. Meadows, et al. Rhabdomyosarcoma complicating multiple neurofibromatosis. J Pediatr 1978;93:992–993.
36. E.J. Stay, and G. Vawter. The relationship between nephroblastoma and neurofibromatosis (von Recklinghausen's disease). Cancer 1977;39:2550–2555.
37. M. Havez, L. Sharaf, S.M.A. El-Nabi, and G. El-Wehedy. Evidence of chromosomal instability in neurofibromatosis. Cancer 1985;55:2434–2436.
38. L. Kopelovich, and R.F. Rich. Enhanced radiotolerance to ionizing radiation in connection with increased cancer proneness of cultured fibroblasts from precursor states in neurofibromatosis. Cancer Genet Cytogenet 1986;22:203–210.
39. R.B. Raney, P. Littman, P.D. Jarrett, et al. Results of multimodal therapy in children with neurogenic sarcoma. Med Pediatr Oncol 1979;7:229–236.

11

Plastic Surgery in Neurofibromatosis

John B. Mulliken, M.D.

Neurofibromatosis (NF) is often associated with a myriad of cutaneous and skeletal anomalies that present unusual problems for the plastic and reconstructive surgeon. Some of these manifest at birth as "congenital malformations," but most soft-tissue and bony overgrowth problems evolve during childhood and adolescence. The surgical treatment of NF must be approached with an understanding that all cells in all tissues carry the abnormal gene. The usual goal of total surgical excision cannot be applied to this disorder because so many cells have the potential to form tumors. Although the surgeon cannot eradicate the underlying disease, surgical procedures can be very beneficial by removing abnormal tissue and reconstructing skeletal defects that interfere with function or cause cosmetic concern.

Most NF-associated tumors grow slowly. It is their location, rather than their size, that determines the indications for surgical intervention. Even a small soft-tissue tumor in a critical position can be a significant problem, whereas large tumors are usually asymptomatic.

Early medical literature is replete with bizarre examples of soft-tissue and bony disfigurement in NF. Fortunately, such problems are exceedingly rare, and today there is no reason for patients to present for medical care with such "end-stage" deformities. This literature also suggested that surgical interference might increase the known risk of malignant degeneration in this disease. This is no longer believed to be true.

Soft-Tissue Manifestations

The dermal tumor, called *molluscum fibrosum* (Latin, *molluscus* meaning soft), is a soft to firm papule that can vary in size from a few millimeters to a centimeter, or more. They are multiple and can assume a myriad of shapes—flattened, sessile, pedunculated, or lobulated (Fig. 11–1). The skin color is variable, from fleshy-pink to violaceous. The molluscum fibrosum lesion is

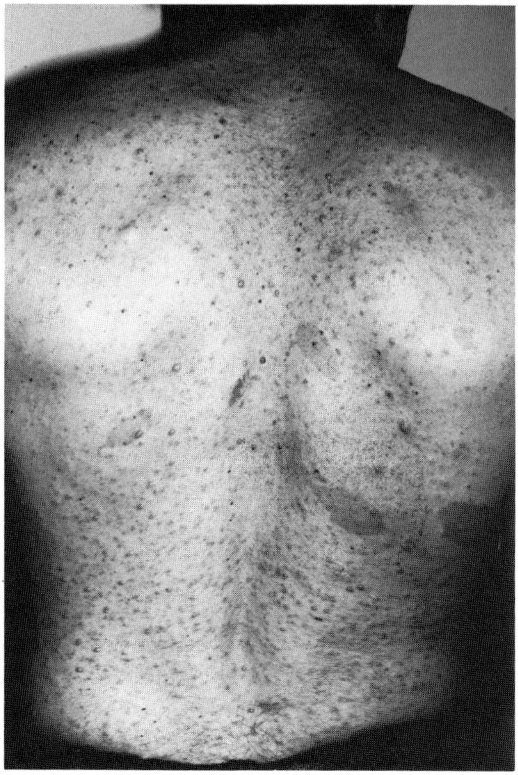

Figure 11–1. Multiple dermal and subcutaneous lesions of NF: molluscum fibrosum, neurofibromas, and café au lait spots.

also distinguished by its spongy center that can be invaginated into the dermal defect by pressure of a fingertip ("button-holding" phenomenon (1).

The subcutaneous tumors, which are multiple, present as either a firm, well-defined nodule attached to a nerve (neurofibroma), or as a diffuse, infiltrating mass in the subcutaneous tissue (plexiform neurofibroma). When there is a grotesque enlargement, the terms pachydermatocele and elephantiasis neuromatosa are used. Such gross or pedunculated skin lesions are generally not seen in childhood, but grow after adolescence over many years. The earlier the onset of soft-tissue changes, the more severe they become. The typical distribution of cutaneous neurofibromas is concentration of tumors on the trunk, head, and neck, with decreasing incidence of lesions in the extremities. However, there is a wide variation in the genetic expression; many patients have no cutaneous tumors, or only a solitary neurofibroma (2).

These soft-tissue tumors rarely cause functional problems. When a neurofibroma is located in a cutaneous nerve, particularly the ulnar or radial nerve, the patient may have pain, muscle weakness, or slight sensory loss. Normally, it is appearance, rather than a functional problem, that causes a patient to consider a surgical procedure.

In the facial region, a swelling is often first noted in the eyebrow, eyelid, temple, or malar area. In time, the involved skin becomes thickened, pigmented, and sometimes hirsute. The soft tissues seem to gradually loosen from their normal position; there is a downward drift of the lateral part of the eyebrow, outer canthus, melolabial fold, or oral commissure. In addition to producing cosmetic deformities, plexiform neurofibroma can interfere with the nasal airway, the eyelids, vision, mastication, and lip competence. NF can involve the motor, sensory, and autonomic nerves in the head and neck region (3). Surgical exploration reveals enlargement of the facial nerve branches or trigeminal divisions prior to demonstration of either motor or sensory deficits.

OSSEOUS MANIFESTATIONS

Bony abnormalities commonly occur in NF. In the Mayo Clinic series, a radiological abnormality of bone was seen in nearly 40% of cases (4). Usually the bony deformations conform, more or less, to the overlying soft-tissue hyperplasias. The skeletal changes are not thought to result from pressure atrophy due to an enlarging soft-tissue mass; but rather, the skeletal abnormalities seem to reflect defective control of neuroectodermal-mesodermal tissue elements.

Fortunately, the skeletal changes in NF are not nearly as severe as commonly believed. The popular vision of the Elephant Man must be modified, for there is strong evidence that Joseph Merrick probably did not have NF (5). Gross bony exostoses and localized hypertrophy of the craniofacial skeleton, as exemplified by the Elephant Man, are more typical of the Proteus syndrome.

THE EXTREMITIES

The most common skeletal changes in NF are kyphoscoliosis, scoliosis, pseudoarthroses, and peripheral bone deformation. Gigantism of the digits, hand, and extremities is also seen in NF. Osteochondral (bone and cartilage) enlargement around the epiphyses of phalanges and metacarpals may interfere with joint motion and flexor tendon function (6). In an affected area, the blood vessels and tendons are of normal size, but the peripheral nerves are often enlarged. Histological sections of these giant nerves show increased fibrous tissue and proliferation of neurilemmal cells (7). Plexiform neurofibromas and periosteal neurofibromas have also been noted at the site of peripheral skeletal bowing and overgrowth (8).

CRANIOFACIAL REGION

Craniofacial skeletal abnormalities, which are less common than the axial peripheral skeleton, include hyperplasia, hypoplasia, bony defects, and intraosseus cysts (9). Many children with NF have a large head; macrocranium occurs in the absence of elevanted intracranial pressure (10,11). Calvarial defects, particularly in the lambdoidal suture area, the pterion, and midoccipital region, have been noted (12). There may be enlargement of the middle cranial fossa, causing a temporal bulge, elevation of the sphenoid ridge, and a decreased anteroposterior diameter of the orbit (12). Expansion of the supraorbital and/or infraorbital fissures and optic foramen is associated with neurofibroma within the orbit, and an enlarged optic nerve. Bone underlying soft-tissue masses in the head and neck more commonly shows hypoplasia than overgrowth. The zygoma may be atrophic, with thinning, bowing, and elongation of the zygomatic arch. Hypoplasia of the mandibular ramus and condyle, and elongation of the coronoid process are associated with the neurofibroma of the inferior alveolar nerve (13,14). Hyperplasia of the mandible or maxilla, and cystic changes in the jaws, have been reported (13). Malocclusion and tilting of the occlusal plane may also occur.

A curious characteristic feature of NF is congenital absence of the posterosuperior orbital wall, involving the greater and lesser wings of the sphenoid bone and orbital section of the frontal bone (4,15) (Fig. 11–2). The absence of the orbital roof allows direct contact between the temporal lobe meninges and orbital contents, and consequently there is transmission of the intracranial vascular pulsation to the globe. Pulsating exophthalmos can be the first presentation of previously undiagnosed NF. There is no suggestion in the literature that pulsating exophthalmos is progressive, or that there is a long-term threat to vision (16). However, neurofibromas within the periocular tissues, even with an intact orbital wall, can result in proptosis, extraocular muscle weakness, and visual impairment. Less commonly, expansion of the orbital cavity may result in enophthalmos. In some instances, the eye itself may be enlarged (buphthalmos); this may be an expression of regional gigantism, or the result of increased intraocular pressure (17). The triad of unilateral buphthalmos, homolateral plexiform neurofibroma of the eyelid, and facial hemihypertrophy is known as François syndrome (18).

OPERATIVE THERAPY

Soft-Tissue Procedures

Indications for a surgical procedure are often cosmetic. However, in rare instances, soft-tissue overgrowth or tumors can cause functional problems, such as interference with eyelid movement. An operation should be recommended when the growth becomes unsightly enough to disturb the patient.

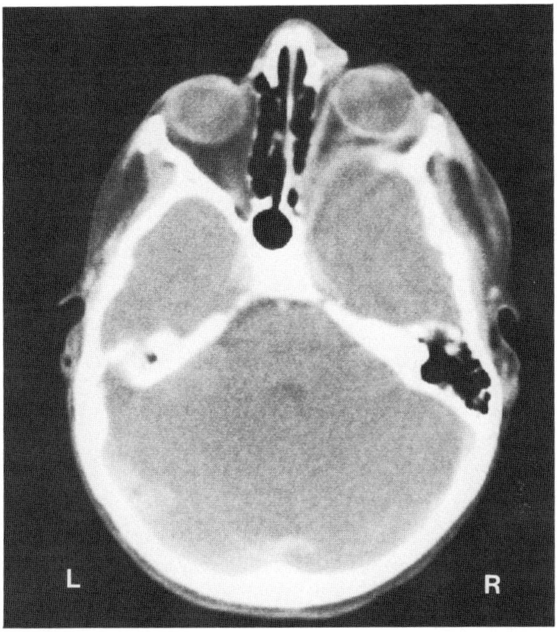

Figure 11–2. Axial CT scan of an 8-year-old girl who presented with mild proptosis of the right globe and expansion of eyebrow hairs. Absence of the greater wing of the sphenoid bone characteristic of NF.

The most common surgical procedure in this disorder is excision of a plexiform neurofibroma. Discrete neurofibromas are also frequently removed from the skin of the face, trunk, or extremities, either as a biopsy or to improve appearance. The length of the scar that will mark the excision site must be about one-third longer than the diameter of the nodule to be excised.

A bulky plexiform neurofibroma is easily removed, and closure of the incision is simplified because of the presence of excess skin. Figure 11–3 shows an example of a young girl who underwent excision of a localized pendant mass hanging from the upper arm. Asymmetrical enlargement of the breast, secondary to NF, can be mistaken as a sign of sexual precocity. Figure 11–4 illustrates the surgical correction of a breast nipple–areolar complex, deformed by plexiform neurofibroma. Localized intraoral tumors can interfere with mastication (particularly those located in the tongue or buccal mucosa) and should be removed.

The most complex soft-tissue problems occur in the head and neck region. There may be well-localized or diffuse involvement of one side of the face. Subtotal excision of plexiform neurofibromas will predictably improve contour (19). Often, multiple procedures are needed (Fig. 11–5). If necessary,

A

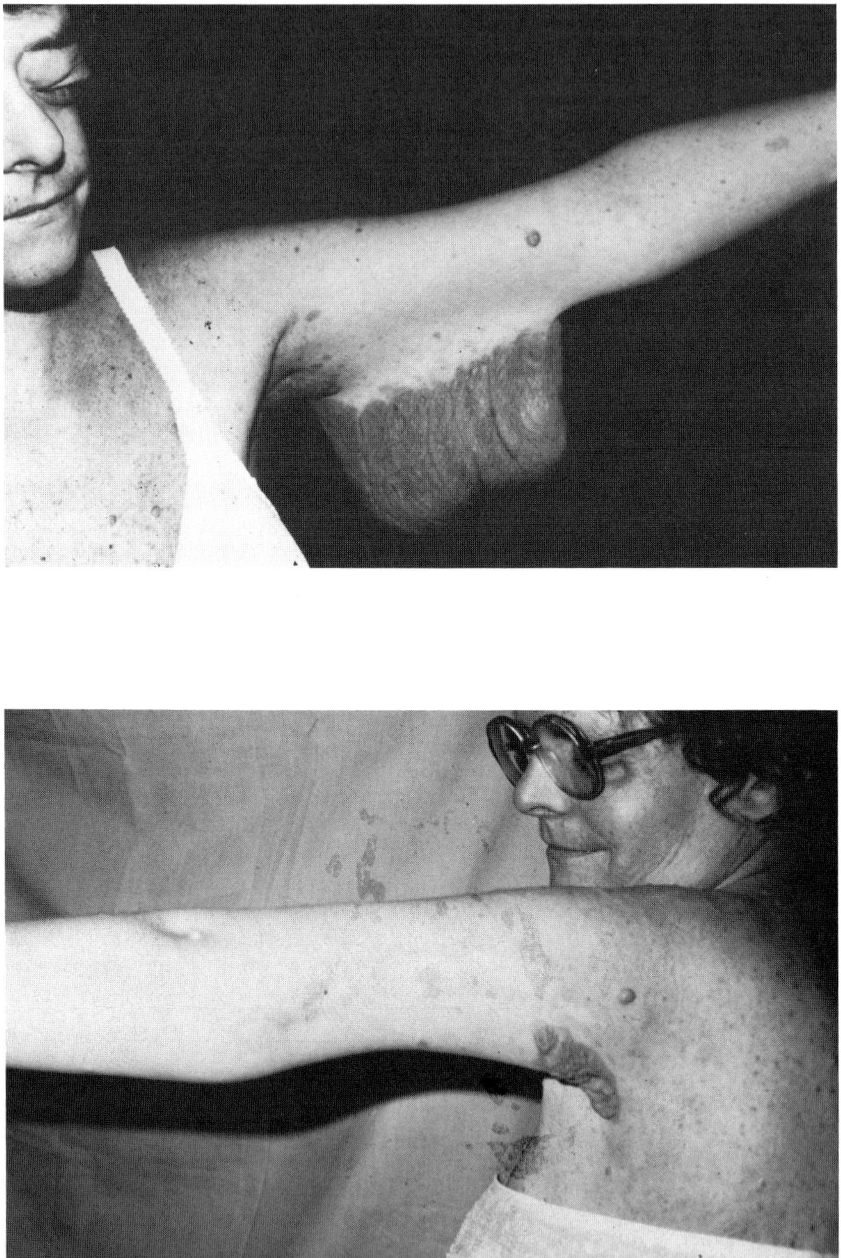

B

Figure 11–3. **(A)** An 18-year-old woman with a large plexiform neurofibroma of the upper arm and proptosis of the left eye. **(B)** Three years following excision of the arm tumor. Another plexiform lesion is seen in the posterior axillary region. Neurofibroma was also removed from the left orbit to correct proptosis.

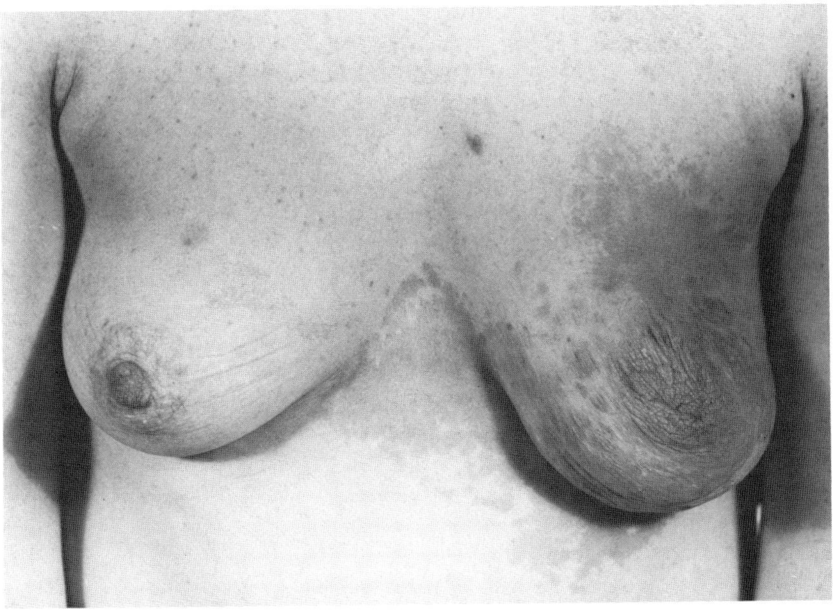

A

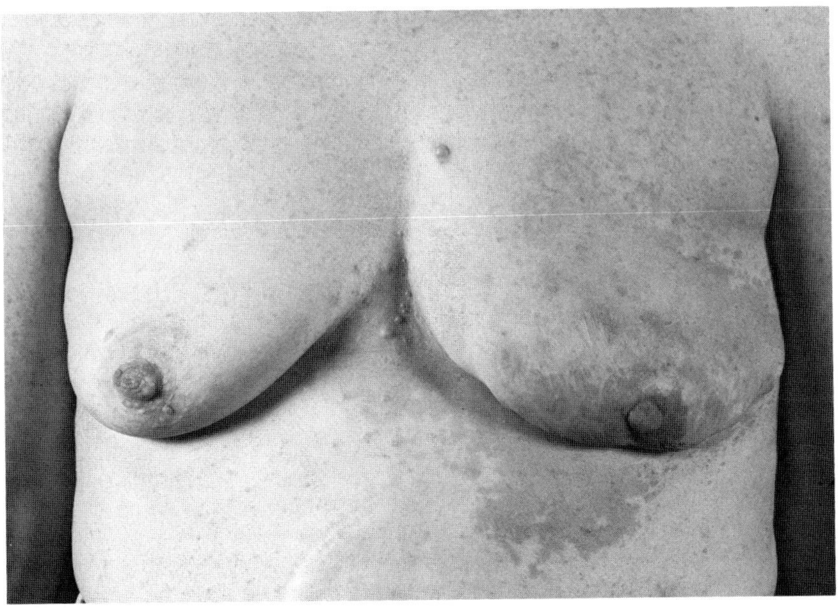

B

Figure 11–4. **(A)** A 24-year-old woman with plexiform neurofibromatous involvement of the left breast. **(B)** Following excision of the tumor and reconstruction of the distorted nipple-areolar complex.

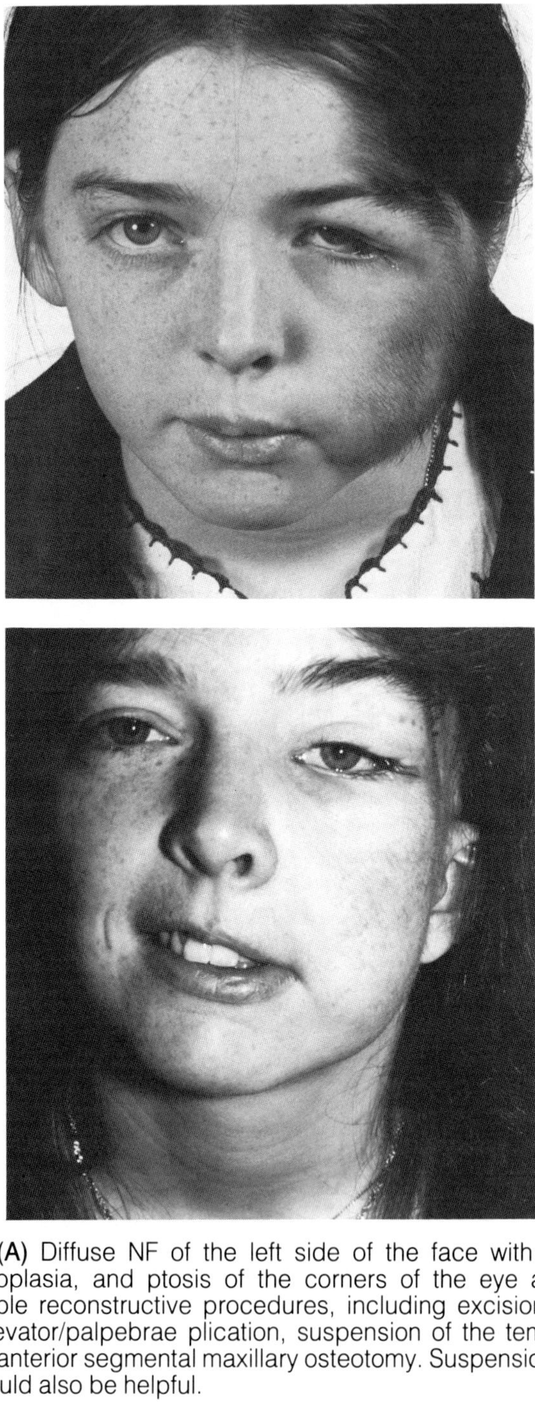

A

B

Figure 11–5. **(A)** Diffuse NF of the left side of the face with hypertrichosis, zygomatic hypoplasia, and ptosis of the corners of the eye and mouth. **(B)** Following multiple reconstructive procedures, including excision of skin in the upper eyelid, levator/palpebrae plication, suspension of the temporal canthus, depilation, and anterior segmental maxillary osteotomy. Suspension of the left oral commissure would also be helpful.

displaced structures, such as the eyebrow, outer canthus, or oral commissure, can be transposed into a more normal position. For example, the patient in Figure 11–6 had a suspension of the ear, combined with a face-lift type procedure to improve facial contour.

Neurofibromas within the eyelids and periorbital tissues are difficult to remove, unless they are small and well localized. Neurofibromas within the eyelids can infiltrate the levator musculofascial complex, causing blepharoptosis; although this ptosis can be improved by levator resection, the end result is often unsatisfactory. Repeated dissections within the periorbital risk damage to sensory nerves to the cornea, and can interfere with the levator apparatus and extraocular muscle function. The general rule is to preserve the globe as long as there is useful sight, because there is always the possibility of loss of vision in the normal eye. If, in time, and following several surgical attempts, the involved globe is proptotic and without vision, then enucleation is justified. In these instances, remodeling of the orbital framework, resection of residual orbital tumor, and prosthetic replacement result in a far better appearance (Fig. 11–7).

Skeletal Procedures

Congenital absence of the bony walls of the orbit may result in pulsatile exophthalmos (20). Although this can be a harmless physical finding, proptosis can be progressive, particularly if there is neurofibroma within the periorbital cone. It is possible to build the bony wall and roof in the orbit to separate the eye from the brain of the anterior cranial fossa. This is accomplished by approaching the orbit via a coronal incision, behind the hairline. The meninges (dura) are separated from the periorbital region, and a cranial bone graft is placed in the orbital defect. To date, the results using this procedure have been somewhat disappointing; the bone graft tends to resorb, with recurrence of exophthalmos (19).

Skeletal overgrowth of the jaws can be managed with standard orthognathic procedures. An example is the young man shown in Figure 11–8 with mandibular prognathism, treated with osteotomy and advancement of the upper jaw, in addition to contour resection of the lower jaw. Bone grafts are used to augment a hypoplastic orbit, zygoma, or malar eminence. Usually the grafts are taken from the outer table of the cranium; ribs and iliac bone grafts can also be used.

Localized gigantism of the extremities presents in a wide spectrum. Debulking of the soft tissue is normally done in staged procedures. Giant fingernails may be narrowed and set into better position. Overgrowth of the digits may be controlled by prompt epiphyseal arrest in childhood. Increased girth of bones requires complex longitudinal osteotomies, and reconstruction of the joints and joint capsule. Amputation may be the last resort in the case of macrodactyly (particularly toes, to allow the wearing of normal shoes).

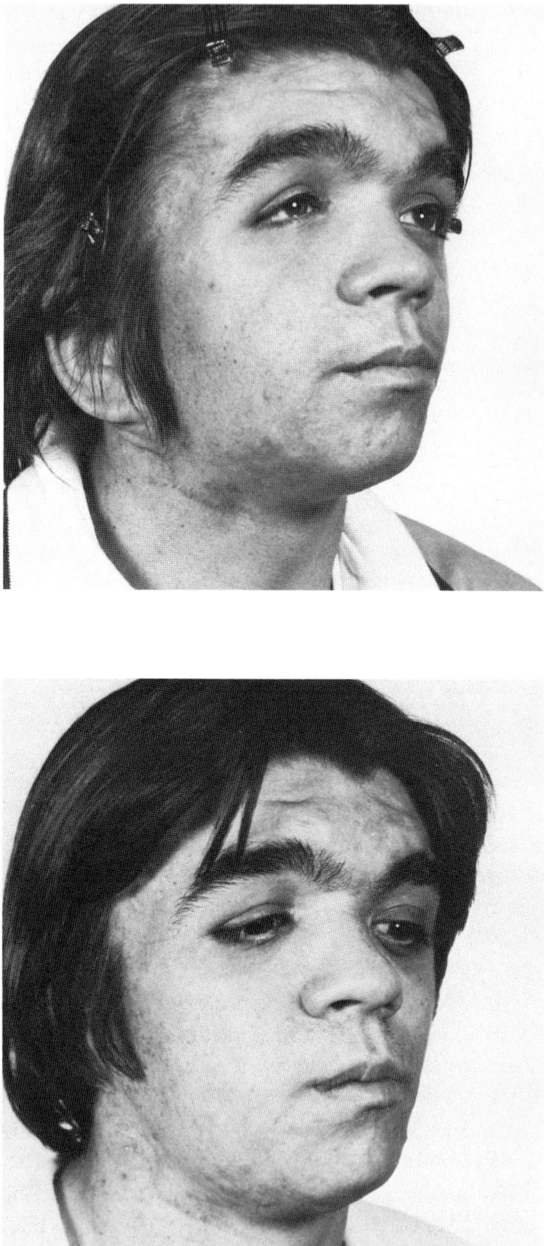

A

B

Figure 11–6. (A) A 19-year-old male with soft-tissue overgrowth of the right side of the face and the right ear. (B) Two years following excision of the plexiform neurofibroma of the eyebrow, forehead, cheek, and postauricular region. The right ear was suspended with fascia lata.

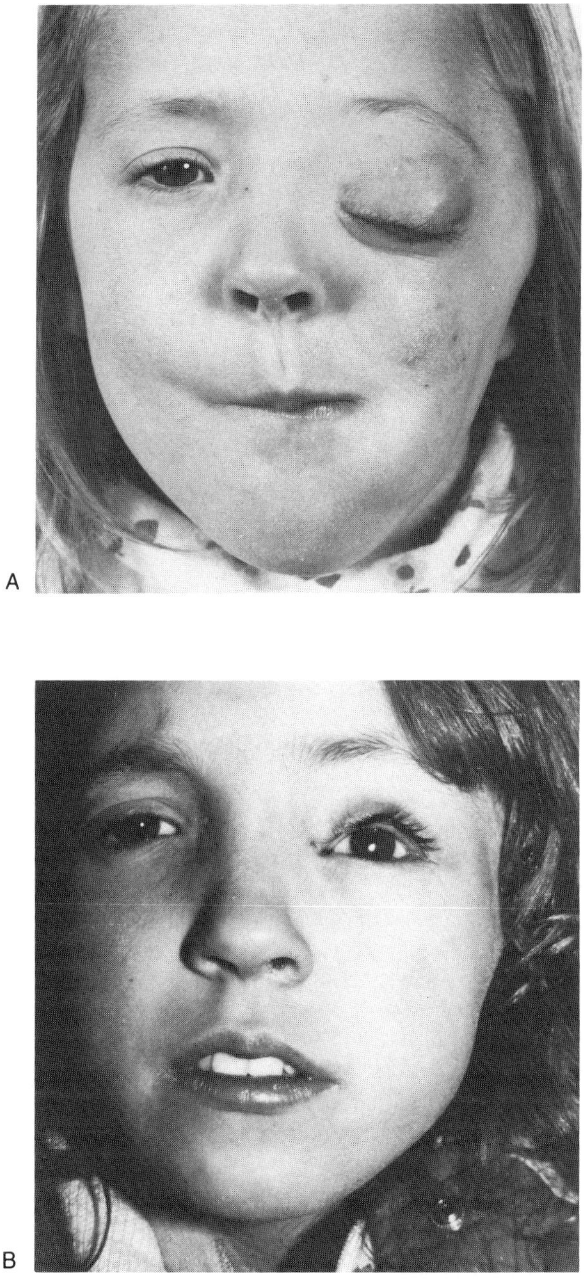

Figure 11–7. **(A)** Five-year-old girl with severe proptosis of the left globe and failing vision. **(B)** At age 9, after several attempts at excision and construction of the orbit with bone grafts, an enucleation was done. She is photographed with an ocular prosthesis.

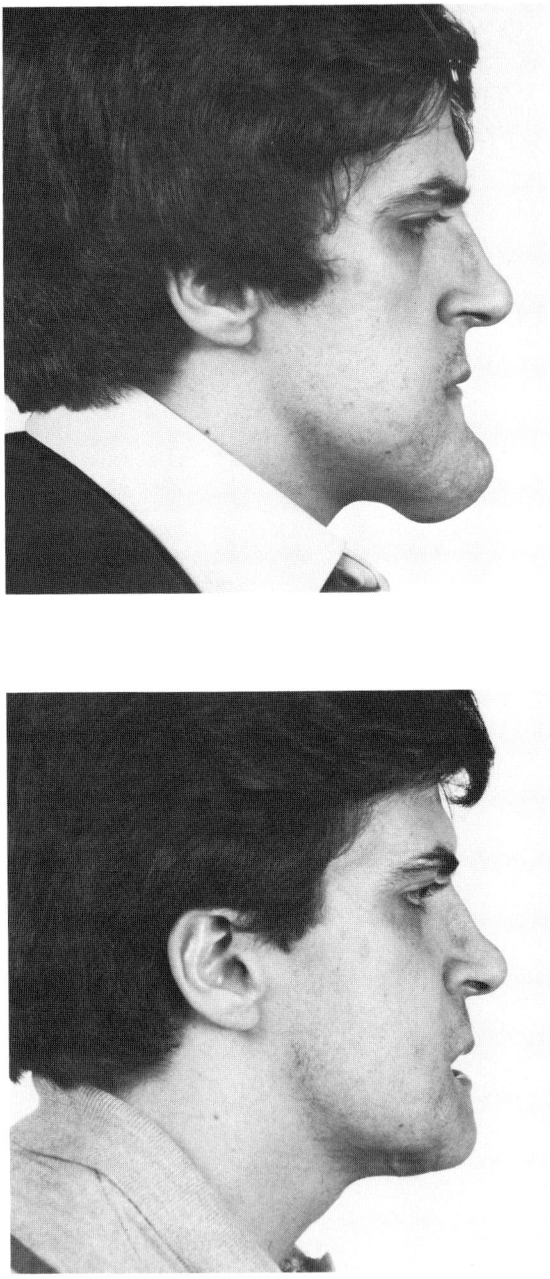

A

B

Figure 11–8. (A) A 24-year-old male with NF causing maxillary hypoplasia and mandibular prognathism. (B) Following osteotomy and advancement of maxilla, contour burring of the hyperplastic mandible, and excision of neurofibromas of the chin.

RESULTS AND COMPLICATIONS

It must be re-emphasized that surgical procedures cannot eradicate this disease, since every cell carries the potential to initiate tumor growth. NF progresses slowly and irregularly, with possible acceleration, especially at puberty and during pregnancy. Nevertheless, carefully planned, and often staged, procedures can improve contour and function. Patients can never be certain of how long the results will last. Fortunately, additional procedures can be done, years to decades later, if necessary.

Bleeding is persistent and insidious during an operation within tissues containing neurofibromas. The bleeding is not massive or life-threatening; however, blood transfusion may be necessary. A cautery knife or carbon dioxide laser can be useful in minimizing blood loss during an extensive resection. Because of this tendency for tissues to bleed, the most frequent postoperative complication is hematoma, a localized collection of blood within the surgical site. For this reason, a suction drain is needed for such procedures and this drain may have to remain in place for several days after the operation.

If the surgical procedure is carried out through abnormal tissue, wound healing of the skin edges may be delayed, because the nutritive blood supply to the skin margins is diminished. Nevertheless, there is generally no abnormality of the wound-healing mechanism. The surgical scars are usually more than acceptable; they remain flat and pale, with minimal tendency to hypertrophy.

Nerve loss is another well-known complication. Nerves that are involved in a plexiform neurofibroma must be sacrificed, often resulting in permanent loss of sensation. More worrisome is loss of motor function; this not infrequently occurs following surgical procedures around the facial nerve, resulting in weakness or loss of facial motion.

CONCLUSION

Every patient with soft-tissue or skeletal abnormalities of NF requires individual consideration. The surgeon and patient must accept the fact that often several operations may be necessary, and that this disease cannot be surgically cured. Patients with cosmetic and functional problems due to NF can definitely be helped by selective, carefully planned and conservative procedures. More radical resection of involved tissue seems justified in patients who already have loss of function.

REFERENCES

1. F.W. Crowe, W.J. Schull, and J.V. Neel. A clinical, pathological, and genetic study of multiple neurofibromatosis. Springfield, IL, Charles C Thomas, 1956.

2. G.S. Bromley, J.E. Sherman, and D. Goulian, Jr. Neurofibromatosis—Distribution of lesions and surgical treatment. Ann Plast Surg 1982;8:272–277.
3. W. Krueger, E. Weisberger, A.J. Ballantyne, et al. Plexiform neurofibroma of the head and neck. Am J Surg 1979;138:517–519.
4. J.C. Hunt, and D.G. Pugh. Skeletal lesions in neurofibromatosis. Radiology 1961;76:1–19.
5. J.A.R. Tibbles, and M.M. Cohen. The Proteus syndrome: The Elephant Man diagnosed. Br Med J 1986;293:683–685.
6. P.C. Dell. Macrodactyly. Hand Clin 1985;1:511–513.
7. M.T. Edgerton, and D.B. Tuerk. Macrodactyly (digital gigantism): Its nature and treatment. In J.W. Littler, L.M. Cramer, and J.W. Smith, ed. Symposium on reconstructive hand surgery. St. Louis, C.V. Mosby, 1972, pp 157–172.
8. M.J. Pitt, J.F. Mosher, and J. Edeiken. Abnormal periostium and bone in neurofibromatosis. Radiology 1972;103:143–144.
9. K.C. Davidson. Cranial and intracranial lesions in neurofibromatosis. AJR 1966;98:550–552.
10. J.F. Hall, and L.R. Kuhns. Macrocranium and macroencephaly in neurofibromatosis. Skel Radiol 1976;1:25–28.
11. K.A. Weichert, M.S. Dine, C. Benlon, and F.N. Silverman. Macrocranium and neurofibromatosis. Radiology 1973;107:163–166.
12. S.K. Gupta, H.V. Nema, P.L. Bhatia, et al. The radiological features of craniofacial neurofibromatosis. Clin Radiol 1979;30:553–556.
13. I. Koblin, and B. Reid. Changes in the facial skeleton in cases of neurofibromatosis. J Maxillofac Surg 1975;3:23–24.
14. H. Muller, and P.J. Slootweg. Maxillofacial deformities in neurofibromatosis. J Maxillofac Surg 1981;9:8911–8912.
15. J. van der Meulen. Orbital neurofibromatosis. Clin Plast Surg 1987;14:123–135.
16. D. Wiesenfeld, and P.L. James. Pulsating exophthalmos associated with neurofibromatosis. J Maxillofac Surg 1984;12:11–13.
17. C.S. Hoyt, and F.A. Billson. Buphthalmos in neurofibromatosis: Is it an expression of regional gigantism?. J Pediatr Ophthalmol 1977;14:228–229.
18. J. Francois, L. Haustrate, and A. Philips. Hydrophthalmie unilaterale et hypertrophie hemifaciale homolaterale (neurinomatose de von Recklinghausen). Ann Ocul 1956;189:186–187.
19. M.M. Mukeriji. Giant neurofibroma of the head and neck. Plast Reconstr Surg 1974;53:1984–1986.
20. B. Linder, M. Campos, and M. Schafer. CT and MRI of orbital abnormalities in neurofibromatosis and selected craniofacial anomalies. Radiol Clin North Am 1987;25:787–802.

12

Orthopedic Aspects of Neurofibromatosis

G. Dean MacEwen, M.D.

Once a child has been diagnosed as having neurofibromatosis (NF), it is important to be aware of the orthopedic complications that may arise in association with the disorder. Most children with NF do not have major orthopedic problems; many have none at all. The severe deformities seen in textbooks are certainly more the exception than the rule, and should not be considered the norm in NF. When they do exist, most orthopedic problems can be treated successfully *if detected at an early stage*. Prompt, appropriate treatment can usually prevent or reduce cosmetic deformity and functional impairment. The key, then, to successful management of orthopedic complications in NF is early diagnosis of the condition.

Health-care providers are likely to recognize skin lesions and any obvious skeletal changes that occur; however, often the orthopedic manifestations of NF are subtle, or occur only as a child approaches adolescence. It is therefore critical, when a diagnosis of NF is made or a family history of NF disclosed, that the patient be followed carefully, with a high "index of suspicion" regarding any orthopedic problems or changes in the musculoskeletal lesions. The orthopedic problems seen in NF vary widely, and each child must be considered individually. The degree of involvement does not follow any pattern, even among affected members of the same family.

The most commonly seen skeletal lesions in NF include spinal deformities and abnormalities related to bone development. Each of these will be considered separately, as well as other, less frequent orthopedic manifestations. It should be noted that orthopedic problems are confined mainly to NF1, and are not common in NF2.

Spinal Deformities

The orthopedic problem most frequently encountered in children with NF is scoliosis, or lateral curvature of the spine (1–5). While incidence of this deformity in the overall population is only 2%, a much larger proportion of preadolescent children with NF have some degree of scoliosis. These children tend to develop scoliosis much earlier than other children, almost always beginning before they reach the age of 10 years. This points again to the need for early and frequent evaluation of the child with NF. The intention is not to frighten the family but rather to emphasize the need for early detection, so as to avoid the complicated treatment that becomes necessary when the problem remains untreated for too long. Also, a delayed therapy is less likely to produce a satisfactory result.

Detection of a minor curve in a patient with scoliosis is accomplished by the same method used for school screening in the general population. The patient bends forward at the waist, and the examiner looks to see if there is more fullness on one side of the thorax (or trunk) than the other (Fig. 12–1). We now regard 5 degrees of angulation or more, as caused by trunk rotation, to be significant enough to warrant an x-ray of the spine. The x-ray is evaluated to detect any specific problem and to determine if treatment aimed at preventing curve progression is in order.

There are two types of lateral spinal curvature in NF. The more commonly seen type is a long, C-shaped curve which involves a significant portion of the spine (eight to 10 vertebrae, or segments) (Fig. 12–2). When this occurs in patients who do not have NF, it is referred to as idiopathic scoliosis, meaning

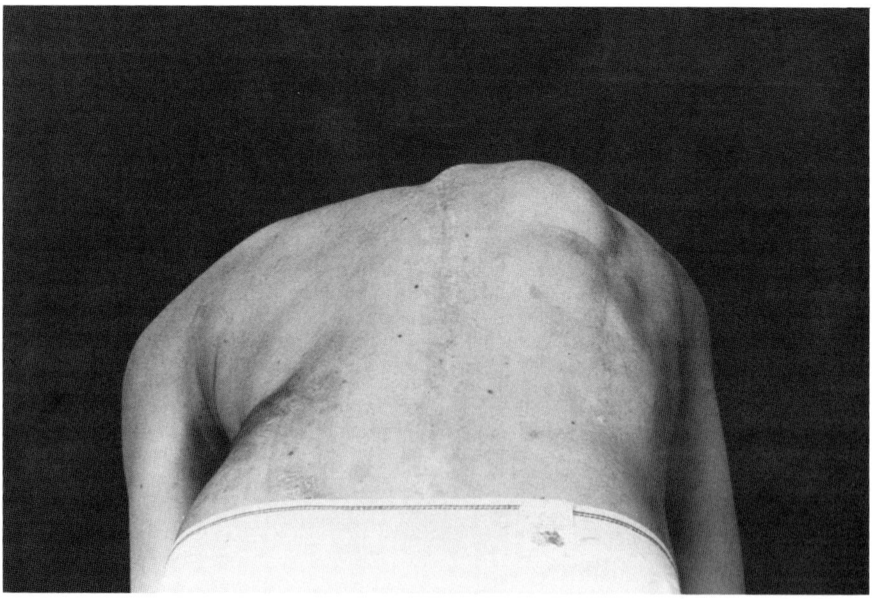

Figure 12–1. To check for scoliosis, the patient is asked to bend forward while the examiner looks for increased fullness on either side of the trunk.

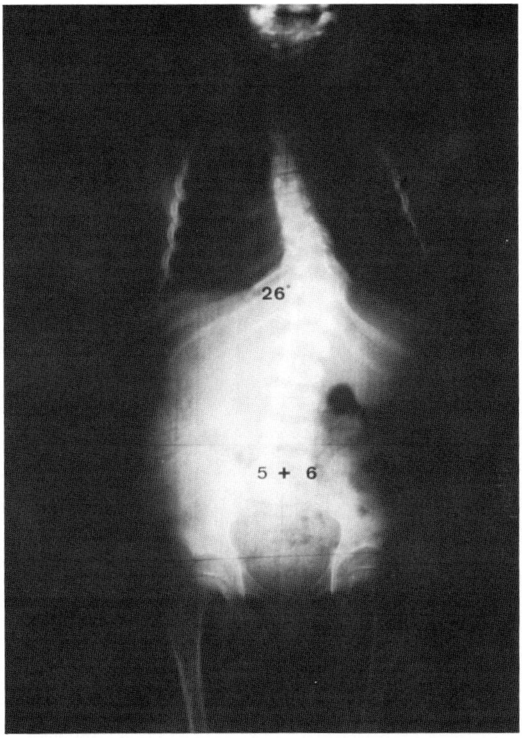

Figure 12–2. This radiograph shows a long, C-shaped curvature of the spine in a 5½-year-old child with NF. While this type of scoliosis is also seen in the general population, usually beginning during adolescence, children with NF tend to develop these curves much earlier.

that the cause of the deformity is unknown. The long, sweeping type of curve may also be associated with many other types of musculoskeletal disorders, and therefore is not in itself an indication of NF.

The second, more unusual type of scoliosis seen specifically in NF is of a more serious nature. It usually involves a smaller portion of the spine (five vertebrae or less), and causes a very sharp, angular curve (Fig. 12–3). This type of deformity is found almost exclusively in patients with NF. In fact, physicians who are accustomed to looking at x-rays of the spine, especially those who deal with scoliosis, can almost determine from this type of curve that a patient has NF even if the diagnosis has not otherwise been made.

In a child with scoliosis, the greatest risk of curve progression exists as long as the patient continues to grow (2). The rate of progression depends on the type of curve as well as the degree of skeletal maturity at the onset of curvature. Treatment consists of conservative measures (observation, bracing, etc.), surgical intervention (usually spinal fusion), or a combination of the two (2,6).

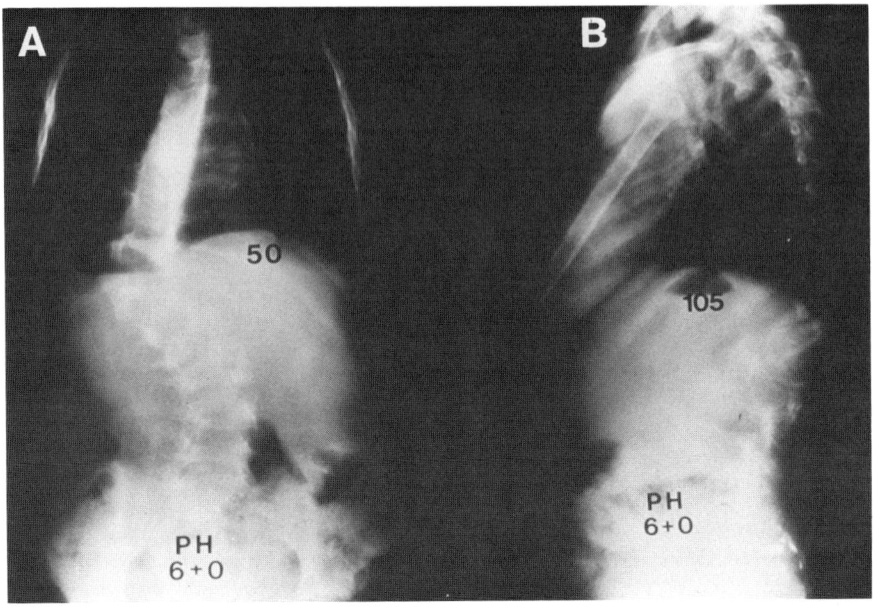

Figure 12–3. **(A)** This radiograph shows the sharp, angular type of scoliosis that is found almost exclusively in patients with NF. Although only a relatively small area of the spine is involved, surgical treatment is usually necessary to avoid severe deformity. **(B)** In the same patient the lateral curvature, or scoliosis, is complicated by a front-to-back curvature known as kyphosis.

For example, in a child with a mild, progressive C-type curve, a small body jacket may be worn under the clothes to keep the curve from getting worse (Fig. 12–4). While this will not correct the spinal deformity, it may obviate the need for surgery, or at least allow surgery to be delayed until the child is closer to skeletal maturity. If a curve is found very early, frequently the child can be placed in this type of orthosis on a part-time or half-time basis and still obtain the desired result.

Another type of conservative treatment that has gained attention in recent years is electrostimulation of the muscles around the spine. There is not yet enough known about this method in regard to NF to justify its use in anything but an experimental basis. However, based on early results, it would seem that this treatment modality will not play an important role in the management of scoliosis associated with NF.

If, in spite of conservative treatment, curve progression cannot be arrested and a significant curve develops, it is best to perform a spinal fusion in the involved part of the spine. Patients with NF are more likely to require spinal fusion if their curves are of the short, angular type rather than the long, sweeping type. This angular type of scoliosis causes the rest of the spine to lean

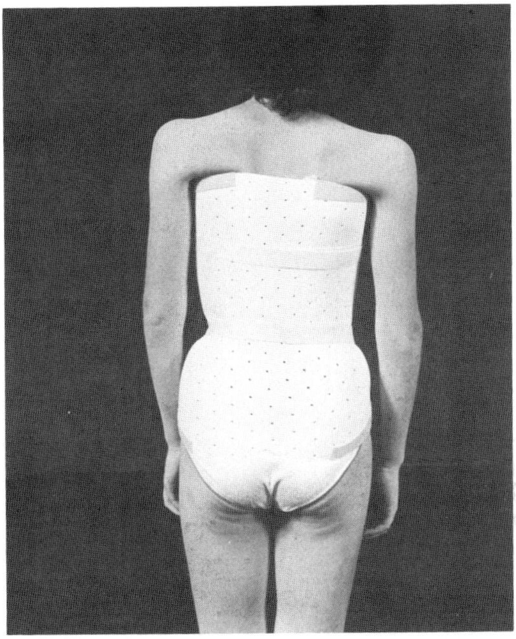

Figure 12–4. A lightweight orthosis worn underneath the patient's clothing may be used to treat mild scoliosis, or to prevent curve progression while the child continues to grow.

toward the opposite side of the body in order to maintain balance. Although there are defects in only a few segments of the spine, the only hope for a satisfactory realignment is to recognize the deformity before it becomes severe. Even then, spinal fusion is usually required to stop curve progression. The risks of neurological involvement or pulmonary compromise are increased with short curves, and conservative treatment is rarely effective.

Spinal fusion is a major operative procedure that is performed to correct spinal curvature as much as possible, as well as to halt curve progression. Although this limits mobility of the spine, since the intervertebral joints are fused together in the corrected position, it remains the treatment of choice in patients with moderate to severe, progressive curves that would otherwise threaten the cardiovascular and pulmonary systems.

Preoperative brace treatment and/or traction are sometimes used, depending upon the degree of curvature, the affected area of the spine, and the type of curvature (Fig. 12–4). Extensive postoperative treatment with a cast and brace is essential in achieving optimal correction of the deformity. The postoperative immobilization, first in a plaster cast and later an orthosis, continues full-time for up to 1 year following fusion. In many instances, full- or part-time brace wearing is continued until the patient reaches full skeletal maturity, in order to avoid deformity in the rest of the spine.

In most instances, a posterior spinal fusion is performed, meaning that the spine is approached through the back of the body. In some patients an anteroposterior (front-to-back) curvature of the spine, known as kyphosis, accompanies the lateral deformity (scoliosis) (Fig. 12–3). When this happens, anterior spinal fusion is often performed through the front of the body in order to correct the kyphosis and to further stabilize the spine. The anterior procedure is usually performed first, followed a few weeks later by the posterior fusion.

There are many different methods for performing spinal fusion, again depending on the degree and location of curvature. The area to be fused generally extends from the vertebra just above the upper end of the curve down to the vertebra just below the lower end of the curve. In some situations the fusion is carried down to the sacrum, or lower end of the spine. The basic principles for fusion are to realign the intervertebral joints so that the spine is straightened and to "fuse" the area by use of bone grafts that maintain the vertebral bodies in the corrected position. Frequently, the bone graft alone is sufficient to achieve fusion. However, in more severe curvatures some type of spinal instrumentation may be used to further stabilize the spine; this may involve placement of a metal rod along the corrected area (e.g., Harrington instrumentation) or a series of wires through each corrected segment of the spine (e.g., Luque instrumentation).

It must be noted that a child or adolescent with NF who does require surgery has more of a risk than most individuals that the bone will not fuse properly the first time, because the quality of the bone is poor. This failure of fusion (pseudoarthrosis) occurs in approximately 15% of NF patients. However, when a second fusion procedure is performed on these patients, the chances of acceptable results are improved.

Many patients with the sharp, angular form of scoliosis seen in NF also have a significant deformity of the cervical region of the spine that gives the impression of a prominence on the back of the neck; this is cervical kyphosis (7). The deformity usually comes slowly and often does not cause pain in the early stages. It can, however, cause pressure on the spinal cord, and is very difficult to correct if not treated early. We have observed in our institution approximately 20% of NF patients with significant deformities of other parts of the spine associated with cervical anomalies (Fig. 12–5). Thus, patients with NF should be re-evaluated periodically for this subtle, painless deformity in order to avoid progression and the need for very involved treatment measures. If the kyphosis is progressive, spinal fusion may become necessary to avoid neurological compromise.

In general, our results with both brace treatment and surgical management of NF patients with mild spinal curvatures have been very successful. We believe it is worthwhile to undertake early aggressive treatment in these

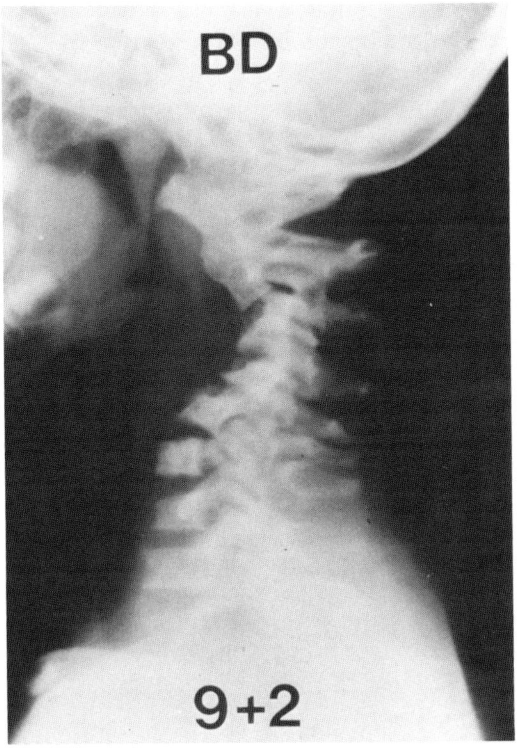

Figure 12–5. Abnormalities of the cervical region of the spine, as seen in this radiograph, occur frequently in patients with NF who have curvatures of other areas of the spine.

patients, rather than wait to see how serious the deformity is likely to become and then settle for a less than satisfactory result.

Often in treating patient with NF, orthopedic problems are considered secondarily while other manifestations of the condition are treated. It is not true that every NF patient who has scoliosis requires definitive care. However, if there is any indication that a curve is starting to progress, reevaluation should be made at 4- to 6-month intervals. Sometimes the increase in curvature is very gradual, with only subtle changes occurring between follow-up visits. However, these minor changes may eventually produce a significant deformity, and should be carefully monitored so that treatment may be initiated at the appropriate time.

ABNORMAL BONE DEVELOPMENT

Musculoskeletal problems in relation to abnormal bone development are also seen in patients with NF. One such problem is bone overgrowth, which is sometimes seen in association with subcutaneous neurofibromas (8). Again, early treatment in the form of removal of associated tumors can lead to very good results, by preventing the tumors from increasing in size and promoting more normal bone growth.

When overgrowth occurs, the upper or lower leg bones become thicker and longer on one side of the body than on the other, producing an inequality in leg lengths (Fig. 12–6). Since bone growth is governed primarily by areas known as physes, or growth plates, which are found at both ends of the long bones of the leg, treatment is directed toward these areas. The growth plates remain active as long as the body continues to grow; at skeletal maturity, the growth plates are considered to be closed, and no further growth occurs. In a child with NF who has overgrowth of one of the long bones, a procedure known as epiphysiodesis may be performed to slow the growth of the involved limb, while allowing the normal side to continue to grow. This procedure involves destruction of the growth plate, which stops growth in that area of

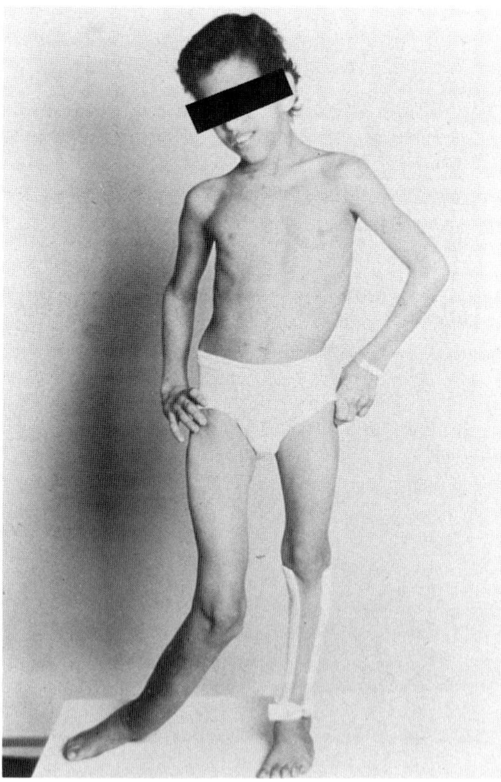

Figure 12–6. Overgrowth of the long bones, as seen in this patient, may result from physeal disturbances caused by neurofibromas.

bone. The timing of an epiphysiodesis is very important, since the amount of remaining growth in the normal limb varies with the patient's age. If the procedure is performed too early, there is a chance that the normal limb will outgrow the operated side; if it is performed too late, the normal limb may not have time to catch up with the overgrown side, since its own growth plate will close naturally.

Fortunately, there are methods for determining the degree of skeletal maturity, or bone age; this does not always correspond with the patient's chronological age, since not everyone grows at the same rate. Based upon bone age, and the use of growth charts which allow the amount of remaining growth to be predicted, it is possible to calculate the best age for performing an epiphysiodesis. In most instances, the procedure is most effective when performed in a patient 10 to 13 years of age; because girls tend to reach skeletal maturity earlier than boys, epiphysiodesis may be indicated at even earlier ages in females than in males. Close follow-up of these patients is necessary in order to ensure that the limb lengths are approaching each other as the child continues to grow.

Another orthopedic problem often seen in children with NF is congenital bowing of a long bone. The most common bone involved is the tibia, which becomes bowed in an anterolateral direction, meaning that the lower part of the leg is curved forward and to the outer side (Fig. 12–7) (9). Other bones, including the ulna (10) and radius (11), are also sometimes involved. This deformity must be carefully watched, since it has been found that fractures in this area tend to result in failure to heal (pseudoarthrosis) if the usual casting techniques are used (Fig. 12–8). Treatment of this type of bowing should consist of early bracing to support the area, with the intention of preventing fractures and avoiding any surgical efforts to straighten intact bones.

Management has been greatly improved by the use of very lightweight orthoses, including the so-called clam-shell brace with easily applied front and back pieces that extend to just below the knee and fit inside the shoe. With careful orthotic fitting and good follow-up care, many NF patients now go safely through an at-risk period of relative bone weakness without fracture and subsequent surgery for pseudoarthrosis. Upon removal of the brace, the bone is usually much stronger, and certainly less vulnerable than it would be following a surgical procedure (Fig. 12–9).

However, even preventive measures sometimes fail, and some patients will sustain fractures with or without braces. Often these fractures fail to unite following traditional treatment measures. In the past, such a situation called for taking bone grafts from the child's opposite, uninvolved limb—or from the mother—and inserting them into the fractured tibia, usually with metallic plates or pins (12). A healing rate of approximately 50% was attained with these methods. However, some of these fractures never completely heal.

In recent years, the use of external and internal electrical stimulation devices has led to improved results in bone healing (13,14). This should not be viewed

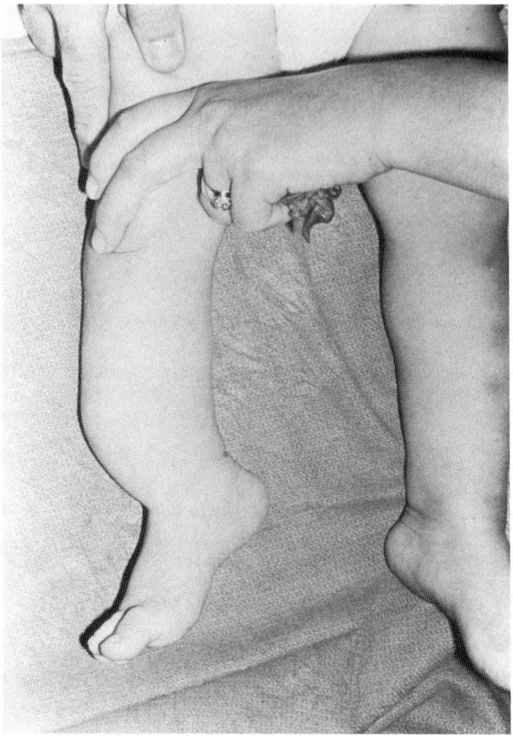

Figure 12–7. Anterolateral bowing of the lower part of the leg is an orthopedic problem that occurs frequently in children with NF.

as a general panacea by any means, as it is not always successful in achieving bony union. Another method that has been used with some success, first in China and now in other parts of the world, involves removing a piece of bone from the opposite limb with the blood supply intact; this graft is then placed at the site of nonunion (15). One disadvantage to this procedure is that it involves scarring of both the affected and unaffected limbs. This method is relatively complex, and should probably be considered only if other methods have been unsuccessful.

In spite of advances in treatment, pseudoarthrosis of the tibia still represents a very difficult problem in children with NF, and there is no single solution that solves every patient's problems. Fortunately, as the patients approach skeletal maturity, the risk of fracture in this area is greatly decreased.

While some children with NF will have overgrowth of the bones, others with very severe involvement may have a gross thinning of the bones, especially the tibia, along with slow skeletal growth (Fig. 12–10) (1,8). In order for these patients to function, some type of brace must be used to support the small,

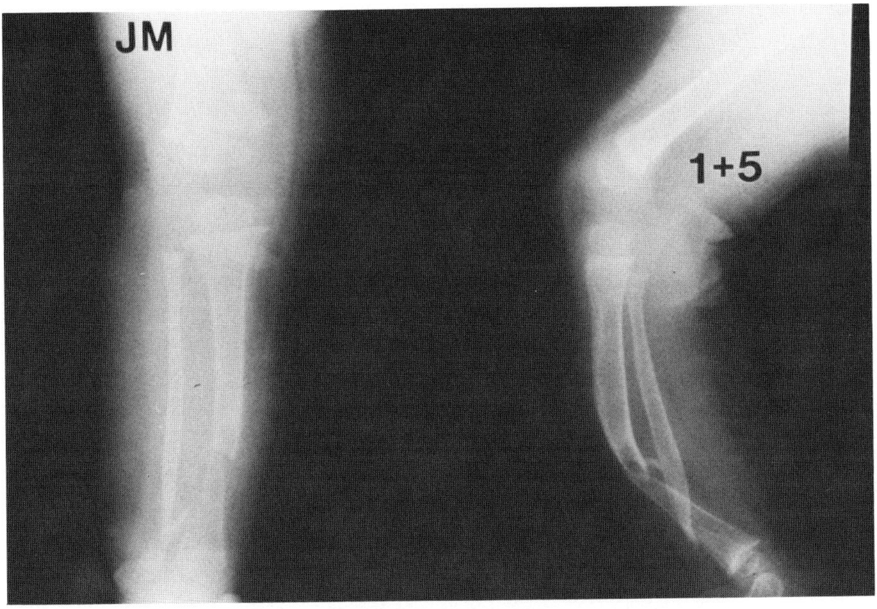

Figure 12–8. Fractures of the tibia in young patients with NF often fail to heal. This condition, known as pseudoarthrosis, may be seen in these radiographs of a 17-month-old child.

underdeveloped skeleton. This type of growth may occur, for example, around the foot; tumors in this area may extend into the joints, often in front of the ankle, causing atrophy and erosion of the small bones and joints. In some patients, localized tumors can be removed successfully to avoid further joint erosion and stiffness. If this problem can be recognized early, the tumor can often be excised to allow the bones to grow in a relatively normal fashion.

OTHER ORTHOPEDIC ANOMALIES

Other orthopedic considerations in the treatment of the patient with NF include subperiosteal problems, which are frequently overlooked. Occasionally, what appears to be phlebitis or just a superficial injury develops on a patient with a relatively large leg. Such a development may indicate a subperiosteal problem, such as a hemorrhage underneath the covering of the bone, which will produce a very thick-looking leg (Fig. 12–11). This condition is sometimes seen in combination with phlebitis or even with a hemorrhage in the soft tissues. While this is not common, it should at least be considered that a NF patient who presents with a swollen leg may have this type of subperi-

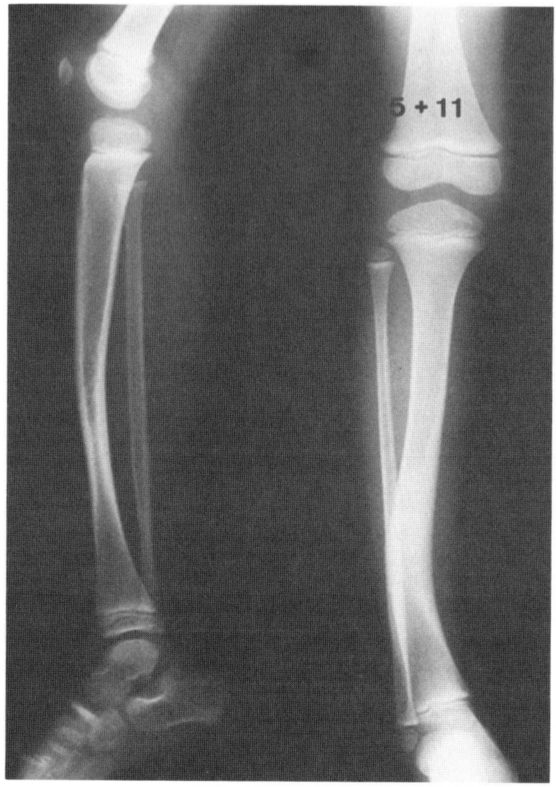

A

Figure 12–9. (A) These radiographs show anterolateral bowing of the tibia in a 5-year, 11-month-old boy with NF. (Figure continues.)

osteal hematoma (16). This rare condition must be recognized early if it is to be corrected. However, the condition is difficult to diagnose since x-rays during the early stages are not likely to be helpful. Treatment calls for a compressive dressing, to avoid a large, seriously deformed leg that will be very difficult to treat.

Patients with NF may develop severe limb deformities, in addition to overgrowth or bowing, due to the effects of neurofibromas on bone development. Angular deformities of the long bones can often be improved by corrective osteotomies. However, if tumors occur in the area of the knee or ankle joints, growth disturbances may lead to serious functional impairment (Fig. 12–12). In some instances, such as a patient with a deformed foot with little hope for functional improvement, it is sometimes best to amputate. While amputation may seem a drastic measure, it may sometimes truly be the

B

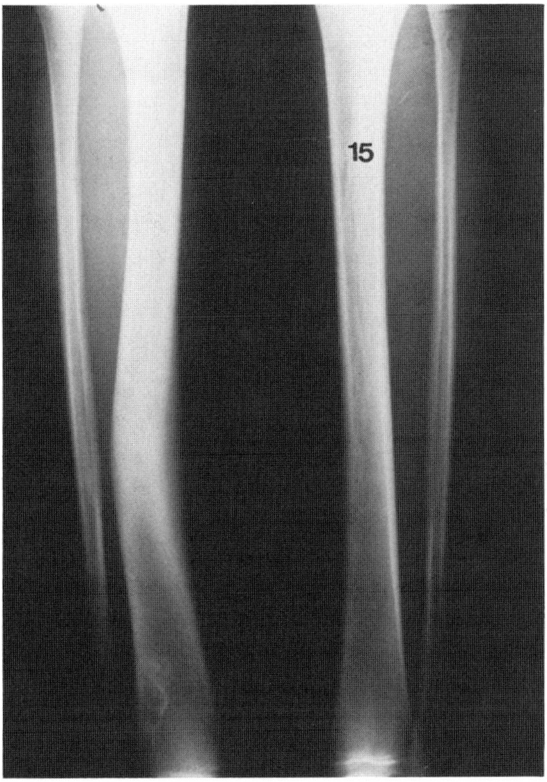

Figure 12–9 *(continued).* **(B)** Following the use of orthoses during growth, the deformity has improved and the bones are much stronger at 16 years of age.

treatment of choice because an extremity that is functioning more poorly than an artificial limb is not of any real value to the patient. However, this type of procedure should not ever be considered without the patient's involvement in the decision, and only rarely before the child reaches adolescence.

There are several other types of orthopedic anomalies, some of which occur in the general population, that are seen with some frequency in patients with NF. In most instances, these problems may be treated as in otherwise normal patients, tailoring treatment to the patient's particular situation and medical needs at the time. If surgical treatment is to be undertaken, it should be remembered that the NF patient is likely to have poorer quality bone, and that pseudoarthrosis may occur following a bony procedure. Some of the other skeletal lesions that occur in patients with NF include: short stature; macrocephaly, or disproportionately large head size relative to the rest of the body;

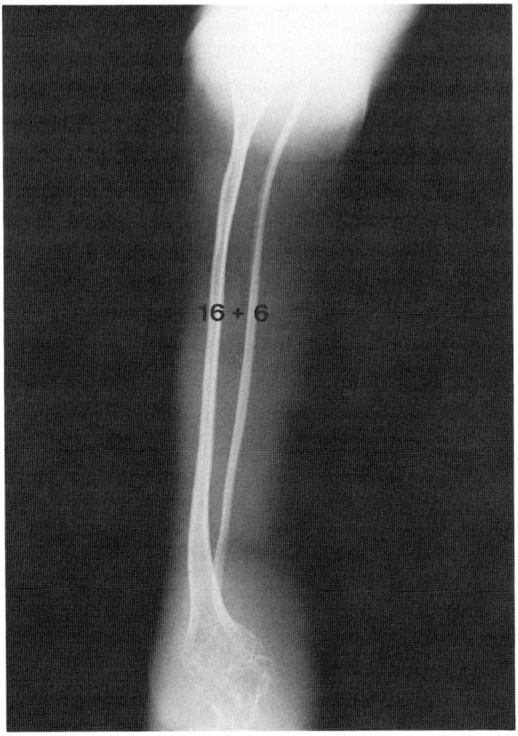

Figure 12–10. This radiograph shows very thin bones in the lower part of the leg, which require bracing and careful observation to avoid fracture and progressive deformity in this area.

spondylolisthesis, or forward slipping of the lower lumbar vertebrae over the sacrum; intrathoracic meningocele, which involves a spinal cord defect in the area of the chest with neurological involvement; and protrusio acetabuli, which is a deformity of the hip joint in which the acetabulum is too deep for the femoral head, resulting in limitation of hip motion.

CONCLUSION

In conclusion, it is important for all those involved in evaluation and treatment to be aware of the way NF can affect the skeletal system. Overall, the key to successful management of orthopedic involvement in NF is early detection and diagnosis. Often, less than satisfactory results of treatment are seen when orthopedic problems are allowed to go untreated for long periods of time, resulting in cosmetic and functional impairment.

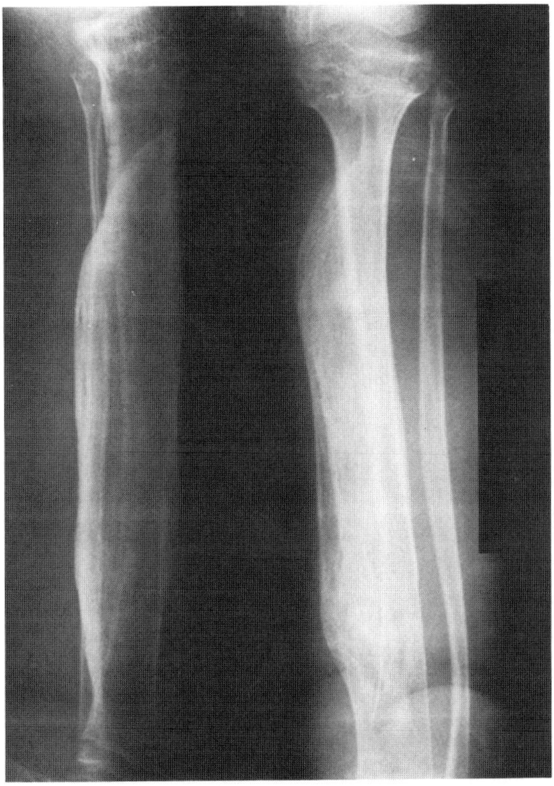

Figure 12–11. A subperiosteal problem may occur in a patient with NF who has some overgrowth of the bone. These problems are rare, but should be watched for, since the consequences can be serious.

The most frequently seen orthopedic problem in NF is scoliosis, of which there are two types. When mild, C-type curves are detected early, conservative treatment (with an orthosis) is usually effective. More severe scoliosis requires early detection and treatment if realignment of the spine is to be attained; spinal fusion is often necessary.

Anterolateral bowing of the tibia is also found among NF patients. Treatment consists of early bracing for support, with fracture and subsequent pseudoarthrosis being the greatest fear. Treatment of pseudoarthrosis varies: grafting techniques, internal fixation, and electrical stimulation have all been used; massive grafting and rigid fixation are frequently successful. Limb overgrowth in the NF patient can be successfully managed with an appropriately timed epiphysiodesis. Skeletal undergrowth requires supportive bracing.

Finally, it should be remembered that many children and adolescents with NF do not have major orthopedic deformities. Most anomalies can be recog-

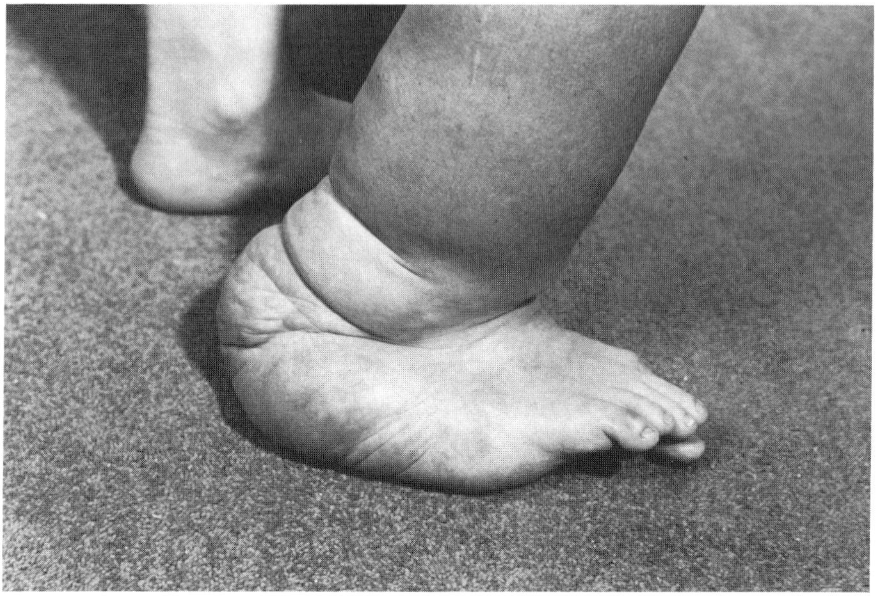

Figure 12–12. Neurofibromas in the foot or ankle may lead to deformities that severely compromise the function of the extremity.

nized early, allowing for the implementation of appropriate treatment, usually with good or excellent results.

REFERENCES

1. A.H. Crawford, and N. Bagamery. Osseous manifestations of neurofibromatosis in childhood. J Pediatr Orthop 1986;6:72–88.
2. J.H. Chaglassian, E.J. Riseborough, and J.E. Hall. Neurofibromatosis and scoliosis. Natural history and results of treatment in thirty-seven cases. J Bone Joint Surg [Am] 1976;58:695–702.
3. A.H. Crawford. Neurofibromatosis in children. Acta Orthop Scand [Suppl] 1986;218:1–60.
4. J.W. Laws, and C. Pallis. Spinal deformities in neurofibromatosis. J Bone Joint Surg [Br] 1963;45:674–682.
5. R.B. Winter, J.H. Moe, D.S. Bradford, et al. Spine deformity in neurofibromatosis. A review of one hundred and two patients. J Bone Joint Surg [Am] 1979;61:677–694.
6. R. Savini, P. Parisini, S. Cervellati, and G. Gualdrine. Surgical treatment of vertebral deformities in neurofibromatosis. Ital J Orthop Traumatol 1983;9:13–24.
7. K. Yong-Hing, A. Kalamchi, and G.D. MacEwen. Cervical spine abnormalities in neurofibromatosis. J Bone Joint Surg [Am] 1979;61:696–699.
8. J.F. Holt. Neurofibromatosis in children. AJR 1978;130:615–639.
9. K.S. Anderson. Congenital pseudoarthrosis of the leg. J Bone Joint Surg [Am] 1976;58:657–662.

10. M.S. Ali and G. Hooper. Congenital pseudoarthrosis of the ulna due to neurofibromatosis. J Bone Joint Surg [Br] 1982;64:600–602.
11. P.J. Gregg, B.A. Price, H.A. Ellis, and J. Stevens. Pseudoarthrosis of the radius associated with neurofibromatosis: A case report. Clin Orthop 1982;171:175–179.
12. H. Hallock. The use of multiple small bone transplants in the treatment of pseudoarthrosis of the tibia of congenital origin or following osteotomy for the correction of congenital deformity. J Bone Joint Surg [Am] 1938;20:646–647.
13. C.T. Brighton, Z.B. Friedenberg, L.M. Zemski, and B.R. Pollis. Direct current stimulation of non-union and congenital pseudoarthrosis. Exploration of its clinical application. J Bone Joint Surg [Am] 1975;57:368–370.
14. L.S. Lavine, I. Lustrin, M.H. Shamos, et al. Electric enhancement of bone healing. Science 1972;175:118–119.
15. P.C. Leung. Congenital pseudoarthrosis of the tibia. Three cases treated by free vascularized iliac crest graft. Clin Orthop 1983;175:45–50.
16. M. Pitt, J.R. Mosher, and J. Ediken. Abnormal periosteum in bone in neurofibromatosis. Radiology 1972;103:143–146.

13

The Endocrine System in Neurofibromatosis

R. Neil Schimke, M.D., F.A.C.P.

The endocrine system is composed of a number of different glands scattered throughout the body. These glands secret a variety of hormones, some of which are steroids (cortisone, estrogen, testosterone), some are peptides (growth hormone, insulin), and still others are peptides to which sugar molecules have been added, e.g., the so-called glycoprotein hormones like thyroid-stimulating hormone (TSH). For many years it was thought that the pituitary gland, located in the middle of the skull right below where the optic nerves cross, was the chief regulator of most of the other glands, chiefly because it has multiple secretory products that stimulated the other glands; e.g., TSH stimulates the thyroid to secret thyroid hormone. A simple feedback system was visualized whereby sufficient secretion of, for example, thyroid hormone was able to turn off the pituitary secretion of TSH. While this remains true to some extent, it is now known that the pituitary is also positively and negatively controlled by still other hormones from the lower middle part of the brain (hypothalamus) and that these hypothalamic hormones can in turn be regulated by nerve connections from higher brain centers.

A condition like neurofibromatosis (NF) with its recognized potential to involve all aspects of the nervous system might be expected to cause a variety of disturbances in hormone secretion. What is surprising is that NF does not do this often; i.e., in actuality, endocrine abnormalities are not common in NF. They do occur, however, and it is important to recognize their patterns for heuristic value.

Hypothalamic-Pituitary Axis

The chief reason for dysfunctional secretion of hormones from the hypothalamus and pituitary is a tumor located in this region. These tumors may compress normal structures as might be the case with an optic nerve tumor or glioma which could develop right over the pituitary gland. Other neural tumors might interfere with the nerve connections between hypothalamus and pituitary or destroy critical cells that regulate hypothalamic secretion, again by mass effect. The end result of this tumorous growth could be either deficient secretion of one or more hormones or, on occasion, excess secretion, with the production of characteristic symptoms.

Excessive Growth or Short Stature

Growth is a complex process that depends on a number of factors: genetic makeup, nutrition, and hormonal growth factors. One of these growth factors is growth hormone (GH), without which individuals remain short in stature, meaning well below 5 feet (152.4 cm) in height, but retain normal proportions. As mentioned earlier, GH, like the other pituitary hormones, is regulated in part by the hypothalamus. Any lesion in the hypothalamus that interferes with the control of GH secretion could result in either excessive tall stature in children (gigantism) or, in adults, after the growth centers of bones have fused and growth has ceased, a disorder known as acromegaly. Both conditions have been seen in NF but they are not common.

When tumors are recognized as causing excessive GH secretion, the usual approach is surgery, or if they are inaccessible, radiation therapy. There are some drugs, like the currently available agent bromocriptine, or the still experimental analogs of a hypothalamic substance that normally inhibits GH (somatostatin), that may prove to be very effective in individual cases.

Excessive short stature or pituitary dwarfism also has been seen in NF, but again, not commonly. Less impressive degrees of short stature were seen in 16% of a series of 137 patients with NF who had no gross evidence for GH deficiency (1). Since children with NF may have short stature for other reasons, it is important to exclude those causes that can be treated. For example, if the children have disproportionate short stature, skeletal x-rays may reveal evidence of an independent growth problem in the long bones, spine, or both. There are a number of such disorders, collectively termed chondrodysplasias, and each has specific clinical and radiographic features.

In other instances, children may be short because of non-NF-related familial short stature or may have what is termed a constitutional delay. In the latter instance the bone age is usually about 2 years behind the chronological age, indicating that the child will likely mature a bit later and grow a bit longer than his or her peers, with the ultimate adult height being in the normal range. In the absence of skeletal disproportion, good screening studies for treatable growth deficiency include blood thyroid hormone level (true thyroxine), a somatomedin-C level (an indirect means of measuring GH secretion), and a bone age determination, which consists of a hand and wrist x-ray and comparison of the timing of appearance of the carpal bones with well-established standards.

Early or Delayed Puberty

Puberty is likewise a complex process that depends upon two pituitary hormones, follicle-stimulating hormone (FSH) and luteinizing hormone (LH), collectively called gonadotropins because they stimulate estrogen and progesterone production in the female ovary and testosterone in the male testes. The gonadotropins in turn are regulated by hypothalamic gonadotropin-releasing hormone (LHRH) that is normally activated in both sexes between 10 and 14 years of age. The steroid hormones are directly responsible for the development of menstruation and breast development in the female and genital enlargement and the characteristic body shape in the male.

Early or precocious puberty has been seen with NF. It is almost invariably caused by tumors in the hypothalamus that interfere with LHRH secretion (Fig. 13–1) (2). In addition to surgery and radiation, a variety of pharmaceutical agents that might interrupt this precocious development are being investigated mainly because of the potential psychological adjustment problems that are engendered by becoming a physical (but not an emotional) adult too soon. One word of caution: on occasion local tumors in NF that have nothing to do with hormonal hyposecretion or hypersecretion may cause enlargement of the female clitoris or male penis (3). In some instances this localized growth is so

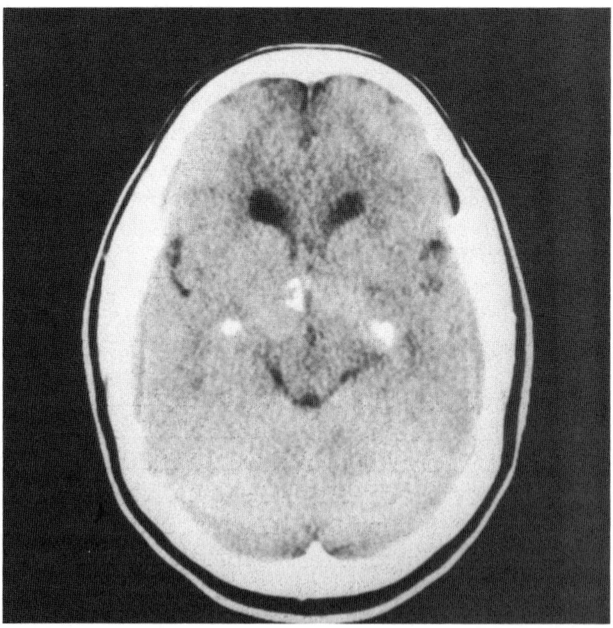

Figure 13–1. CT scan showing calcified optic glioma in child with NF and precocious puberty.

unusual that an intersex state is suspected, as for example in a female with clitoral enlargement so extensive that it simulated a penis. She also had groin masses that were considered to be undescended testes but were at surgery found to be neurofibromas. These were localized, not systemic changes.

Delayed development in both sexes has also been recognized in NF. As there are many causes of delayed puberty, it is not appropriate to ascribe such an occurrence to NF without more extensive investigation. In general, if puberty is either excessively early or unduly delayed, an endocrinologist should be consulted so that systemic evaluation can be undertaken.

Galactorrhea-Amenorrhea

Another hormone of the pituitary is prolactin, a substance important in milk release in the nursing mother. Prolactin production is normally tonically inhibited by hypothalamic prolactin-inhibiting factor (PIF). When secretion of PIF is interfered with, excessive secretion of prolactin results, which can stimulate inappropriate milk secretion by the breasts of both sexes, although more commonly in the female. Excessive prolactin also has the ability to turn off pituitary LHRH release so that menses frequently cease abruptly in the female. In the male the changes of decreased testosterone secretion such as loss of libido are more subtle and may be easily overlooked. The galactorrhea-amenorrhea syndrome has been seen, albeit rarely, in NF.

The therapeutic approach is similar to that of other hypothalamic-pituitary tumors. If no overt tumor is found, bromocriptine may be quite useful as it has an action very similar to PIF. Here again, a note of caution is in order. Both liver and kidney disease can result in elevated blood levels of prolactin. By the same token, a variety of drugs such as sedatives and tranquilizers can interfere with PIF secretion with resultant excess prolactin. Not infrequently individuals with NF might be ingesting prescription drugs that will produce the syndrome quite independent of NF.

THE THYROID

The thyroid is composed of two types of cells, the follicular cells that secrete thyroid hormone in response to pituitary TSH and the parafollicular cells that secrete calcitonin, the latter a hormone whose normal function remains unknown. Hyperthyroidism and hypothyroidism are both sufficiently common in the general population that no statistically significant relationship has been established between either of these states and NF.

On the other hand, one might expect a stronger association between NF and parafollicular cell activity, since this cell is embryologically derived from neural tissue, the so-called neural crest, whereas the thyroid follicular cell is not. Tumors of the parafollicular cell are called medullary thyroid carcinomas and they have been occasionally seen in NF. They are more common in other conditions involving endocrine tumors in multiple glands, the so-called multiple endocrine neoplasia (MEN) syndromes. These conditions are likewise inherited and at least one of them shows some overlapping features with NF, i.e., café au lait or freckle-like pigment spots or on occasion peripheral neurofibromas. However, these conditions are genetically distinct from NF.

PARATHYROIDS

The parathyroid glands, four in number, are located in the neck close to the thyroid. Unlike the thyroid, they are not regulated by the pituitary but by serum calcium levels. Parathyroid hormone (PTH) in turn regulates calcium absorption from the gut and resorption from the kidney and bone. Excessive autonomous secretion of PTH leads to high blood calcium levels that may be toxic to the heart, kidneys, etc. There is a passing relationship between NF and the parathyroid glands since neural crest tissues contribute to the glandular superstructure; however, the secretory parts of the glands are from another embryological source. Only a few patients with NF and hyperparathyroidism have been described and the association should best be considered coincidental.

PANCREAS

The pancreas has the ability to secrete many hormones—insulin, glucagon, pancreatic polypeptide, etc. The most important of these is insulin because a relative or absolute deficiency of this peptide gives rise to diabetes mellitus. Diabetes mellitus is common. No statistical excess of diabetes has been seen in NF over that expected by chance.

Excessive insulin secretion as would be occasioned by islet cell tumors of the pancreas (the source of insulin) leads to profound and refractory hypoglycemia. For some time the islet cells were thought to be of neural crest origin, but the bulk of present evidence is to the contrary. Islet cell tumors are not part of the NF tumor spectrum.

ADRENAL GLANDS

The adrenal glands are paired structures located above the kidneys. In actuality, each gland is itself two glands, the outer cortex being responsible for steroid hormone secretion (mainly cortisone) while the inner portion or medulla secretes epinephrine, more commonly known as adrenaline. The cortex and medulla are from different embryological sources; only the latter is

related to NF as it is derived from neural crest. Not unexpectedly, there is no known relationship between hyposecretion or hypersecretion of cortisone and NF.

On the other hand, tumors of the adrenal medulla, called pheochromocytomas, have long been known to be present in a small proportion of people with NF (4). Hypersecretion of adrenaline leads to a fight or flight reaction—elevated blood pressure, fast heart rate, a feeling of fear or intense anxiety, and so forth. The symptoms are usually episodic and appropriate laboratory tests can quickly confirm the diagnosis. The best method for diagnosing the presence of pheochromocytoma is measurement of the metabolites or breakdown products of adrenaline as they are excreted in the urine. A 24-hour urine sample analyzed for catecholamines, metanephrines, and vanillomandelic acid (VMA) will generally suffice for the diagnosis.

The most prominent symptom is hypertension and a diagnosis should be considered in any individual with NF and high blood pressure. However, in two extensive series of patients with NF, pheochromocytoma occurred in less than 1% (1,5). The incidence might be higher in hypertensive NF individuals but is still probably no more than a few percent. In other words, a hypertensive patient with NF is far more likely to have independent, so-called essential hypertension than tumor-related blood pressure elevation. Pheochromocytomas virtually never occur in children with NF and the usual onset is in the 30s, about the same age as a sporadic; i.e., non-NF-related pheochromocytoma would develop. The tumors when they do occur are generally only on one side and are benign. Malignant pheochromocytoma tumors are uncommon. Surgical removal of the pheochromocytoma results in prompt resolution of the symptoms.

CARCINOID TUMORS

There are unusual tumors generally located in the gastrointestinal tract. There is not a normal carcinoid gland but the tumors are mentioned for completeness because they may develop in individuals with NF, and they may be hormonally active. A favored location for carcinoids is the appendix where they are usually found incidentally at appendectomy or autopsy. They can occur in the upper bowel such as the duodenum where they cause symptoms of obstruction or bleeding. Rarely are they found in the respiratory tract. Occasionally carcinoid tumors cause symptoms because they secrete excessive quantities of a substance called serotonin. Serotonin causes blood vessels to dilate, giving rise to episodes of flushing and dizziness due to low blood pressure. Tumors in the bronchial tree may cause obstruction or, if they secrete serotonin, bronchospasm and wheezing.

There appears to be a significant association between carcinoid tumors and NF (6,7). In fact, patients have been reported with NF, a pheochromocytoma, and a carcinoid tumor. The carcinoid itself is, like the adrenal medulla and the thyroid parafollicular cells, also derived from the neural crest, so the relationship is logical. The tumors may become malignant and the associated symptoms depend on tumor mass, location, and presence or absence of serotonin secretion.

GONADS

Generally speaking, involvement of the gonads in either sex in NF is secondary to disordered central gonadotropin secretion as discussed earlier. There is a subgroup of individuals who have the physical signs of NF along with other physical features including characteristic facial appearance, stenosis or narrowing of the pulmonary valve on the right side of the heart, short stature, and other minor problems, all of which independently have been called Noonan syndrome (8). Some of the individuals with this constellation of findings have primary gonadal deficiency. Whether such individuals represent the simultaneous occurrence of two relatively common genetic conditions, an independent condition with overlapping features, or part of the broad spectrum of developmental anomalies that occur in NF remains uncertain. In any case, save for these special circumstances, ovarian or testicular failure is not a conspicuous feature of NF, and fertility is ordinarily unimpaired.

There is controversy surrounding the use of oral contraceptives (birth control pills) in NF. Some women claim their neurofibromas have grown while they are on these agents. However, most of the so-called evidence is anecdotal. In other words, peripheral tumors grow in no predictable fashion normally in NF, so it is virtually impossible to establish a cause-and-effect relationship between tumor growth and oral contraceptives. In my experience and in the experience of the directors of three large NF clinics, there is no firm evidence that birth control pills enhance the growth of peripheral tumors. Increases in skin pigment may accompany birth control use in people with NF, but whether this increase is related to an interaction of NF and birth control pills or is coincidental is also an open question. Many women without NF have increased skin pigment with birth control pills.

There is concern, however, that the brain tumors in individuals with the central form of NF who have acoustic neuromas, meningiomas and so forth may respond inappropriately to the estrogen component in the birth control pill (9). It is probably wise to use other contraceptive measures for such individuals whereas those with peripheral tumors likely can take the pills, providing careful observation is possible.

The effect of pregnancy on growth of neurofibromas is likewise the subject of numerous case reports, but has not been studied systematically. The growth of existing neurofibromas, and the appearance of new ones, have been well documented to occur during pregnancy, but the risk of this occurring is not known (10). Hypertension during pregnancy, which can have an adverse effect on the growth of the fetus, appears to be increased in women with NF.

SUMMARY

Some components of the endocrine system share an embryological relationship with NF. However, except for pheochromocytomas, involvement of the endocrine system in NF is uncommon. Central lesions may interfere with normal growth and normal pubertal development, but even this is unusual. Careful attention should be paid to all aspects of the dysfunctional endocrine state in a patient with NF, because except for the few instances cited, it is likely the hormone problems and NF are unrelated the vast majority of the time.

REFERENCES

1. K.M. Saxena. Endocrine manifestations of neurofibromatosis in children. Am J Dis Child 1970;120:265–271.
2. L. Laue, F. Comite, K. Hench, et al. Precocious puberty associated with neurofibromatosis and optic gliomas. Am J Dis Child 1985;139:1097–1100.
3. J. Kaneti, E. Lieberman, P. Moshe, and R. Carmi. A case of ambiguous genitalia owing to neurofibromatosis—Review of the literature. J Urol 1988;140:584–585.
4. V. Kalff, B. Shapiro, R. Lloyd, et al. The spectrum of pheochromocytoma in hypertensive patients with neurofibromatosis. Ann Intern Med 1982;142:2092–2098.
5. W. Andler, K. Roosen, U. Kohns, and L. Stolecke. Endokrine Storungen bei Kindern mit Neurofibromatose von Recklinghausen. Monatschr Kinderheilk 1979;127:135–138.
6. D.R. Hough, A. Chan, and H. Davidson. Von Recklinghausen's disease associated with gastrointestinal carcinoid tumors. Cancer 1983;51:2205–2208.
7. Y. Dayal, K.A. Tallberg, G. Nunnemacher, et al. Duodenal carcinoids in patients with and without neurofibromatosis. Am J Surg Pathol 1986;10:348–357.
8. J.M. Opitz, and D.D. Weaver. The neurofibromatosis-Noonan syndrome. Am J Med Genet 1985;21:477–490.
9. R.L. Martuza, D.T. Maclaughlin, and R.G. Ojemann. Specific estradiol binding in schwannomas, meningiomas, and neurofibromas. Neurosurgery 1981;9:665–671.
10. I. Blickstein, M. Lancet, and Z. Shoham. The obstetric perspective of neurofibromatosis. Am J Obstet Gynecol 1988;158:385–388.

14

THE CHILD WITH NEUROFIBROMATOSIS

Angela C. Obringer, Ph.D., Anna T. Meadows, M.D., and Elaine H. Zackai, M.D., Ph.D.

The child with neurofibromatosis (NF) requires a comprehensive multidisciplinary approach for medical care. This need reflects the nature of the NF gene itself—its variable expressivity and effect on multiple systems. Since the condition has been reported to occur in 1 in 3000 births, the average pediatrician will see several during a professional lifetime. While many of the children we have examined and followed for the past 5 years are healthy and have no serious medical problems, parents and health professionals need to be aware of the potential consequences of this disorder.

Concern that early identification and recognition of the unique problems of NF and appropriate referral are of primary importance in the management of this disorder led to the establishment of a specialty clinic at the Children's Hospital of Philadelphia (CHOP). Diagnosis, genetic counseling, and long-term follow-up of the pediatric patient with NF and his or her family are the functions of the clinic. It is the purpose of this report to review our experience and to make suggestions and recommendations regarding the care of children with NF.

THE NEUROFIBROMATOSIS CLINIC AT THE CHILDREN'S HOSPITAL OF PHILADELPHIA

The Neurofibromatosis Clinic of the CHOP was established in 1979 as a joint effort of the Clinical Genetics Center and the Division of Oncology. It arose from the realization that the medical care of the child with NF often required the intervention of many areas of specialization, which needed coordination and open lines of communication. With the cooperation and recommendations of all the medical specialties, guidelines were developed for the evaluation and follow-up of the pediatric patient with NF, affected and unaffected siblings and parents, and these will be discussed.

The clinical objectives of the Neurofibromatosis Clinic include:

1. Diagnosis and early identification of NF and associated problems
2. Genetic counseling of probands, parents and siblings
3. Appropriate referral to departments such as orthopedics, ophthalmology, neurology, surgery, neurosurgery, plastic surgery, child development and rehabilitation, and dentistry
4. Long-term follow-up of children with NF.

The Neurofibromatosis Clinic also provides resources for clinical and basic research scientists who are studying the pathophysiology and molecular genetics of NF. The permanent staff of the Neurofibromatosis Clinic include a pediatric oncologist and a clinical geneticist, both of whom are pediatricians, and a clinic coordinator, who has training in human genetics. The composition of any Neurofibromatosis Clinic staff will vary in an institution depending on the professionals who are interested in this disorder. However, since NF is the single most common genetic disorder associated with cancer, it was only natural that the two disciplines—genetics and oncology—should promote the establishment of a multidisciplinary clinic for children with NF. The clinic coordinator acts as a liaison between the medical staff, the patient and his family, and the medical specialists. Besides obtaining the medical and family history and coordinating medical services, the clinic coordinator is available to the NF family to answer questions and address the specific concerns of the patient and his family.

The other medical specialists do not normally attend clinic. However, their expertise and advice are always available. Most specialists, e.g., neurologist, ophthalmologist, or orthopedist, prefer to see patients in their own offices or clinic settings where the appropriate diagnostic instruments are readily available. However, in an emergency, an immediate consultation can always be obtained.

Medical students, pediatric residents and fellows in human genetics, and other health professionals rotate through the Neurofibromatosis Clinic regularly. Through teaching health-care professionals who will be practicing in the community, we expect to promote the education of the medical community about NF, and to make them aware of the variable manifestations of NF, particularly as they apply to children.

REFERRAL

Families are referred to the Neurofibromatosis Clinic from various sources including the hospital's medical and specialty clinics, private physicians, or health-care facilities in the community as well as the National Neurofibromatosis Foundation.

When a child is referred to the Clinic a complete medical history and family pedigree are obtained. The reason for the referral is ascertained. The concerns and questions of the family are elicited during the telephone interview. An ophthalmological evaluation and skeletal survey are arranged. These are included as part of the initial evaluation protocol for several reasons. Both of these examinations may provide diagnostic information when clinical manifestations of NF are not definitive, e.g., the presence of Lisch nodules, vertebral scalloping, or rib thinning. The information obtained by these studies is incorporated into the baseline assessment as a reference for future evaluations and clinical concerns. Along with the physical examination, the eye exam and skeletal survey often provide important clinical information for referral to a specialist. A patient, particularly a young child, with scoliosis diagnosed by clinical examination and x-ray may need to be referred to an orthopedist for follow-up, depending on severity. A specific example illustrating the important role of these two examinations in the initial evaluation is given by the following case history.

> A 15-year-old black female was referred to the Neurofibromatosis Clinic by the Adolescent Clinic at CHOP. She was not aware of the diagnosis of NF, but had come to the Clinic for a referral to a plastic surgeon for removal of a "lump" on her lip for cosmetic reasons only. When the skeletal survey was performed, the skull x-ray revealed an enlarged sella and macrocephaly. Papilledema and enlarged corneal nerves were observed at the ophthalmological evaluation. Her visual acuity was normal. She was totally asymptomatic, and had no other signs of increased cranial pressure. A computed tomography (CT) scan revealed massive hydrocephalus. She was referred to the neurosurgeon for evaluation. During the next 3 weeks her papilledema increased and visual acuity deteriorated. She was admitted to the hospital and underwent ventriculoperitoneal shunting. Further imaging studies have not delineated the exact cause for the hydrocephalus, although there is a distinct fullness on the posterior fossa. She continues to be followed by the neuro-oncologist for the possible development of tumor.

Although this is an extreme example, it points to the need for comprehensive baseline diagnostic studies, even in the clinically mildly affected child.

When a family is seen in the Neurofibromatosis Clinic, the initial conference aims to review the medical and family history, and to determine parental concerns and level of knowledge about NF—its genetics and manifestations. These are subsequently addressed during the discussion with the family following the examination. Ideally, all family members (proband, siblings, and parents) are examined. Height, weight, head circumference, and blood pressure are recorded. Number and sites of café au lait spots are noted, as well as presence or absence of axillary and inguinal freckling, neurofibromas, and other masses. Other clinical observations include presence or absence of asymmetry, scoliosis, gross neurological function, Tanner stage, and the other parameters of a normal well-child examination. Recommendations for appropriate referral and follow-up are made to the patient and the family based on the results of the physical examination, skeletal survey, and eye exam. The spectrum of clinical manifestations of NF is explained, and appropriate genetic counseling is given to the family.

It is essential that ample time be spent with the family at the initial session to assure that information is transmitted completely and specifically (depending on the presenting problems), but also with sensitivity (being aware of the patient's and/or family's level of anxiety). Our most important task, beyond making a diagnosis and providing genetic counseling, is to develop a solid ongoing relationship with parents so that they will feel free to discuss concerns at any time.

Most children with NF return annually for follow-up visits. This visit is important for maintaining contact with the family, and providing reassurance through re-evaluation of clinical status.

At an appropriate time, depending on the age and maturity, the genetics of NF should be discussed with the child, and the clinical manifestations and importance of routine medical follow-up as an adult should be reviewed. Adolescents with NF are a very special group. We are just beginning to address the needs and issues that concern them, e.g., sex education and birth control, their reproductive options, and self-image, particularly if there is physical disfigurement.

RESULTS

In the 5 years of the Neurofibromatosis Clinic at CHOP, data documenting the spectrum of clinical manifestations seen even in the very young child attest to the variability of expression of the gene. In addition, the longitudinal data obtained by annual follow-up visits illustrate the unique and progressive nature of this genetic disorder.

We examined 606 individuals from 196 families. A definite diagnosis of NF was made in 259, including 175 probands, 25 siblings, 59 parents, and numerous other relatives. In addition, there were three families with NF2 (bilateral acoustic neuromas) and three probands with segmental NF. Two patients had congenital nevi with associated neurofibromas. In the remaining individuals (303), the diagnosis of NF could not be made. The clinical manifestations are summarized in Table 14–1.

Demographic Data

Equal numbers of males and females were found to be affected, and approximately 70% of the probands were white. This proportion reflects the racial distribution of the region.

The probands ranged in age from several months to the early or middle twenties. Seventy-five percent were 15 years old or younger at the time of the initial visit.

Almost one-half of the patients have been followed for at least 2 years. There is also a small group who were followed by other multidisciplinary clinics within the hospital, e.g., craniofacial, oncology or neuro-oncology, and neurol-

Table 13–1. Clinical Findings in 200 Children with Neurofibromatosis

	FREQUENCY (%)
Cutaneous Manifestations	
Café au lait spots, axillary freckling only	
< 6 years old	60
> 15 years old	5
Café au lait spots, axillary freckling, neurofibromas	
< 6 years old	25
> 15 years old	90
Ophthalmological findings	
Lisch nodules (> 6 years old)	34
Multiple problems	10
Other associated findings	10
Optic glioma	
Ptosis alone	
Plexiform neurofibromas of eye or orbit	
Congenital glaucoma	
Corneal neurofibroma	
Skeletal findings	
Scoliosis	20
Pseudoarthrosis or tibial bowing	8
Other radiological findings	20
Pectus excavatum or carinatum	
Kyphoscoliosis	
Rib thinning	
Vertebral scalloping	
J-shaped sella	
Cortical bone cysts	
Absence of sphenoid wing	
Growth parameters	
Head circumference (> 95 percentile)	38
Short stature (below 5 percentile)	10
Other	5
Precocious or delayed puberty	
Failure to thrive	
Malignancy	11
Other	44
Learning disabilities	
Mental retardation	
Communication disorders (speech, language, voice)	
Fine- and gross-motor coordination	
Seizures	
Asymmetry—segmental or somatic	
Dental problems, e.g., jaw cysts, oral neurofibromas	

ogy. Those patients who were over 20 years at the time of the initial visit received appropriate genetic counseling and were then referred to an internist for medical follow-up. Unfortunately some families, for whatever reason, were lost to follow-up. Twenty percent failed to return for 2 years.

Inheritance Pattern

Although the literature reports that approximately 50% of individuals with NF receive the NF gene from a parent, with the remainder being the result of a sporadic mutation, the inheritance pattern in this population differs somewhat from the published data.

There were 91 probands (60%) with a negative family history including a negative parental exam. A positive family history was documented in 60 probands. In 41 the origin of the NF gene was maternal and in 19, paternal. These proportions differ markedly from the published data and may represent a referral bias. There was no differential fertility noted. A comparison between those families in which the father or mother had NF revealed no difference in the mean number of offspring. Nor was there an increase in the frequency of spontaneous abortions or stillbirths in either group. In addition, no differences in severity of the clinical manifestations were noted when offspring of sporadic cases were compared to those inheriting NF from either sex parent.

There were 24 individuals in whom the mode of inheritance could not be determined. Four children were adopted. In all but three of the remaining 20 cases, one or both parents were not examined nor was sufficient documentation available to ascertain the mode of inheritance.

Only 25 of 68 siblings at risk (i.e., those with affected parents) had NF. Their clinical manifestations did not differ from the probands as a group, but were usually less severe; 16 were younger than the proband and this age difference or selection bias based on medical need may account for the difference in severity.

Cutaneous Manifestations

Only 60% of the children under 5 years of age had six or more café au lait spots and/or bilateral axillary freckling. In this age group, the presence of six or more café au lait spots, axillary freckling, and more than one neurofibroma occurred in only 25% of the probands. As older age groups were evaluated, there appeared to be a linear increase in the frequency of the three cutaneous diagnostic signs, so that by 15 years 90% of the population demonstrated the classic criteria for diagnosis.

The frequency of cutaneous manifestations of NF by age did not differ significantly by the manner in which the NF gene was acquired.

Head Circumference

Besides the cutaneous manifestations, another parameter which is useful in the diagnosis of the pediatric patient is head circumference. Holt (1) and Weichart (2) found 44% and 30%, respectively, of patients with NF had macrocephaly confirmed by radiological measurements. In our population, 38% of the probands had a head circumference greater than the 95th percentile. Longitudinal records of head circumference are also useful for detecting abrupt increases in head circumference measurement, an indicator of intracranial involvement.

Ophthalmological Findings

Lisch nodules or hamartomas of the iris have been reported by Lewis and Riccardi (3) as diagnostic in 77% of patients older than 6 years. Forty-four percent of our probands older than 6 years had negative exams, 34% were positive for Lisch nodules, and 10% had multiple ophthalmic problems, e.g., optic gliomas, congenital glaucoma, neural hypertrophy, optic atrophy, corneal neurofibromas, and ptosis with and without plexiform neurofibromas of the eyelid or optic glioma. Exophthalmos may result from a neurofibroma within the orbit, optic glioma, or abnormality of the bony structure of the orbit (4). We have seen four children with congenital absence of the sphenoid wing, but only one demonstrated the classic clinical manifestations of NF, including a positive family history. Two children had isolated plexiform neurofibromas in the orbital area and the fourth child had an orbital teratoma.

It is important that children with NF have regular eye examinations, because of the myriad of ocular manifestations of the NF gene (5).

Radiological Findings

Skeletal changes occur in many patients with NF (1,6,7). These may be the result of a mesodermal dysfunction or bony erosion by tumor. The most common radiographic findings include: scoliosis and kyphoscoliosis, anterior bowing of the tibia with subsequent pseudoarthrosis in some cases, growth abnormalities, posterior scalloping of vertebrae, twisted-ribbon rib deformity, absence of the sphenoid wing, J-shaped sella, cortical bone cysts, and macrocranium. Erosion of the bone by tumor can be seen radiographically and contributes to the frequency of findings, e.g., J-shaped sella, vertebral scalloping, rib abnormalities, and erosion or absence of the orbital bones. Appropriate radiographic studies, obtained because of clinical indication, can also determine involvement of the genitourinary, gastrointestinal, or cardiovascular systems, which occur infrequently.

Although 50% of our patients had a negative skeletal survey, the remaining probands had findings that were diagnostic of NF or important for orthopedic follow-up, including scoliosis (20%) and pseudoarthrosis or tibial bowing (8%). Vertebral scalloping and rib thinning are often isolated findings, although some were associated with plexiform neurofibromas.

In five children, there were chest deformities associated with extensive neck and mediastinal neurofibromas, which have compromised pulmonary function or impinged on the integrity of the spinal cord. These patients have required extensive medical and/or surgical intervention, although they participate in most school and extracurricular activities.

Developmental (Neurological) Findings

As we see more school-age children, we have become more aware that children with NF are at risk for learning disabilities, hyperactivity, developmental delay, poor fine- and gross-motor coordination, speech delay, and mental retardation.

The role of the NF gene in developmental and/or cognitive dysfunction has yet to be elucidated. We have been involved in research related to communication disorders in children with NF. The preliminary findings are discussed elsewhere in this volume. However, the frequency of language problems is impressive, and we have found it useful to employ a speech and language evaluation as a screening technique and indicator for more general learning problems (see Chapter 6). Evaluation of neuropsychological function should also be part of an ideal comprehensive assessment for all NF children.

Specific neurological problems were present in 5% with seizures the most common of these. Other neurological problems may arise as specific consequences of central nervous system tumors and plexiform neurofibromas impinging on cranial or spinal nerves, or are the result of the treatment children receive for these tumors.

Malignancy

NF is the single most common genetic disorder associated with cancer in childhood, although the incidence of malignancy in NF during the pediatric years is not known (see Chapter 10). It is for this reason that we stress yearly comprehensive follow-up of the pediatric NF patient. We have seen 19 children with NF who have developed cancer. Central nervous system tumors were most common: optic gliomas (six), astrocytomas (two), and meningiomas (two). Soft-tissue sarcomas were seen in seven: malignant schwannoma (five) and rhabdomyosarcoma (two). There was also one child with chronic myelogenous leukemia (CML) and one with Wilms tumor. Four of these patients were diagnosed as a direct result of a Neurofibromatosis Clinic visit. One set of siblings with similar tumors and one patient who has had two primary tumors were included in our clinic population. There were 22 additional pediatric patients with NF registered in the CHP Tumor Registry on whom we have compiled data. These cases included another set of siblings with concordant brain tumors and a patient with four histologically distinct neoplasms.

Awareness that there is an increased risk of malignancy in children with NF enables parents to communicate any concerns about their child's health to the Neurofibromatosis Clinic staff, so that prompt diagnosis and treatment can be initiated if and when necessary.

Other Manifestations Requiring Special Care

Dental problems, e.g., oral neurofibromas and jaw cysts or neurofibromas, occur infrequently. These could, however, cause problems requiring oral surgery, orthodonture, or even speech therapy.

Facial asymmetry may be an early indicator of the presence of a diffuse neurofibroma. Plastic surgery may be required to reduce the cosmetic consequences of this manifestation and other noticeable manifestations such as ptosis. Children with somatic asymmetry or hemihypertrophy should be carefully monitored, because of the association of hemihypertrophy and intraabdominal embryonal tumors such as Wilms tumor.

Although 87% of the children had linear growth (height) between the fifth and 95th percentiles, short stature and delayed puberty occurred in approximately 10% of the children. No organic cause has been found in the majority of cases. Failure to thrive has also been reported in the medical histories of several children with NF.

SUMMARY

The clinical criteria for diagnosis of NF were defined by Crowe et al. in their classic monograph (8). The multifaceted nature of this genetic disorder has also been well documented. Several extensive reviews on the effects of the NF gene on multiple organ systems have been published (9–14); some are concerned principally with childhood manifestations (15–18). However, except for the data of Carey et al. (14) and Huson et al. (13), the information detailed in these publications is from retrospective analyses of selected populations of hospitalized patients. The authors do emphasize the marked variability of NF, the need for a multidisciplinary approach to evaluation of the NF patient, the unpredictability of the prognosis in NF, and the necessity for careful long-term follow-up of individuals with this disorder. However, these literature reviews of multiple organ systems describe patterns of NF in childhood among populations selected on the basis of medical need.

The variability of the NF gene appears to be more pronounced in the child with NF than in the adult, in that a large fraction appears to be totally asymptomatic. The data presented here confirm the wide spectrum of clinical manifestations of NF in the pediatric population. However, the child with NF may develop serious medical problems at any age. It is impossible to present an exhaustive list of these medical problems associated with NF in childhood. The majority of children with NF have no major health problems, but often have minor chronic physical, health, or school problems and parents are usually excessively concerned because of the underlying diagnosis. It cannot be stressed enough that early diagnosis with a baseline skeletal survey and eye examination, plus annual follow-up evaluations, are important for the continuing care of the pediatric NF patient.

As children with NF reach adolescence and young adulthood, the concerns of the parents become the concerns of the child. The psychological impact of learning that they have a genetic disorder which can be progressive, physically debilitating or disfiguring could be devastating. It is important that the genetics and prognosis of NF be approached gradually, with sensitivity and reassurance.

Support groups for these children and their parents can play a vital role in terms of improving self-image and channeling their strengths and weaknesses into positive productive activities. The family and patient need support through the Neurofibromatosis Clinic, support groups, and psychological and genetic counseling. Families should be encouraged to avail themselves of these services to meet their specific needs and those of the children.

ACKNOWLEDGMENTS—The authors wish to thank Mr. Jack L. Elias for his assistance in the preparation of this manuscript. Supported in part by grants from the National Neurofibromatosis Foundation and the Canuso Foundation.

REFERENCES

1. J.F. Holt. Neurofibromatosis in children. AJR 1978;130:615–639.
2. K.A. Weichert, M.S. Dine, C. Benlon, and F.N. Silverman. Macrocranium and neurofibromatosis. Radiology 1973;107:163–166.
3. R.A. Lewis, and V.M. Riccardi. Von Recklinghausen neurofibromatosis: Incidence of iris hamartomas. Ophthalmology 1981;88:348–354.
4. P.J. Savino, J.L. Glaser, and M.N. Luxenberg. Pulsating enophthalmos and choroidal hamartomas: Two rare stigmata of neurofibromatosis. Br J Ophthalmol 1977;61:483–488.
5. S.M. Huson, D. Jones, and L. Beck. Ophthalmic manifestations of neurofibromatosis. Br J Ophthalmol 1987;71:235–238.
6. E.S. Casselman, W.T. Miller, S.R. Lin, and G.A. Mandell. Von Recklinghausen's disease: Incidence of roentgenographic findings with a clinical review of the literature. CRC Crit Rev Diag Imaging 1977;9:387–419.
7. E.C. Klatte, E.A. Franken, and J.A. Smith. The radiographic spectrum in neurofibromatosis. Sem Roentgen 1976;11:17–33.
8. F.W. Crowe, W.J. Schull, and J.V. Neel. A clinical, pathological, and genetic study of multiple neurofibromatosis. Springfield, IL, Charles C Thomas, 1956.
9. R. Brasfield, and T.K. Das Gupta. Von Recklinghausen's disease: A clinicopathological study. Ann Surg 1972;175:86–104.
10. J.V. Wander, and T.K. Das Gupta. Neurofibromatosis. Curr Prob Surg 1977;14:1–81.
11. V.M. Riccardi. Von Recklinghausen neurofibromatosis. N Engl J Med 1981;305:1617–1626.
12. V.M. Riccardi, and J.E. Eichner. Neurofibromatosis: Phenotype, natural history, and pathogenesis. Baltimore, Johns Hopkins University Press, 1986.
13. S.M. Huson, P.S. Harper, and D.A.S. Compston. Von Recklinghausen neurofibromatosis. A clinical and population study in south-east Wales. Brain 1988;111:1355–1381.
14. J.C. Carey, J.M. Laub, and B.D. Hall. Penetrance and variability in neurofibromatosis: A genetic study of 60 families. Birth Defects 1979; Original Article Series 15, No. 5B:271–281.
15. D.H. Chao. Congenital neurocutaneous syndromes in childhood. I. Neurofibromatosis. J Pediatr 1959;55:189–199.
16. B.H. Griffith, P. McKinney, C.W. Monroe, and A. Howell. Von Recklinghausen's disease in children. Plast Reconstr Surg 1972;49:647–653.
17. R. Pollnitz. Neurofibromatosis in childhood: A review of 25 cases. Med J Aust 1976;2:49–52.
18. E.G. Chalhub. Neurocutaneous syndrome in children. Pediatr Clin North Am 1976;23:499–516.

SECTION II

GENETIC ASPECTS

15

The Genetics of Neurofibromatosis

John C. Carey, M.D., M.P.H.

Knowledge of the genetic basis of the well-established forms of neurofibromatosis (NF) is key to any presentation of the medical, biological, and causal aspects of the conditions. Von Recklinghausen NF, or NF1, is one of the most common of heritable disorders in humans and serves as a prototype in any discussion of the basic principles of human genetics and their application to health care. In addition, NF1 is of general significance because it is probably the most common disorder due to a spontaneously occurring gene mutation and because its associated features involve several organ systems. The diversity of clinical manifestations in NF1 range from a child with multiple congenital anomaly (birth defect) syndrome to an adult with malignancy.

The purpose of this chapter is to: (1) review the basic principles of human genetics that apply to medical disorders, and (2) Discuss these principles of human genetics in relation to NF in particular. This chapter will lay the groundwork for the presentation of the principal themes in the genetic counseling in families who have the various forms of NF. The following chapter will extend the discussion of genetics in NF to include recent knowledge gained from molecular genetic studies.

Basic Principles and Concepts of Human Genetics

Genes and Chromosomes

The widespread application of the science of genetics to human disease and medical care is a relatively recent event. In the last three decades, technological advances in the field of genetics have paralleled a decline in morbidity and mortality from infectious diseases and helped precipitate recent interest of medical investigators in genetics. It was only in 1956 that the actual number of human chromosomes was accurately determined. This finding led to the discovery that Down syndrome, which had been recognized almost 100 years before, was due to an abnormality in the actual number of chromosomes. The 1960s witnessed a blossoming in the field of biochemistry, the development of prenatal diagnosis of some genetic disorders, and the description of many previously unrecognized syndromes. In the 1970s an actual subspecialty in medicine, medical genetics, evolved from these advances and led to the development of genetic counseling clinics in most universities and centers in North America.

Although the entrance of genetics into medical care is a recent event, the history of genetics as a part of the biological sciences dates back to the 1800s. In 1865, Gregor Mendel, an Augustian priest, laid down the basic principles regarding the units of heredity, which we now call genes, in his experiments with plants. Although his work was unrecognized at the time, Mendel's contributions are now honored by our referring to single gene conditions as mendelian disorders. In this century, population geneticists and eventually molecular biologists developed the classic principles of genetics that apply to the study of human variation and disease.

The basic unit of heredity is the *gene*, a tiny chemical structure that codes for a particular protein essential to the body's correct functioning. Genes come in pairs. It is believed that man has over 100,000 gene pairs and every cell in the body contains the paired sets. Genes are transmitted directly from one generation to the next in egg and sperm cells, germ cells, with each parent contributing half—one of each pair—of a child's genes. Which gene of each pair a mother or father passes on to a child is a matter of chance (Fig. 15–1).

The basic chemical structure of the gene is the complex molecule called *DNA* or deoxyribonucleic acid. The chemical structure of DNA has been delineated in the last 30 years and this molecular work represents the important groundwork for the recombinant DNA technology that will be discussed in the next chapter. Genetic disorders are thought to result from alterations in the actual chemical structure of this DNA. In some disorders these alterations, or *mutations*, are well understood at the level of the chemicals in the DNA molecule. It is presumed that all genetic defects, even though the actual knowledge of the DNA level defect is not known, are due to such changes.

A gene, then, represents a specific segment of the DNA molecule. This chemical structure of DNA comprising a gene encodes the structure of a particular protein (Fig. 15–2). The actual process involved in "translating" the DNA into proteins will not be discussed in this chapter and the reader is referred to the basic texts in genetics and molecular biology (1–3).

Genes are carried on structures inside the nucleus of the cell called *chromosomes* (Fig. 15–3). While genes cannot be seen with a microscope, chromosomes can be visualized and have been studied in great detail. There are 23 pairs of chromosomes, each composed of thousands of genes arranged along the length of the chromosome like beads on a string. These chromosomes are numbered 1 through 22, with the 23rd pair being the sex

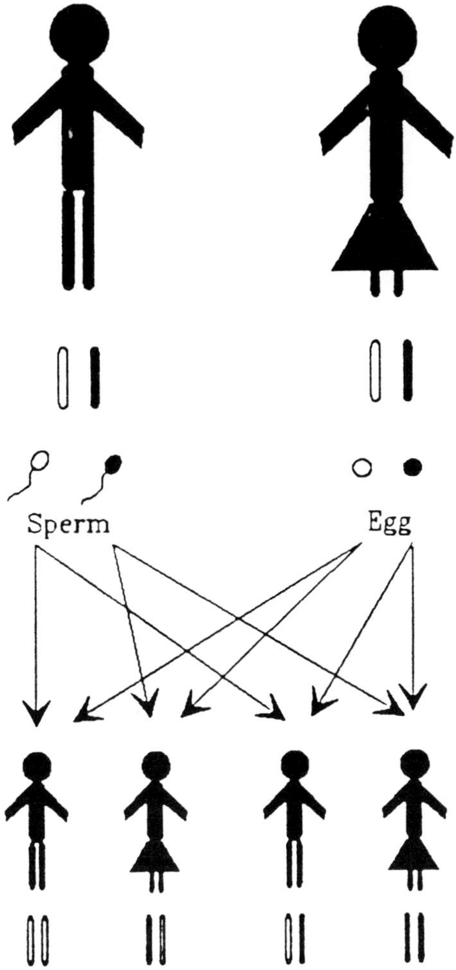

Figure 15–1. Each individual has two copies of every gene. Alternative gene copies are depicted in the figure as the dark and light bars. Only one of these copies is transmitted to the germ cells (sperm or egg). The combination of genes passed on to a child is therefore a matter of chance, depending on the particular forms of the gene carried by the sperm and egg.

chromosomes. Males have the sex chromosome constitution of an X and a Y, while females have two X chromosomes. The 22 nonsex chromosomes are referred to as *autosomes*.

As can be seen from Figure 15–3, each chromosome pair differs from the other pairs by size, the placement of the central constriction (called the *centromere*) and by a specific banding pattern that is due to a chemical stain

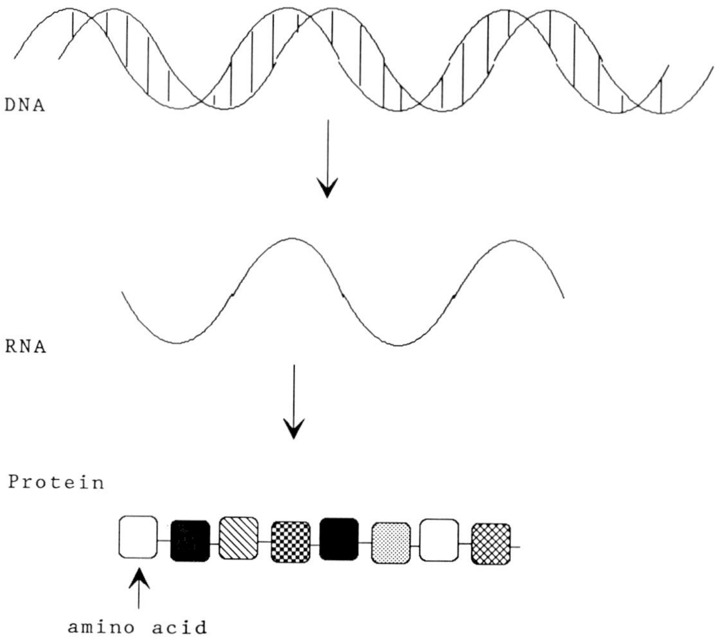

Figure 15–2. The flow of genetic information is from DNA to RNA to protein. The sequence of base pairs in the DNA is transcribed into the sequence of complementary bases in RNA, which is in turn translated into the sequence of amino acids in protein.

placed on the chromosomes during the process of preparing the chromosomes. The chromosomes are divided into two arms: the upper arm in the photograph of the individual chromosome is called the short arm (or p arm), while the lower arm is called the long arm (q arm). The various bands of the chromosome are actually numbered in a complex way that will not be discussed here and the reader is referred to a basic genetic textbook for specific details of chromosome nomenclature.

When cells divide in the process referred to as *mitosis* (Fig. 15–4), the chromosomes are precisely copied so that a complete set of genetic information is provided for each daughter cell. During the development of germ cells, i.e., sperm or egg, the chromosome pairs split up through a special process called *meiosis* (Fig. 15–4). In this way each germ cell receives only a single copy of each chromosome pair so that when fertilization occurs the normal situation of two copies of each chromosome is restored.

Two other concepts will be introduced at this point to assist in a further discussion of the relationship of genes to human diseases and development. The first of these terms is *genotype*, which refers to the genetic constitution of the individual or organism under discussion. The term that has been used by

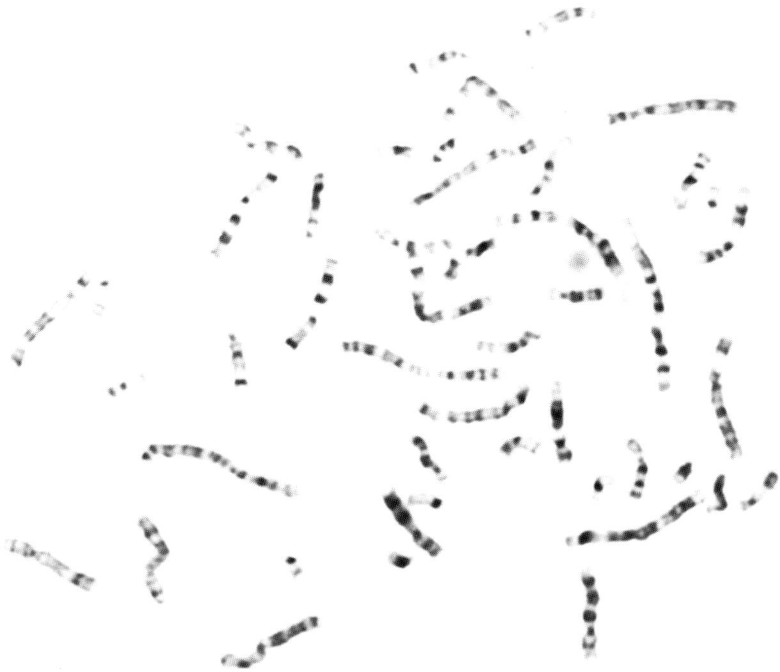

Figure 15–3. The 46 chromosomes from a male are displayed in a standard form known as the karyotype. The chromosomes have been stained so that a distinctive banding pattern appears, allowing each chromosome to be unequivocally identified. Homologous chromosomes are paired together in this array, which was produced by cutting out the image of each chromosome from a photograph of the chromosomes in a dividing cell and then pasting the individual chromosomes onto the karyotype form. There are 22 pairs of autosomes and two sex chromosomes. A male, as depicted, has an X and a Y chromosomes; a female would have two X chromosomes. (Figure continues.)

geneticists to refer to the actual clinical or physical finding in the person at hand is *phenotype*. Thus, the various physical signs of NF are sometimes referred to as phenotypic manifestations. Up until recent years most of the studies of the NF syndromes were at the phenotypic level. It has been through recent advances in DNA technology that now the area of genotypic investigation can occur.

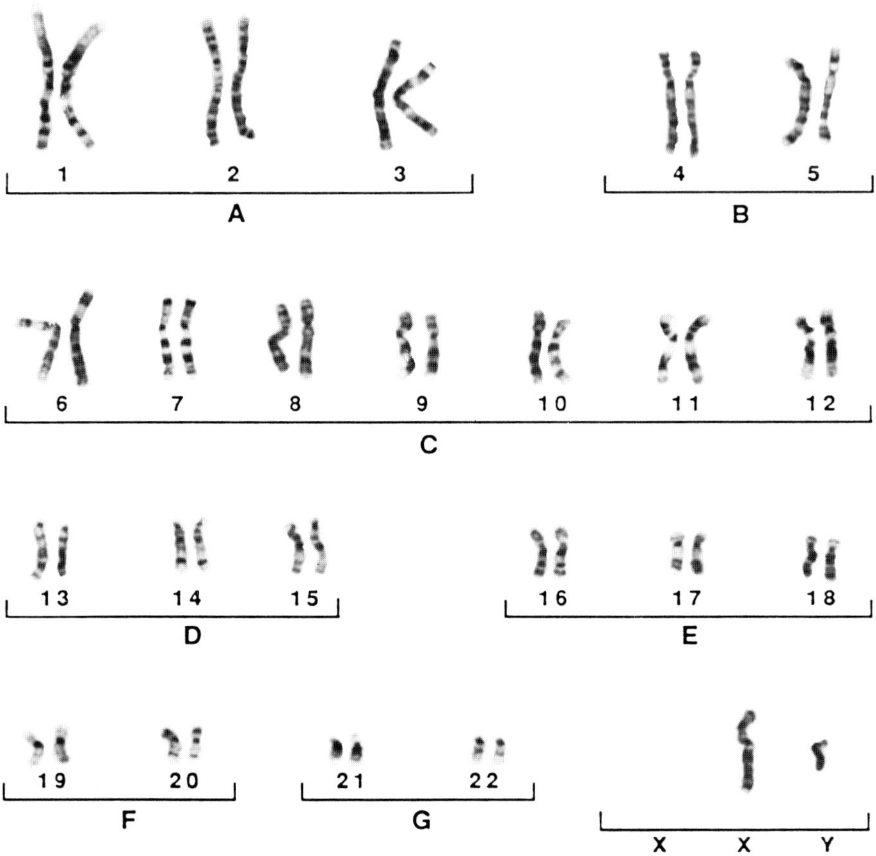

Figure 15–3 *(continued).*

Genetic Disorders

How is it determined that a disorder is genetic? Certainly not all conditions that are familial are necessarily due to altered genes. For example, many infectious disorders run in families and are certainly not due primarily to gene abnormalities. Scientists who study the factors and causes of human disease (epidemiologists) look for certain signs and evidence in their decision to label a condition as genetic. These include comparison of the frequency of the condition in identical versus nonidentical twins (since identical twins have the same genetic material). Comparison of the frequency of the disorder in question in close and distant family members in relation to the general population, and review of the evidence that the condition follows a known pattern of inheritance are other signs useful in considering the genetic causation (etiology) of a disorder.

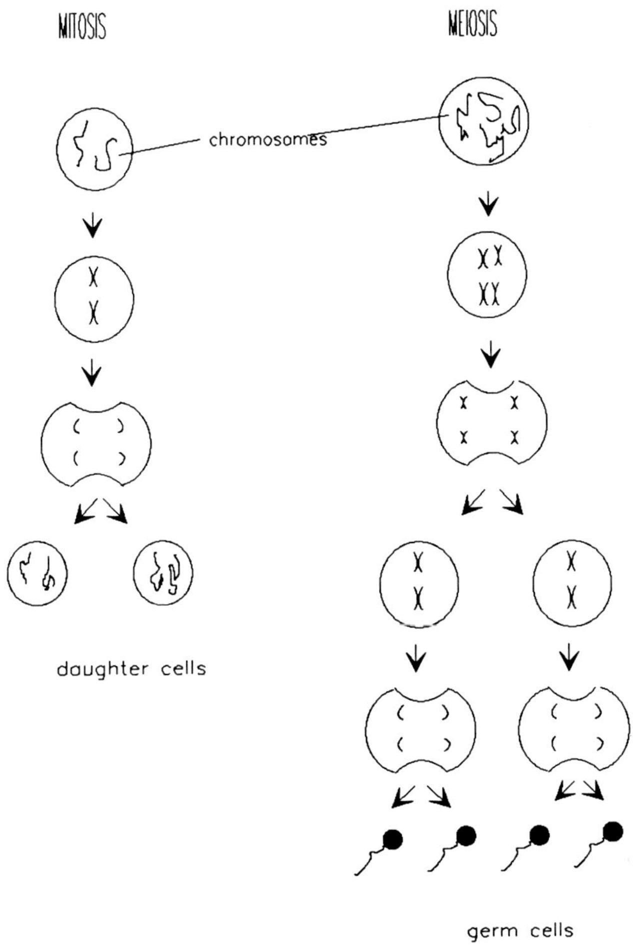

Figure 15–4. In the process of mitosis, the chromosomes are replicated and a copy of each chromosome is passed on to each daughter cell as the cell divides. The number of chromosomes in the cell does not change. Meiosis is the special process of cell division, which occurs only in the formation of sperm or eggs. In this case the chromosomes are replicated and homologous copies pair. The homologues then separate to opposite cells in the first meiotic division. A second division then ensures in which the replicated chromosomes segregate to daughter cells. The result is four germ cells, each containing only one copy of each homologous chromosome, thus reducing the chromosome number in the germ cells from 46 to 23.

Another term that is important to introduce at this point in the discussion is the label *congenital*. This refers to a disorder that is present at birth; this term does not connote etiology but only tells the timing of medical presentation. Because the root of the word has letters that are similar to the word genetic, the term congenital is often inappropriately equated with meaning genetic. Many, but not all, congenital disorders are due to genetic causation, and many, but not all, genetic disorders exhibit their manifestations at birth. The term genetic, used here, refers to the involvement of genes and chromosomes in the causation of the disorder. In this sense of the word genetic does not even necessarily imply familial since many genetic disorders rarely occur in families (example, Down syndrome).

In the previous discussion it was mentioned that one of the points of evidence used to decide if a condition is genetic is that it follows a known pattern of inheritance. The three well-established modes of inheritance of a single gene in genetic disorders are (1) autosomal dominant, (2) autosomal recessive, and (3) X-linked.

Autosomal dominant conditions are those in which alteration of the gene is assumed to be on an autosome (i.e., 1–22 chromosome) and involves only one gene of a gene pair (Fig. 15–5). Thus in autosomal dominant conditions individuals who have involvement of one of the genes of the gene pair will show signs of the condition. This is in contrast with *autosomal recessive* inheritance in which a person who has the condition needs to have involvement of *both* genes in the gene pair (Fig. 15–5).

In autosomal dominant disorders the person who has the condition has the gene on one chromosome in the pair while the other chromosome has the usual or normal form of the gene. Thus, when this person makes germ cells, half will carry the altered gene while the other half have the usual type of gene. Thus autosomal dominant conditions are transmitted from generation to generation (Fig. 15–6). Since the gene is on an autosome there is equal involvement of males and females. Autosomal dominant disorders show vertical transmission because one often can see the condition transmitted through several generations. On the other hand there is always a progenitor who is the first person with the condition in the family; in this situation it is assumed that the person has the condition through spontaneous mutation of the gene.

The proof that a condition is inherited in a certain fashion is based on the examination of a large number of family trees of persons who have the condition or trait. Criteria that would indicate autosomal dominant inheritance of a trait or condition include:

1. Similar frequency of males and females with the condition
2. Generation to generation transmission of the trait, i.e., vertical transmission
3. On the average of 50%, or half, of offspring of an affected individual having the trait
4. Evidence of a male to male (father to son) transmission of the trait through generations. This particular concept has to do with the demonstration that the condition is on an autosome; if a gene is on the X chromosome it cannot be transmitted from father to son since a father gives his Y chromosome to

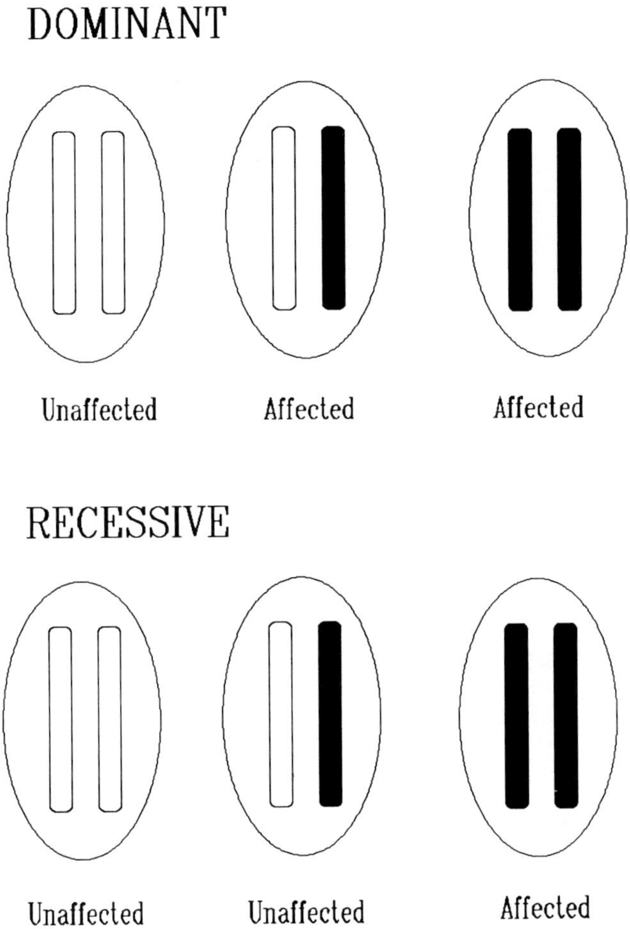

Figure 15–5. Alternative forms of a gene are depicted as dark or light bars, the dark representing a mutant form. For dominantly transmitted traits, both the heterozygote (having one dark and one light), and the homozygote (having both dark) will manifest signs of the mutation. In contrast, for recessively transmitted traits, only the homozygote having both copies of the gene being mutant will express the trait. The presence of a single copy of the nonmutant form in this case is sufficient to suppress the expression of the mutant form.

his sons, not an X chromosome; thus if there is father to son transmission of a trait, X-linked inheritance has been eliminated and location of the gene on an autosome is assumed.

The evidence that a condition is inherited in an autosomal recessive fashion utilizes a similar line of reasoning. This will not be considered in detail since

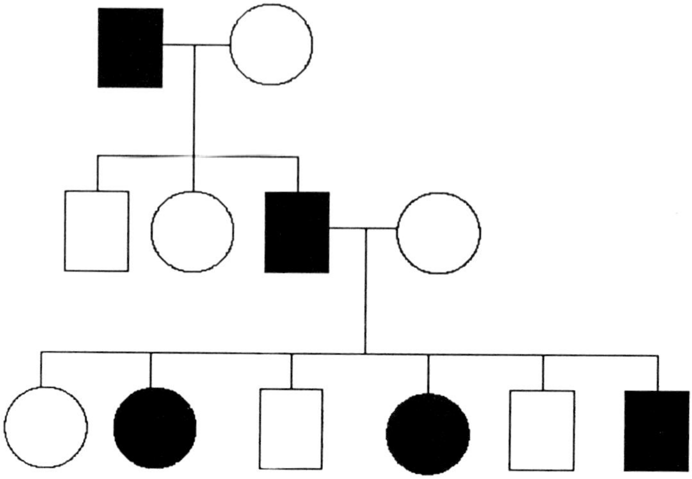

Figure 15–6. A pedigree illustrating dominant transmission of a genetic trait. Square symbols represent males, circles females. The darkened symbols represent individuals affected by the trait in question, for example NF. Affected individuals transmit the condition to approximately one-half their offspring. Both males and females are affected, and can transmit the condition to either sons or daughters. Individuals in each generation are affected, as the trait is passed from generation to generation.

the information does not apply to any of the well-established forms of NF. In addition, X-linked inheritance will not be discussed.

Another concept that is useful to introduce at this point is that of *heterozygote*. This refers to an individual who has two different forms (*alleles*) of a gene at a particular *locus* (position) on a chromosome. People who have an autosomal dominant trait are generally heterozygous since they have the trait in question as well as the usual form of the gene. The term *homozygote* refers to a person who has the same form of the gene at both copies of the particular gene locus.

Genetic disorders can be defined as those that are caused by abnormalities of the chromosomes and/or genes. The use of the term in this context is a broad one. Genetic conditions include three classes of disorders:

1. Mendelian or single gene disorders: These conditions have been discussed already and NF1 is certainly the prototype of autosomal dominant conditions. As mentioned, other types of single gene disorders include autosomal recessive disorders and X-linked conditions.
2. Chromosomal disorders: These conditions are due to structural and numerical aberrations of the chromosomes. These disorders are defined simply by examining the chromosomes under the microscope and detecting a visible defect. The most common example of a chromosomal disorder in humans

is Down syndrome which is due to having an extra 21 chromosome. Chromosomal disorders will not be discussed in any further detail as they do not fit into our discussion of the NF syndromes.

3. Multifactorial/polygenic disorders: This type of human genetic disorder is a complicated one and basically refers to the fact that many diseases in human beings have some genetic predisposition or genetic basis. Multifactorial disorders are conditions that are *not* due to an obvious chromosome abnormality nor is the condition inherited through a well-established mode of transmission. Rather, there appears to be familial clustering and some evidence of genetic etiology but not in a straightforward manner. Multifactorial inheritance is mentioned in this context only to underscore the importance of genetic mechanisms in the causation of most variations and disease in human beings. Examples include diabetes and spina bifida.

Other Classic Principles and Concepts in Human Genetics

The evidence that a particular condition is transmitted in an autosomal dominant fashion has been explained. The following discussion will detail some of the other concepts that have been used to help in the understanding of genetic conditions. It has long been recognized that dominant conditions are extremely variable in the degree of involvement of affected individuals. A number of concepts have been derived to explain the complexities of the phenotypic and clinical aspects of genetic disorders. These concepts include *expressivity*, *penetrance*, *mutation*, *pleiotropy*, and *heterogeneity*.

Expressivity is a term that is used to characterize the degree of variation in manifestations or severity in people with genetic conditions. Individuals with autosomal dominant conditions even within the same family often have marked variation in the range of involvement of the particular manifestations. The reason for variable expression of a genetic disorder is unknown.

Penetrance is the term that applies to a gene's ability to be expressed at all; it is an all or none situation and is contingent on the methods for studying the genotype and phenotype. Penetrance in autosomal dominant disorders is calculated by observing a three-generation family tree and noting the middle individual in the three-person chain. Thus it is obvious from the family tree that this person has the genetic trait in question since his (or her) parent and child both have the disorder. If, in a large population study, every interlocking person in this chain of three people manifests the gene, then the penetrance is considered to be 100%. If, on the other hand, there is an occasional skipped generation, then the penetrance is less than 100%. The key point in examining penetrance is to make certain that the individuals are examined in an up-to-date fashion to ensure that very mild signs of the disorder in question are documented.

The term mutation has already been discussed. It refers to both the process and the end point of the alteration of the gene. In some autosomal dominant disorders (example, NF2), most of the individuals who enter the medical setting have inherited the condition from a parent and only a small number represent a new mutation for the gene. In other conditions the overwhelming majority of people who come to the medical setting are the first person in their family and have their condition as a result of a new mutation. An example of this latter situation is achondroplasia, a skeletal disorder involving short limbs. NF1 falls somewhere in between, whereby about 50% of the individuals who come to clinic have inherited the gene from one of their parents while the other 50% have the condition presumably due to a spontaneous mutation (4). Of course the assumption that a person has the gene as a result of a new mutation depends on the accuracy in eliminating the possibility that one of the parents has a mild expression of the trait.

The term pleiotropy refers to the fact that a single gene mutation has several different consequences in an individual. The clinical correlate of this basic genetic concept is encompassed in the term syndrome. For example, the various pleiotropic manifestations of a condition like cystic fibrosis include the lung disorder involving chronic pulmonary disease, the lack of absorption of foods resulting in the gastrointestinal disorder, and the excessive production of salt in sweat. The pleiotropic manifestations of NF1 consist of the presence of café au lait spots early in life with neurofibromas later in life, as well as the occasional occurrence of one of the more medically serious manifestations. Understanding pleiotropy in genetic disorders is basically understanding the way in which all of the manifestations come about, i.e., the mechanism or pathogenesis of the disorder.

The final term that will be discussed in this section involves the concept of heterogeneity. This refers to the fact that certain genetic disorders may initially appear to be a single condition but after closer investigation, the disorder turns out to be a more general designation for multiple distinct genetic conditions. In the initial description of a syndrome the variety of manifestations may be ascribed to variable expressivity. However as a disorder is more completely studied, it may appear that there are subsets of families or individuals who have their own set of findings, suggesting that they represent an entity similar to the original condition, but separate from it on a genetic basis. An example of this concept is typified in albinism. Persons with albinism have a combination of lightly pigmented skin and hair along with visual disabilities. Initially all people with albinism were lumped under the single category of the disorder, which was known to be inherited in autosomal recessive fashion. Now it is thought that there are several different forms of this condition, with disorders overlapping yet having distinguishable manifestations.

NEUROFIBROMATOSIS AND THE BASIC PRINCIPLES OF HUMAN GENETICS

As has been noted elsewhere in this book, there are at least two distinct forms of NF, now referred to as NF1 and NF2 (5). That these are genetically distinct has long been suspected on the basis of the fact that individuals who have features of both NF1 and NF2 rarely, if ever, occur in the same family. (To some extent the features of these two conditions do overlap, perhaps accounting for rare individuals said to have both NF1 and NF2.) The recent discovery that the gene for NF1 is on chromosome 17 (6,7) and that for NF2 is on chromosome 22 (8,9) provide final proof that the disorders are distinct. Therefore, there is true genetic heterogeneity for NF.

Neurofibromatosis Type 1

Based on extensive family studies and investigations of populations of people with NF1, this disorder is clearly an autosomal dominant disorder with variable clinical expression and close to 100% penetrance. In fact NF is often considered to be the prototype of the autosomal dominant disorder. Several population studies have been done in different parts of North America and Europe on the genetic aspects of NF1. The most extensive of these studies was carried out by Crowe et al. (10) who studied over 200 individuals with NF in the 1950s. This study documented more than 12 families with three- or four-generation transmission of NF as well as a number of families with two-generation transmission. This evidence, as well as that of Borberg (11), documents the autosomal dominant causation of NF1. This means that when a person has the gene for NF1, there is a 50% or half chance with each pregnancy that the gene will be transmitted to the child. Since the evidence that NF is due to an autosomal dominant gene is so well documented, this risk figure is based on sound information.

In the population studies that have been performed on NF1, it is consistently noted that approximately half of the individuals who are evaluated by an investigator are the only person in their family with NF. The studies do vary on how well the parents of these apparently nonfamilial or sporadic cases were examined for signs of NF. It is assumed that, if the parents are carefully examined and have no signs of NF, the child must have NF due to a new mutation of the gene. That particular individual would be at a 50% risk with each pregnancy to have an affected child with NF like any person with a dominant gene. If one were to carry this line of reasoning one step further, then the brothers and sisters and parents of this sporadic case would not be at an increased risk over the general population to have a child with NF.

However, the above conclusion cannot be stated with 100% certainty since it is possible that the gene may not be completely penetrant. Although the gene appears to be fully penetrant, there are a few isolated reports of what appears to be a skipping of generations in the gene for NF. Thus, conventional wisdom indicates that penetrance for NF is probably very close to 100% but perhaps just under it. This means that parents of a sporadic case can never be 100% sure that they do not have the gene for NF. For all practical purposes, if the parents of an apparently sporadic individual have been examined by someone familiar with NF and *none* of the medical complications, cutaneous findings, or eye findings (especially Lisch nodules) are present, the individual can be assumed to be a sporadic case and the family can be assumed to be near the population risk for another child to have the gene.

The clinical manifestations of NF1 are extremely variable in expression (12). Within the same family there can be persons with minimal expression, and individuals with more serious manifestations of the condition. It appears that when someone has the gene for NF1, that person is at risk for the different manifestations but the factors that enter into the development of each manifestation are completely unknown. More than half of all people with NF will only have café au lait spots and cutaneous neurofibromas. The remaining 30 to 40% of individuals will have one or more of the more medically serious complications that are summarized in many of the chapters in this book. As emphasized in the chapters, a number of these manifestations or complications are treatable and once taken care of will not occur again. Thus for these reasons the majority of people with NF will have a trait that puts them *at risk* for problems rather than causes a disease.

The specific aspects of the concepts of pleiotropy and heterogeneity in NF were discussed in the previous section as examples of those particular terms. Thus, they will not be explained in this section.

Neurofibromatosis Type 2

Details of the clinical features and genetics of NF2 are provided in Chapter 3 of this book. NF2 is considerably less common in the population than NF1. It is also transmitted as an autosomal dominant trait with high penetrance but variable expression. The rate of new mutation at this locus appears to be much lower than for NF1, although the manifestations in a parent may be subtle.

SUMMARY

Both NF1 and NF2 are genetically transmitted as autosomal dominant traits, although the two disorders are due to distinct mutations located on different chromosomes. NF1 is a prototypical autosomal dominant disorder, displaying substantial variability of expression, even within a family. About 50% of individuals with NF1 do not have affected parents and are apparently the results of new mutation of the NF1 gene. The principles of mendelian genetics form the basis for genetic counseling of individuals with NF, and have led to new approaches to identify the responsible genes.

REFERENCES

1. F. Vogel and A.G. Motulsky. Human genetics. Problems and approaches. Berlin, Springer-Verlag, 1986.
2. J.S. Thompson and M.W. Thompson. Genetics in medicine. Philadelphia, W.B. Saunders, 1986.

3. F.C. Fraser and J.J. Nora. Genetics of man. Philadelphia, Lea & Febiger, 1986.
4. J.C. Carey, B.J. Baty, J.P. Johnson, et al. The genetic aspects of neurofibromatosis. Ann NY Acad Sci 1986;486:45–56.
5. D. Stumpf. Consensus Development Conference of Neurofibromatosis. Arch Neurol 1988;45:575–578.
6. D. Barker, E. Wright, K. Nguyen, et al. Gene for von Recklinghausen neurofibromatosis is in the pericentromeric region of chromosome 17. Science 1987;236:1098–1102.
7. R.R. Seizinger, G.A. Rouleau, L.J. Ozelius, et al. Genetic linkage of von Recklinghausen neurofibromatosis to the nerve growth factor receptor gene. Cell 1987;49:589–594.
8. G.A. Rouleau, W. Wertelecki, J.L. Haines, et al. Genetic linkage of bilateral acoustic neurofibromatosis to a DNA marker on chromosome 22. Nature 1987;329:246–248.
9. W. Wertelecki, G.A. Rouleau, D.W. Superneau, et al. Neurofibromatosis 2: Clinical and DNA linkage studies of a large kindred. N Engl J Med 1988;319:278–283.
10. F.W. Crowe, W.J. Schull, and J.V. Neel. A clinical, pathological, and genetic study of multiple neurofibromatosis. Springfield, IL, Charles C Thomas, 1956.
11. A. Borberg. Clinical and genetic investigations into tuberous sclerosis and Recklinghausen's neurofibromatosis. Contributions to elucidation of interrelationship and eugenics of the syndromes. Acta Psychiatr Neurol Scand 1951;71(Suppl):1–239.
12. J.C. Carey, J.M. Laub, and B.D. Hall. Penetrance and variability in neurofibromatosis: A genetic study of 60 families. Birth Defects 1979; Original Article Series 15, No. 5B:271–281.

16

MOLECULAR GENETICS OF NEUROFIBROMATOSIS

Bruce R. Korf, M.D., Ph.D., and John C. Carey, M.D., M.P.H.

Although modern medical knowledge about neurofibromatosis (NF) dates back more than 100 years, little is known about the basic pathogenesis of the disorder. Recent advances in molecular genetics, however, offer a fresh, very promising, and already productive approach to this problem. This approach is sometimes referred to as "reverse genetics" because it involves the study of a gene in order to learn about a condition, as opposed to the traditional approach of first understanding a condition and then learning about the gene that causes it. This chapter will provide an overview of molecular genetic studies of NF types 1 (NF1) and 2 (NF2), and describe some recent exciting findings which are having an impact on clinical practice.

FINDING THE GENES FOR NEUROFIBROMATOSIS TYPES 1 AND 2

As described in the previous chapter, all genetic information is encoded in the DNA molecules, which reside in the nucleus of cells. There are estimated to be over 100,000 different genes in humans, each of which encodes the information for a specific protein molecule. Genetic disorders such as NF represent changes, or *mutations*, of the coding sequence, resulting in the production of deficient or aberrant proteins. A major goal of research therefore is to identify the protein molecules that are normally encoded by the NF1 and NF2 genes, and to understand the manner by which the genetic mutations upset the function of these proteins. It is hoped that this will lead to understanding of the basic mechanisms of each form of NF, and perhaps will eventually suggest new forms of treatment.

The traditional genetic approach of studying various body proteins in the hope of finding one that is abnormal in persons with a genetic disorder has been completely unsuccessful for NF. There are hundreds of thousands of proteins in the body, and there is no clue even where to look for the protein products of the NF genes. For this reason, researchers have turned to the reverse genetics approach. Here, the first step is to locate the NF genes on the human chromosomes, and then to identify those genes and study their structure. From the structure of the genes scientists can readily read the genetic code and thereby infer the structure of the protein products, both in their normal and abnormal forms (Fig. 16–1).

Gene Mapping

Locating the genes for NF1 and NF2 would still seem to be a formidable task, since there are over 100,000 genes spread over the 22 autosomes and the pair of sex chromosomes. As noted in the previous chapter, it has long been known that neither form of NF resides on the X or Y chromosome, but until recently there was no idea where else these genes might be located. A technique known as genetic linkage analysis has answered this.

Genes are arranged in linear order on the chromosomes, like rungs of a ladder, and the location of specific genes in relation to one another is the same in all people (Fig. 16–2). Genes that are located close to one another on the chromosome are said to be *linked*. A gene such as the one for NF1 or NF2 can therefore be mapped if it can be shown that it is linked to another gene that has already been mapped.

Genes that can serve as references for mapping by linkage analysis are known as *markers*. The essential feature of these marker genes is not only that they have previously been mapped (by means to be described in the next section), but also that these genes exist in several specific forms, or *alleles*, which are common in various members of the population (Fig. 16–3). Since all

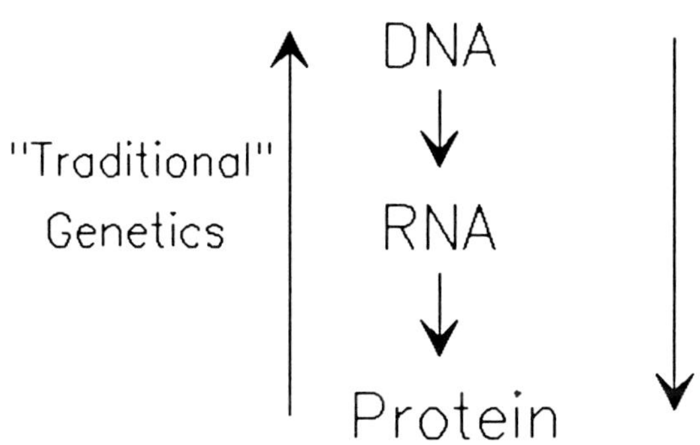

Figure 16–1. The "traditional" approach to studying human genetic disorders is to identify the protein product of a gene, and then to use that information to isolate the gene that encodes that protein. The "reverse" genetics approach starts with the DNA sequence comprising the gene. This is usually identified by knowledge of its location in the genome. After the gene is isolated, study of the structure of the gene can be used to infer the structure of the protein it encodes. This provides a means of identifying the protein product responsible for a genetic disorder based solely on knowledge of the location of the gene.

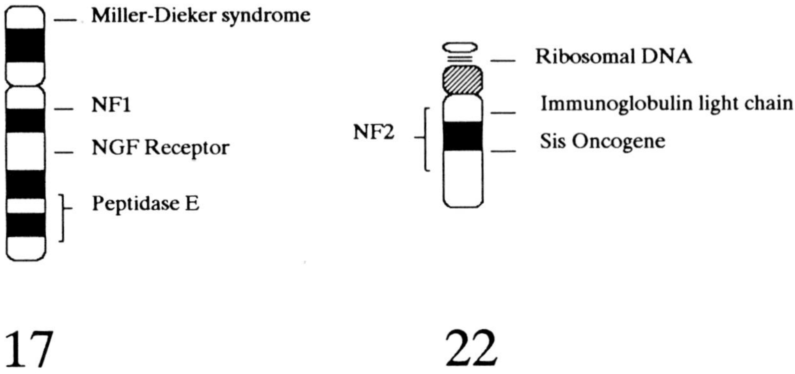

Figure 16–2. Maps of chromosomes 17 and 22, indicating the approximate locations of the genes for NF1 and NF2, and some other genes that have been mapped to these chromosomes.

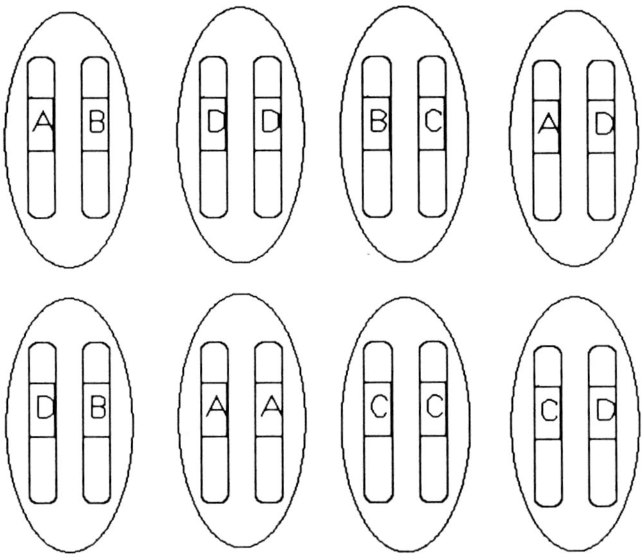

Figure 16–3. Genotypes of eight individuals with respect to a gene locus with four alleles, designated "A," "B," "C," and "D." Since each individual has two copies of the gene on a pair of homologous chromosomes, a variety of possible combinations of alleles, or *genotypes*, is possible. For example, one individual has the genotype "AB," another "DD," another "BC," etc. Individuals with two different alleles on the two chromosomes, such as "AB," are *heterozygous*. Individuals who have the same allele on each chromosome, such as "DD," are *homozygous*. The gene locus in question can be said to be *polymorphic* since there are a number of possible alleles at the locus, and different people have different combinations of these alleles.

persons have two copies of every gene (having received one from each parent), this raises the possibility that an individual might be heterozygous for a marker locus; that is, the gene copy on one chromosome is represented by one allele, and the copy on the other homologous chromosome by another allele. Genetic loci such as this, with many alleles that are common in the population, are said to be *polymorphic*. An example is the ABO blood group locus, different alleles of which are responsible for type A, B, or O blood.

If an individual is heterozygous for a marker gene and his or her spouse is homozygous, the marker alleles can be used to distinguish the two homologous chromosomes in the heterozygous parent. The specific homologue that is transmitted from the heterozygous parent to any offspring can be determined by noting which allele for the marker gene the child has received. Each child gets one or the other form of the marker from the heterozygous parent, and always the same form from the homozygous parent.

If the heterozygous parent also carries a defective gene such as NF in heterozygous form, and if the defective gene is linked to this marker gene, it is possible to track the segregation of the defective gene by following the segregation of the marker (Fig. 16–4A). One chromosome of this parent carries

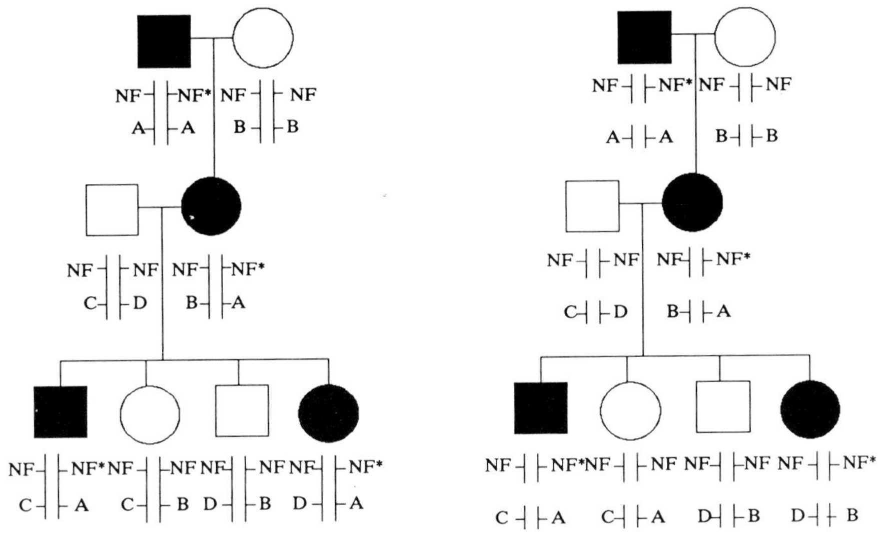

A) Marker Linked to NF1 B) Marker Not Linked to NF1

Figure 16–4. **(A)** Pedigree demonstrating segregation of NF in relation to a marker locus that is closely linked. Four alleles at the marker locus are "A," "B," "C," and "D." In this family allele "A" is transmitted along with the NF mutant gene (designated NF*). **(B)** Pedigree demonstrating random segregation of NF and another locus that is not closely linked to NF. In this family no particular allele of the nonlinked marker locus consistently occurs together with NF* in affected individuals. Dark symbols in both pedigrees represent individuals affected with NF.

the defective form of the NF gene nearby one allele of the marker, and the other chromosome carries the normal form of the NF gene nearby the other marker allele. A child who inherits the chromosome carrying the marker allele that is associated with the gene defect should likewise inherit the defect. If, on the other hand, the marker gene and the defective gene of interest are not linked, the segregation of marker and disease alleles to offspring will be random (Fig. 16–4B).

It should be stressed that the marker gene is not the disease gene; it is a separate genetic locus which happens to be nearby, and which serves to distinguish the two homologous chromosomes. It should also be stressed that the particular marker allele that is on the same homologous chromosome as the disease gene allele will differ from person to person in the population. What is always true for all people is that a pair of closely linked genes will always be nearby one another.

The main requirement for mapping a gene by linkage analysis is that markers be available along the entire genome; with sufficient markers virtually any gene can be mapped. To map a gene one would test markers from various locations in the genome looking for one whose alleles regularly segregate with an allele of the gene of interest. (One complicating feature of this analysis, genetic recombination, will be discussed later when the diagnostic use of linked markers is considered.) Until recently, there were very few such markers, but advances in molecular genetics have generated a potentially unlimited number.

Marker Genes Derived by Recombinant DNA Methods

The technical advance that has revolutionized genetics research is the ability to *clone* sequences of DNA by recombinant DNA methods. To clone a DNA sequence means that a short stretch of DNA is separated from the remainder of the genome and placed in a system which allows the generation of unlimited amounts of that sequence. This makes it possible to study that particular sequence in isolation from all the millions of others. In practice (Fig. 16–5), one usually begins with DNA isolated from cells such as white blood cells. The DNA is then cleaved into fragments using special enzymes, to be described in detail. The fragments are then attached to bits of DNA which have the ability to infect bacterial cells and replicate themselves inside the bacteria. Since each bacterial cell incorporates a recombinant DNA molecule containing only a single fragment of human DNA, a colony of bacteria grown from one cell contains millions of copies of that same fragment; moreover a different human DNA fragment will be represented in each colony.

DNA prepared from these bacterial colonies contains purified fragments of human DNA for further study. It is possible that one of these fragments contains a gene of interest, for example the NF1 gene, but it is difficult to know which fragment that is without having any prior knowledge about the structure of the gene. Yet one thing can be done with cloned fragments of human DNA even

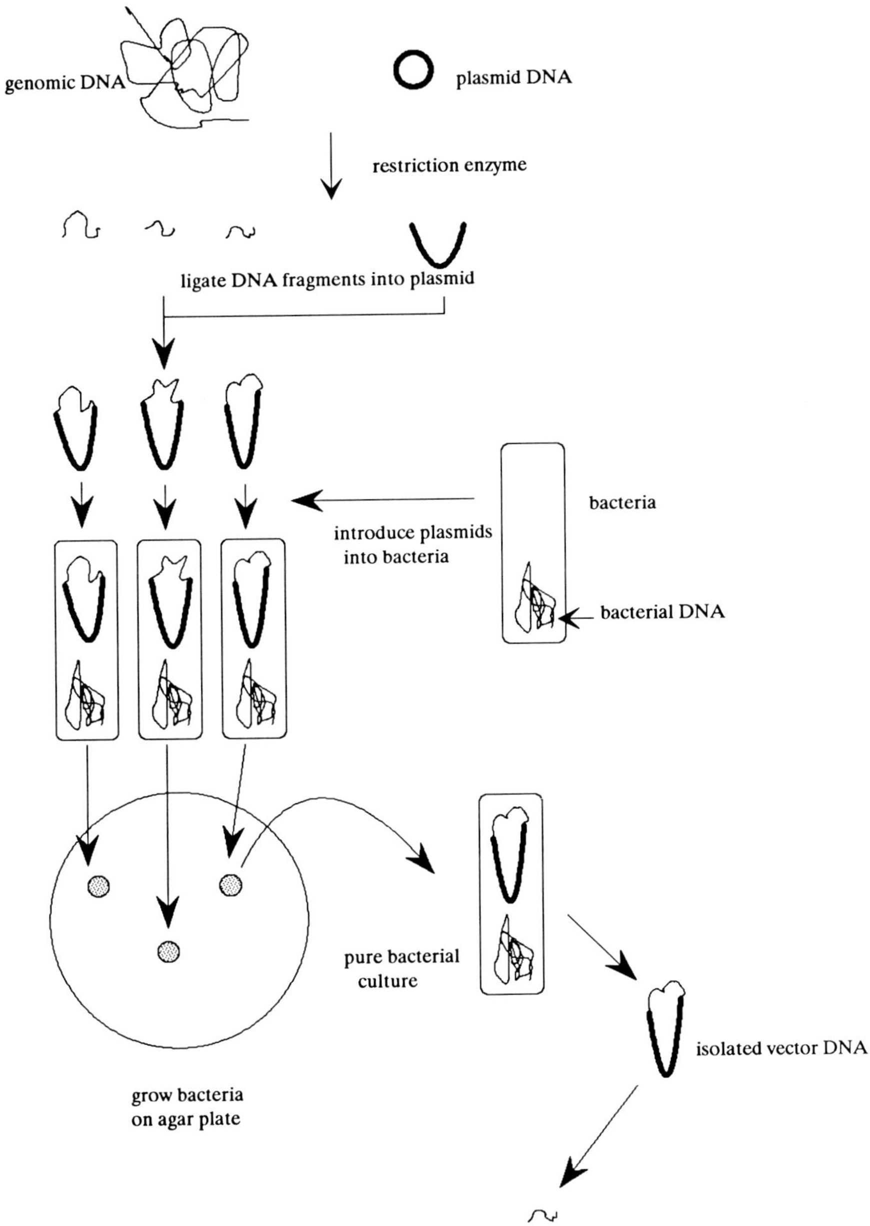

Figure 16–5. Diagram illustrating steps in cloning a DNA sequence. Genomic DNA is cleaved into fragments using a restriction enzyme. A bacterial plasmid DNA, normally circular, is opened with the same enzyme. Fragments of genomic DNA are then ligated at random into the plasmid DNA, closing the circle. These recombinant plasmids are then introduced into bacterial cells, which are then grown on agar plates as colonies. Each colony is derived from a single bacterium which has incorporated a single recombinant plasmid. When a colony is isolated and grown up, the plasmid DNA that is purified from the bacterial culture contains a single piece of human genomic DNA, which represents a cloned sequence.

when we do not know which represent specific genes. That is to map the genes, and therefore use them as markers for linkage analysis. Strategies for gene mapping are beyond the scope of this chapter, but it can be said that a variety of approaches now permit cloned DNA sequences to be easily located on the chromosome map.

DNA Sequence Polymorphism

The map of marker genes greatly facilitates the task of linkage analysis, but to be useful, a marker must exist in distinguishable forms in the population, i.e., be polymorphic. That is required so that the two homologous copies of a chromosome can be distinguished in a heterozygous individual. Each cloned DNA fragment will differ from another by the specific sequence of building blocks known as *bases*. It is the sequence of these bases that encodes the sequence of amino acids, the building blocks of proteins. Different fragments have different base sequences and one would expect that a particular fragment cloned from any two persons would have the same base sequence. For the most part this is true, but in fact it is not unusual for the base sequence of specific fragments to differ slightly from individual to individual. Some of these differences represent differences in the base sequence of genes, and therefore in the amino acid sequence of proteins. Such differences are the basis for genetic differences among people. Not all of the sequence differences necessarily correspond with differences in protein structure, however. Some DNA does not encode genetic information; for example, some serves a structural role, as spacers between adjacent genes. Differences in base sequence in such regions are common because the spacer function is accomplished equally well regardless of the exact base sequence.

For purposes of linkage analysis it is fortunate that DNA base sequence variation is so common. Yet it would be difficult to use polymorphic markers if it were necessary to determine the base sequence for a given cloned marker in every individual being studied for linkage. Fortunately, an alternative and very rapid method of detecting base sequence differences has been devised. This is the technique of detecting *restriction fragment length polymorphisms* (RFLPs).

The tool on which this technique is based is the *restriction enzyme*. Restriction enzymes are found naturally in microorganisms, and have the property of recognizing specific sequences of bases in DNA and cutting the DNA at these sites. Most enzymes recognize runs of four to eight bases, and are very precise in their ability to cleave only at this exact sequence. Even a single base pair change is sufficient to prevent the enzyme from cutting a given site. If a base pair difference between two individuals happens to occur within an enzyme recognition site, the enzyme will cut that site in one individual but not the other (Fig. 16–6).

Restriction enzyme recognition sites are widely distributed through the genome, since any run of four to eight bases will occur every so often due to chance. Any DNA sample exposed to a restriction enzyme will therefore be cut

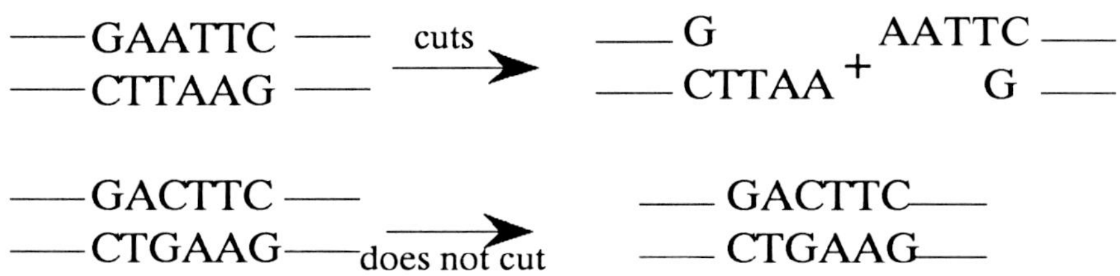

Figure 16–6. The restriction enzyme *Eco*RI cuts DNA whenever the six base pairs GAATTC (on one strand of DNA) occur. If there is even a single base pair change in this sequence, such as GACTTC as shown, the enzyme does not cut. The bases of DNA are guanosine (G), thymine (T), adenine (A), and cytosine (C).

into a set of fragments of different sizes, the size of any particular fragment depending on the distance between enzyme recognition sites. The fragment size that corresponds to a piece of cloned DNA will depend on the distance between the enzyme recognition sites that flank that sequence. The fragment size should be the same from one person to the next, unless one of the recognition sites happens to be polymorphic. In that case, the enzyme will not cleave one of the sites in some individuals, and the cloned segment will be located on a longer fragment, resulting from cleavage at the next restriction site some distance away.

Such RFLPs therefore constitute two allele systems. Individuals can be homozygous for having or not having an intact recognition site near the marker sequence or can be heterozygous. In heterozygotes, the nearby recognition site is intact on one chromosome, but disrupted by a base sequence change on the other (Fig. 16–7).

Southern Analysis

How are RFLP alleles detected in DNA from an individual? This is done by a technique known as *Southern analysis*, named for its inventor, Edwin Southern (Fig. 16–8). The goal is to determine the size of a DNA fragment which includes some cloned piece after DNA from an individual has been cleaved with a particular restriction enzyme. The cleaved DNA is first loaded into a slot in a flat gel, and allowed to migrate in an electrical field, a procedure known as *electrophoresis*. Smaller fragments migrate faster than larger, and this results in a separation of fragments by size. The DNA in the gel is then blotted onto a filter, so that the location of each fragment in the filter is the same as it was in the gel. The DNA in the filter is treated chemically to "expose" the base sequence of each fragment (actually by separating the two strands of the double helix of DNA in each fragment). Meanwhile, the piece of cloned DNA (not necessarily cloned from the same individual) is also treated to expose its base sequence, and chemically "tagged" with radioactivity. The filter paper is

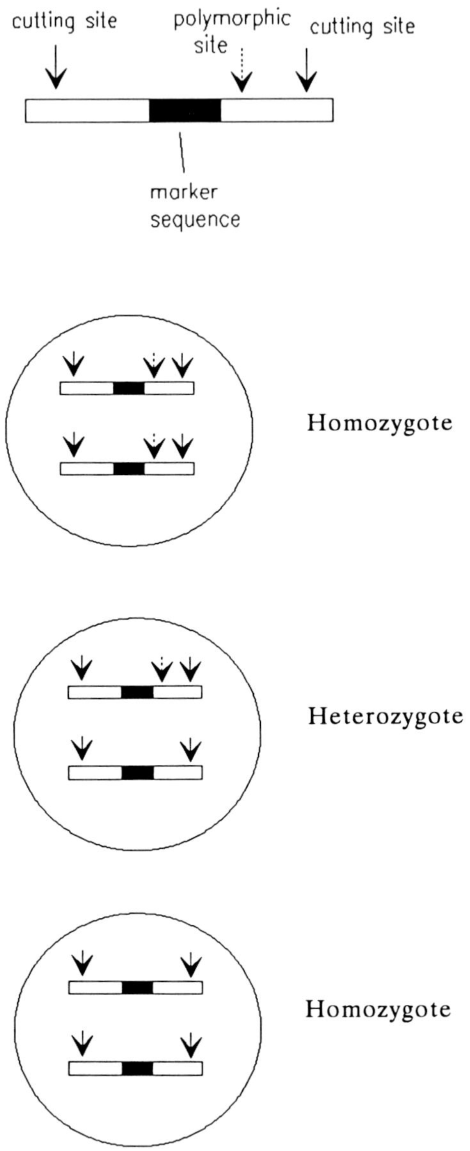

Figure 16–7. The map at the top shows a marker sequence and flanking enzyme recognition sites. To the left of the marker is a site that is present in all people. Immediately to the right is a site that is only present in some people, and therefore constitutes a polymorphism. To the far right is another site present in all people. The three circles below indicate genotypes in different individuals with respect to this polymorphism. The top individual is homozygous for the nearby cutting site, and the bottom individual is homozygous for lacking that site. The middle individual possesses one chromosome with the nearby site and one without it, and therefore is heterozygous.

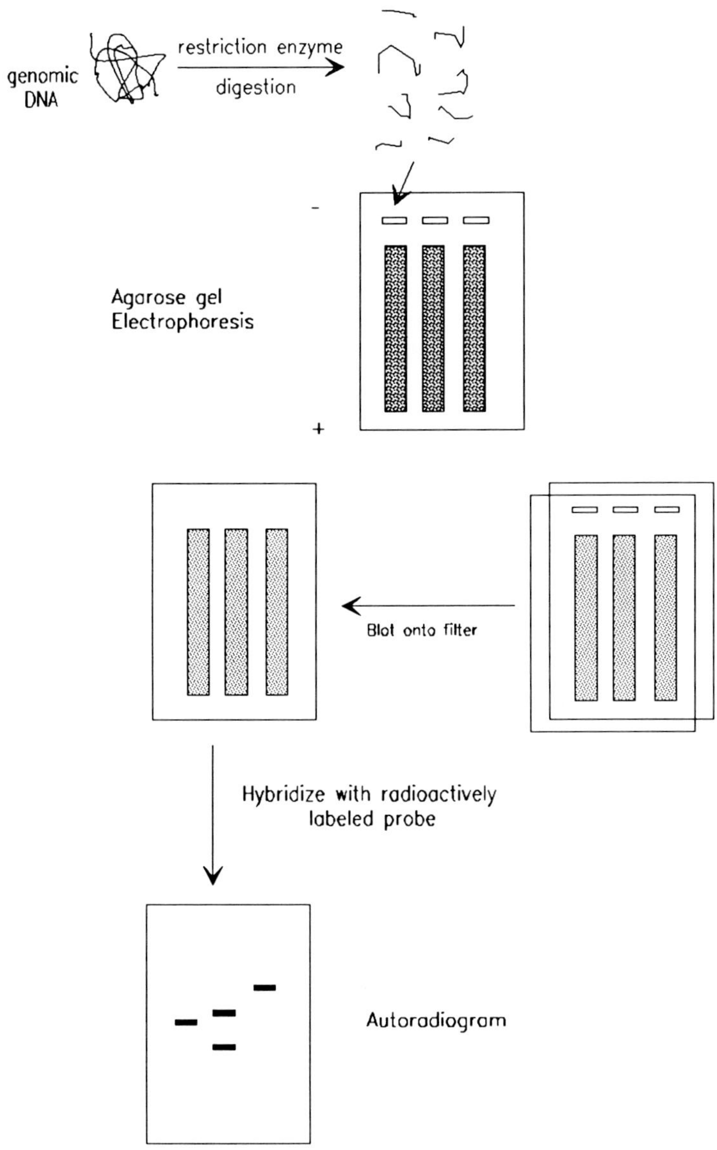

Figure 16–8. Diagram of Southern analysis. A sample of genomic DNA is cleaved into fragments with a restriction enzyme. The fragments are then loaded into an agarose gel and subjected to electrophoresis so that molecules are separated by molecular weight. The negatively charged DNA molecules migrate toward the positive electrode of the electrophoresis apparatus. The DNA in the gel is then blotted onto a filter (nitrocellulose or nylon) so that the position of any fragment of DNA in the filter is the same as it was in the gel. The DNA in the filter is also treated so that the two strands of the double helix are separated. The filter is then bathed in a solution containing single stranded, radioactively labeled cloned "probe" DNA. Wherever the probe finds a homologous copy of DNA in the filter a stable double helix forms. Exposing the filter to an x-ray film results in the appearance of dark bands on the film corresponding to the location of bound probe DNA.

then bathed with a solution containing millions of copies of this tagged DNA sequence. DNA molecules with the same base sequence have a tendency to stick together if their base sequences are exposed, and therefore the tagged molecule will stick to the filter wherever it finds a fragment with a similar sequence. If the unbound molecules are then washed off and the filter exposed to a piece of film, a dark band will appear on the film wherever a radioactive molecule has bound. Since the location of DNA in the filter indicates size, the position of these bands can be interpreted to determine the size of any DNA fragment which includes a base sequence corresponding to the cloned DNA.

Individuals who are homozygous for the presence of a restriction fragment recognition site near a sequence that has been cloned have a single band visible on a Southern blot. Heterozygotes usually have two bands, one corresponding to each fragment size. Using this method it is easy to determine which alleles are present in a given individual for some RFLP. Multiple members of a family can be tested in adjacent lanes on the same Southern blot, making the technique rapid and relatively inexpensive.

Southern blot technology has truly revolutionized genetic diagnosis. Even newer approaches, mostly based on a technique known as the polymerase chain reaction (PCR), are under development. Although these may eventually replace Southern analysis, they are conceptionally similar, and technically beyond the scope of this book.

The Location of the Genes for Neurofibromatosis Type 1 and Type 2

The process of mapping genes such as those for NF1 and NF2 involves examining many large families for the segregation of the NF genes in relation to many polymorphic marker loci. The goal is to find a locus whose alleles segregate together with an NF allele. In practice, this involves preparing DNA from members of many families, cutting the DNA with a variety of restriction enzymes, and performing Southern analysis of this cut DNA with a variety of marker genes located at various sites throughout the genome. Segregation patterns can be tracked by computer, looking for those that indicate linkage of NF to a marker.

Using this approach, both of the NF genes have been mapped. NF1 is located on chromosome 17 (1–4), and NF2 on chromosome 22 (5,6) (Fig. 16–9). The fact that these two forms of NF map to different chromosomes is the final proof that they are genetically distinct disorders. Moreover, it has been found that, at least so far, all people with NF1 seem to have the defective gene on chromosome 17, and likewise for NF2 on chromosome 22. Thus, although NF1 and NF2 are clearly the result of changes in different genes, all people with a given form of NF have a change in the same gene (or at least a gene in the same region).

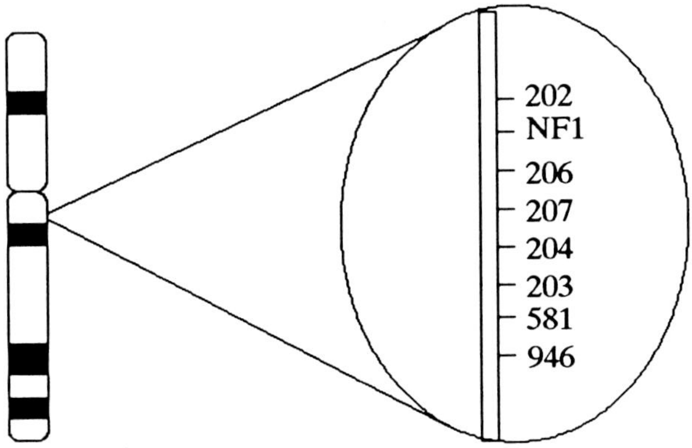

Figure 16–9. Map of the region near the NF1 gene on chromosome 17. The numbers correspond to cloned fragments of DNA that flank the NF1 locus.

MOLECULAR DIAGNOSIS OF NEUROFIBROMATOSIS

The diagnosis of NF has heretofore been made entirely on clinical grounds. Yet because the clinical features of these conditions can be extremely variable, and because many of the features are not present early in life, it is often impossible to be sure whether a specific person at risk actually has NF. A reliable diagnostic test that can be performed early in life would identify those who require follow-up or screening for NF-related problems, and relieve the anxiety of uncertainty.

Another area where a reliable diagnostic test would be helpful is for prenatal testing. Techniques exist for sampling fetal tissues, but until recently there was no way to test these tissues to determine if a fetus has inherited NF. There are many reasons why a family might like to have such information. One is to relieve anxiety surrounding the uncertainty of whether the fetus is affected. Another is the need to plan for the medical needs of a child who has inherited the condition. A final, and very controversial area is the possibility of termination of pregnancy if the fetus is affected. This is an issue that generates strong feelings on both sides, regarding both the ethics of pregnancy termination in general, and the issue of whether NF represents a disorder for which termination might in some cases be considered. It is not appropriate for such arguments to be considered here. It is a canon of modern medical genetics, however, to provide a family with as much information as possible about their medical condition and available options, and to leave the final decision of what action to take to them.

Diagnosis by Linkage Analysis

Until the NF genes are cloned, molecular approaches to diagnosis will rely on genetic linkage analysis. The principle and basic approach is the same as was described for gene mapping. The same genetic markers are used, in this case to track the mutant gene through a family.

The most important requirement for this testing, and its major limitation, are that the couple being tested be part of a family in which many individuals are affected with NF, and that these individuals are willing to be involved in the testing process. This eliminates all families in which NF has occurred in only a single individual as a new mutation. The reason is that the testing is based on genetic linkage, rather than direct detection of the mutant gene.

The basic approach is illustrated in Figure 16–10. By testing the affected mother and her sister it is found that a specific pair of marker alleles from loci that flank NF1 on chromosome 17 are on the same chromosome with the NF mutation. The father is homozygous for different alleles for these marker loci, making it possible to follow the chromosome carrying the NF gene as it is transmitted to any offspring. For example, the child who has received the

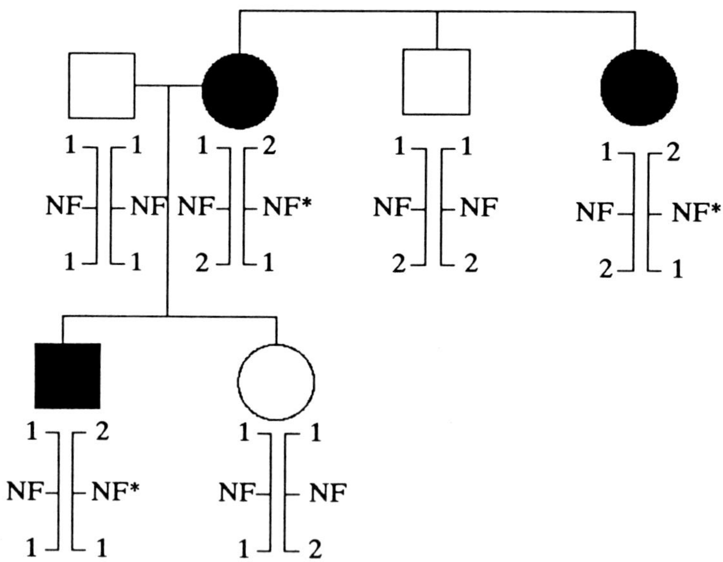

Figure 16–10. Pedigree illustrating the use of flanking markers to track the NF1 gene through a family. Both the bottom and top markers have two alleles, designated "1" and "2." (Note that allele "1" for the top marker is not the same as allele "1" for the bottom; the numbers are just arbitrary ways of distinguishing the markers.) The abnormal copy of the NF gene in affected individuals is designated NF*. In this family, the NF* is located on the copy of chromosome 17, which carries the "2" allele of the top marker and the "1" allele of the bottom.

maternal chromosome that does not carry the mutation is predicted to be unaffected.

There are many important limitations to this mode of testing. First, as has already been noted, linkage testing is only applicable to familial cases of NF. Testing is also not possible if DNA samples cannot be obtained from the necessary relatives required to track the marker genes. In the illustration given, for example, samples were not only from the parents required, but also from an affected sib of the mother. Without information from this individual there would have been no way of knowing which of the mother's marker alleles was on the same chromosome as the NF mutant allele.

A further limitation is that not all individuals will be "informative" for every marker. The ideal scenario is that the affected parent is heterozygous for the marker alleles, and the spouse is homozygous. This allows unequivocal assignment of specific marker alleles to the two homologous chromosomes in the affected parent, and determination of which chromosome has been transmitted to any child. For any particular marker, though, it is a matter of chance that an individual will be heterozygous. To offer reliable molecular diagnosis, then, it is necessary that a variety of markers be available in the vicinity of the mutant gene, in the hope that at least some will be informative in the family. Although many marker genes are available near the NF genes (particularly NF1), there are still occasions in which family members cannot be offered diagnosis because they are uninformative for the available markers.

A final limitation is that the diagnosis is not 100% reliable. This is due to a process known as *genetic recombination*. Recombination is a natural process that occurs during the formation of the sperm and egg cells, in which the two homologous chromosomes of each of the 23 pairs come together during this process, and may exchange segments (Fig. 16–11). When such exchange occurs, the order of loci on the chromosome is unchanged, but the association of particular alleles on a given homologue is altered. Specifically, a particular marker allele that was on the same chromosome as the NF mutant allele may be

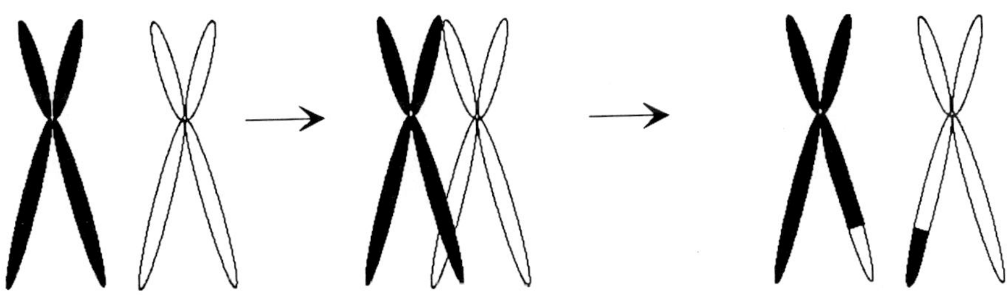

Figure 16–11. Genetic recombination. Two copies of a homologous pair of chromosomes pair during meiosis and may exchange a segment. This does not alter the order of genes on the recombinant chromosomes, but does shift alleles from one member of a pair to the other.

exchanged with the marker allele on the other chromosome 17. Since one is following the markers to infer which chromosome has been transmitted to a child, if the relationship of the marker alleles to the mutant allele has been switched due to recombination, an error in diagnosis can be made.

This would seem to be a serious problem, but in practice it can be overcome in most cases. First, the likelihood of recombination occurring between any two loci is lower the closer the loci are to one another. Diagnosis will therefore be most accurate when the markers are very closely linked to NF. In fact markers exist that recombine with the NF1 locus less than 1% of the time, and therefore afford accurate diagnosis (4). The second safeguard against diagnostic errors due to recombination is the use of markers that flank the mutant gene. A recombination event between one of these markers and the disease gene will necessarily result in recombination between the markers themselves, and can be easily detected. Only a double recombination event, between each marker and NF, a very rare event, would lead to possible erroneous diagnosis.

Process of Molecular Diagnosis

A flow chart depicting the process of molecular diagnosis is shown in Figure 16–12. The first step is to obtain a complete family history, and to confirm the diagnosis of NF in the individuals requesting counseling. Obviously, if the diagnosis is not actually NF, linkage studies will not be helpful. It is also important to confirm the diagnosis in any relative who will be involved in the testing. An erroneous clinical diagnosis in any one of these individuals can lead to misleading or erroneous results in molecular diagnosis. It will usually be necessary for these relatives to be thoroughly evaluated by a physician who is familiar with NF; it will not be sufficient to rely on family hearsay.

After the family history and clinical information are collected and confirmed, DNA samples must be obtained. These are usually prepared from white blood cells isolated from samples of blood drawn from a vein. Usually about 4 to 5 teaspoons (20–25 ml) of blood are obtained, although the laboratory usually can get by with less from young children. DNA prepared from these samples is cut with appropriate restriction enzymes and analyzed by Southern blotting as described in the previous section of this chapter. The entire process requires about 4 weeks, but varies with the size of the family, and the number of marker genes that must be tested in order to find loci that are informative in the family.

If the test is being done for presymptomatic diagnosis, the next step would be for the laboratory and physician to interpret the results and then explain these to the family. If the test is being done for eventual prenatal diagnosis, it is usually desirable to first test the family prior to a pregnancy. This allows the informative markers to be identified without the time pressure of an ongoing pregnancy.

Obtain family history
and confirm diagnosis

↓

Collect blood samples
and isolate DNA

↓

Prepare Southern blots
and determine informative
markers

↓

Prenatal or presymptomatic
diagnosis

Figure 16–12. Flow diagram indicating the steps in performing molecular diagnostic studies on a family with NF.

Methods of Prenatal Diagnosis

Prenatal diagnosis is possible with molecular testing because such testing is done on DNA. All cells of the body contain the same DNA, and therefore the NF mutation is detectable even if the cell type being tested would not normally express the mutant gene. There are currently two methods of sampling fetal tissues for genetic studies.

The older method is that of amniocentesis. This involves the withdrawal of a small amount of the fluid that bathes the fetus. It is usually carried out between 16 and 20 weeks of pregnancy, although it can sometimes be done as early as 14 weeks. The fluid is obtained from a needle passed through the mother's abdomen and uterus into the amniotic cavity (Fig. 16–13A). Contained in the fluid, which is mostly derived from fetal urine, arc some cells of fetal origin, which can be grown in culture and then used as a source of fetal DNA. There is a vast experience in performing amniocentesis at most medical centers, and the test is known to be quite safe. Risk of major complications is generally less than 1 in 200 (7). The major limitation to this approach is that it is carried out fairly late in pregnancy, and the cells must be grown for about 3 weeks before testing can be done. This means that DNA studies may not be performed until after the 20th week of gestation, which leaves little time for performing these tests if a termination is being considered. Also, it means waiting a fairly long time into the pregnancy before the answer is known.

The second major approach to prenatal diagnosis is relatively new, and is referred to as *chorionic villus sampling* (CVS) (Fig. 16–13B). In this procedure, a tiny piece of the fetal placenta is sampled either via a catheter inserted through the cervix or via a needle passed through the mother's abdomen. This can be done as early as 9 weeks of pregnancy, and the material obtained can often be immediately used as a source of fetal DNA. This allows for obtaining information quite early in pregnancy, often before the pregnancy is apparent to

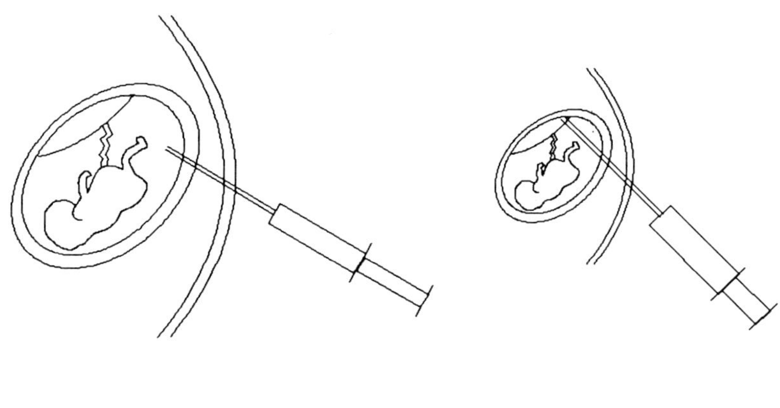

A. Amniocentesis B. Chorionic Villus Biopsy

Figure 16–13. **(A)** Amniocentesis, usually performed between 16 and 20 weeks of gestation, in which a needle is inserted within the amniotic cavity to withdraw some amniotic fluid. **(B)** Chorionic villus sampling, performed in the first trimester, in which a needle is inserted near the placenta to withdraw a small sample of fetal tissue. Chorionic villus sampling can be performed through the mother's abdomen as shown, or via a catheter inserted through the cervix.

family and friends. The major drawback is a higher complication rate—in the range of 3%—than is the case for amniocentesis (8). This higher rate may be partly due to the more invasive nature of the sampling technique. In part, however, it may reflect the fact that miscarriage is a common event in pregnancy, and some of these natural miscarriages do not occur until after 9 weeks' gestation. Therefore at least some of the miscarriages that occur after CVS are not due to the procedure but are fated to occur anyway.

Cost and Availability of Molecular Diagnosis

It is difficult at this point to estimate the cost of this testing or identify all the centers that provide the tests. The application of such testing is just beginning as this chapter is being written. By comparison with other tests which have been available for some time, however, it is likely that the cost will be in the vicinity of $1000 per family, and that a number of commercial and academic laboratories will offer testing. Questions about molecular diagnostic testing are best referred to a local genetic counseling center.

INSIGHTS INTO PATHOGENESIS OF NEUROFIBROMATOSIS

As noted in the introduction, it is hoped that molecular studies will eventually lead to the identification of the NF genes and elucidation of their function. This will provide the tools needed to understand the pathogenesis of these disorders. Some insights into pathogenesis are being obtained even with the closely linked markers now available.

The major progress has come from analysis of linked marker genes in tumor tissue. Tumor cells often differ from normal cells by having acquired a number of changes in the structure of their genetic material. These changes seem to upset normal gene regulation in these cells, which is responsible for their abnormal behavior in a tumor. Studies of tumor material from NF patients have revealed changes in the NF genes in these tumors.

The major observation was initially made in tumors from patients with NF2. It was found that DNA from the tumor cells had lost copies of marker alleles adjacent to the NF2 gene (9). Thus, for individuals who were heterozygous for a nearby marker, and who therefore had two alleles detected in DNA obtained from white blood cells, the tumor tissue had only one of the alleles. This indicates deletion of DNA near, and probably including NF2 from tumor tissue but not from normal tissue. It has been more difficult to detect similar deletions in tumors from those with NF1. Research along these lines is continuing.

A definitive explanation for how NF gene deletions contribute to tumor formation must await isolation of the genes and study of their mode of action. There is one system in which the mechanism of gene deletion leading to tumor formation has been well studied. This precedent is retinoblastoma, a tumor of the retina of the eye, which has no relationship to NF, and involves gene deletions on chromosome 13, far from the NF genes (10,11). Some cases of familial retinoblastoma, in which the tendency to develop tumors segregates as an autosomal dominant trait just like NF, are known. It has been found that affected members of such families have a mutant form of a gene known as Rb-1 on one of their copies of chromosome 13. Their other copy of this gene is normal. In retinoblastomas from these individuals, however, the normal gene copy has been lost (Fig. 16–14). This leaves the tumor cells with no functional copy of the Rb-1 gene, which somehow apparently leads to tumor formation.

It appears now that there are a number of genes whose activity seems to suppress tumor formation, and therefore the loss of whose activity leads to tumor growth (12). Exactly how these tumor suppressor genes work is not yet known, but molecular studies, particularly of the Rb-1 gene, will likely uncover this mechanism in the near future. The NF genes are promising candidates to function in an analogous manner, although our knowledge of this area is very sketchy, and this hypothesis may well be replaced by others as more is learned.

Toward Cloning the Genes for Neurofibromatosis

The major goal of molecular biologists studying NF is the cloning of the genes for NF1 and NF2. As has been noted many times in this chapter, this

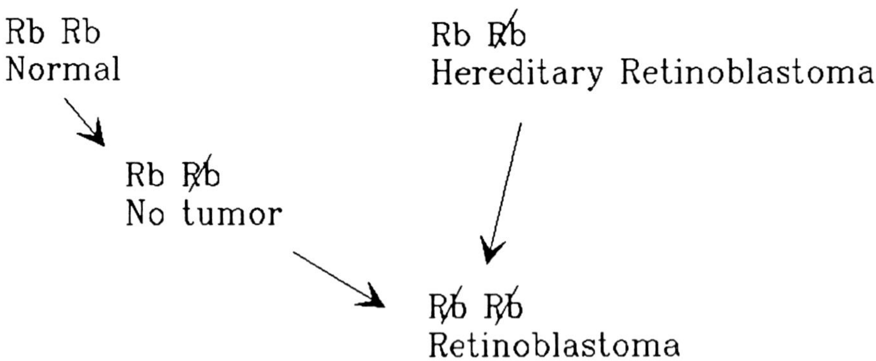

Figure 16–14. The Rb-1 gene, present in two copies in each individual, must be damaged (indicated by a slash through the Rb symbol) in order for a retinoblastoma to develop. Individuals with sporadic retinoblastoma start with two normal copies of the gene, and must sustain damage to both copies in order to develop a tumor. Individuals who inherit a damaged copy only must lose the function of their one remaining intact copy to develop retinoblastoma, and so have a high frequency of retinoblastomas.

accomplishment will go far toward gaining a fundamental understanding of these disorders.

The reverse genetics approach, as noted previously, attempts to identify the product of a gene by first cloning the gene, then determining its coding sequence, and finally inferring the protein structure from the coding sequence (13). The most challenging part of this process is the cloning of the gene. When human DNA is cut up and the fragments are cloned into bacterial cells, the resulting collection of bacterial colonies is referred to as a *genomic library*. Each colony in this library contains a different bit of human DNA. The question is which one contains the DNA corresponding to a region of interest.

One way to determine this is to take advantage of knowledge gained through genetic linkage analysis. Such analysis, described earlier in this chapter, reveals that specific cloned fragments, referred to as markers, are located nearby the gene of interest. With the technique of *gene walking*, it is possible to use these markers to identify cloned fragments even nearer that gene, and eventually the gene itself (Fig. 16–15).

To perform gene walking it is necessary to prepare a genomic library in which the inserted human DNA fragments are relatively long. The lengths of DNA cloned in such a system may be more than 10 times larger than the fragments used to generate marker probes. One then tests the DNA from bacterial colonies in this library to find one whose sequence includes the nearby marker gene, but being larger also contains DNA to either side. Some of this DNA to either side of the marker sequence is then isolated and again used to identify colonies in the library that include this sequence plus DNA to either side. By repeating this process several times the DNA between adjacent linked markers can be gradually filled in. Eventually, the DNA corresponding with the gene of interest will be cloned. Recent progress in gene walking near NF1 on chromosome 17 indicates that cloned fragments exist extremely close to the disease gene (14,15).

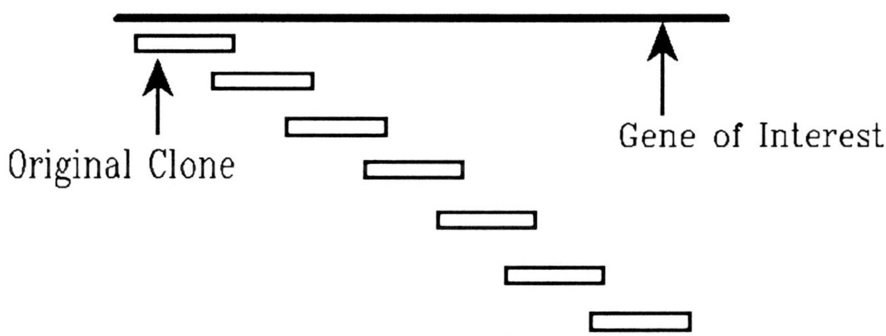

Figure 16–15. Gene walking, in which one begins with a clone some distance from a gene of interest. By using this clone to identify others progressively nearer the gene of interest, one eventually isolates DNA corresponding to the gene of interest.

Identification of a Disease Gene

How can one know when the gene is cloned if one has no prior knowledge of its structure? This is a difficult problem, for which a number of approaches have been tried. The ultimate proof that a cloned piece of DNA represents a gene responsible for a particular disorder involves the demonstration of a number of properties. First, the DNA must be genetically linked to the disease gene locus. This is easily established by linkage analysis. Second, individuals having the disease should have a different sequence from those who are unaffected. This difference would represent the mutation responsible for the disease. Third, the DNA sequence should be expressed in cells that are affected by the disease. A final criterion that the DNA sequence represents some important gene is that its structure is preserved through evolution. Most DNA sequences that encode information tend to be similar in various animal species. DNA sequences that are located between genes, on the other hand, are less conserved. Testing blocks of DNA for species conservation is therefore a shortcut to identifying important genes represented in cloned DNA.

Another shortcut to cloning a disease gene is to test "candidate genes." These are already cloned genes whose normal function may be known, but which have not been identified as being responsible for specific diseases. Many such cloned sequences now exist, and it is relatively easy to test these as candidates to represent the disease gene. The first test, which eliminates most candidates, is to decide whether the sequence is genetically linked to the disease locus. Sequences that are not linked are immediately ruled out as being the same as the disease gene.

The shortest route to cloning a disease gene such as NF1 or NF2 is to use a wide variety of cloning and searching strategies, using knowledge of the location of the genes and of the biology of the disorders. The map locations of NF1 and NF2 are being rapidly refined, and several plausible candidate genes have so far been ruled out (2,16).

Application of Knowledge Gained from Gene Cloning: Diagnosis

Many of the benefits that will result from cloning the genes for NF1 and NF2 have already been alluded to. Probably the first of these will be the availability of better tools for diagnosis. Diagnosis by linkage analysis, as already noted, has many limitations. A test based on analysis of the cloned gene would be free of these limitations. Once the mutation or mutations responsible for NF have been characterized, a diagnosis would be made simply by looking for such a mutation in DNA from the individual or fetus at risk. As knowledge about the mutations increases, such testing can be made precise, reliable, and inexpensive.

In addition to providing diagnostic information, molecular analysis may eventually provide prognostic information. Although all individuals with NF1 have a mutation linked to a locus on chromosome 17, it is likely that the specific mutations will differ in different individuals. This reflects the fact that there are many ways of altering a gene so as to interfere with the function of its product. Some mutations may result in more profound disruption of function than others. For example, in some cases the protein product may not be formed at all, whereas in others the product may be formed, but in smaller quantities than usual. It is possible that these differences may correlate with different levels of severity of the disease, or different types of medical complications. Eventually, then, it may be possible to predict at least some aspects of the clinical course from knowledge of the specific type of gene mutation present in an individual.

Application of Knowledge Gained from Gene Cloning: Treatment

Most individuals with NF are born with few or no signs of the disorder, and only develop difficulties as they grow older. This fact opens the possibility of preventing these problems from occurring. The hope of providing treatment to prevent or reverse the manifestations of NF is the ultimate aim of research into the disorder.

The cloning of the NF genes will be a prelude to studies of the gene products. The first step will be to determine the structure of the protein products, which can be inferred from the structures of the genes. It may turn out that these proteins will be similar to or identical with already known proteins; alternatively they may be unique and previously undiscovered proteins. Research will then focus on understanding how these proteins function in normal cells, and how the abnormalities in NF upset cell functions. It is impossible to say just when we will reach this point, and whether this will result in the development of new treatments. One can only hope that a thorough understanding of the pathogenesis of NF will suggest ways of modifying the effects of the abnormal gene products on the cell.

A more distant possibility for treatment involves the replacement of the abnormal gene with a normal copy. In principle it is possible to insert genes into cells in a way that results in their expression, and this has been proposed as a means of treating certain genetic disorders (17). In practice there are many technical obstacles, and this approach of gene therapy remains in a purely experimental phase. For NF it is difficult to see how gene defect could be corrected in a large number of cells that are very widely distributed in the body. On the other hand, we will have to wait for more knowledge of the nature of the defect in NF to be sure exactly what would need to be achieved to effect such therapy. By that time additional technological possibilities for gene therapy may exist.

SUMMARY

Recent progress in molecular genetics has opened a new approach to the study of NF. This is the reverse genetics approach, in which a genetic disorder is studied by first locating and then isolating the responsible gene. For NF, the genes for both NF1 and NF2 are now localized, to chromosomes 17 and 22, respectively. This has opened the possibility of presymptomatic and prenatal diagnosis for familial cases of NF, and has begun to provide insights into the pathogenesis of the disorders. The current focus is on identification of the genes themselves, which will in turn provide information about their protein products. Such knowledge would result in the development of accurate diagnostic testing, and may suggest novel means of treatment.

REFERENCES

1. D. Barker, E. Wright, K. Nguyen, et al. Gene for von Recklinghausen neurofibromatosis is in the pericentromeric region of chromosome 17. Science 1987;236:1098–1102.
2. R.R. Seizinger, G.A. Rouleau, L.J. Ozelius, et al. Genetic linkage of von Recklinghausen neurofibromatosis to the nerve growth factor receptor gene. Cell 1987;49:589–594.
3. F.S. Collins, B.A.J. Ponder, B.R. Seizinger, and C.J. Epstein. The von Recklinghausen neurofibromatosis region on chromosome 17—Genetic and physical maps come into focus. Am J Hum Genet 1989;44:1–5.
4. D.E. Goldgar, P. Green, D.M. Parry, and J.J. Mulvihill. Multipoint linkage analysis in neurofibromatosis type I: An international collaboration. Am J Hum Genet 1989;44:6–12.
5. W. Wertelecki, G.A. Rouleau, D.W. Superneau, et al. Neurofibromatosis 2: Clinical and DNA linkage studies of a large kindred. N Engl J Med 1988;319:278–283.
6. G.A. Rouleau, W. Wertelecki, J.L. Haines, et al. Genetic linkage of bilateral acoustic neurofibromatosis to a DNA marker on chromosome 22. Nature 1987;329:246–248.
7. NICHD National Registry for amniocentesis study group. Mid trimester amniocentesis for prenatal diagnosis: Safety and accuracy. JAMA 1976;236:1471–1476.
8. G.G. Rhoads, L.G. Jackson, S.E. Schlesselman, et al. The safety and efficacy of chorionic villus sampling for early prenatal diagnosis of cytogenetic abnormalities. N Engl J Med 1989;320:609–617.
9. B.R. Seizinger, R.L. Martuza, and J.F. Gusella. Loss of genes on chromosome 22 in tumorigenesis of human acoustic neuroma. Nature 1986;322:644–647.
10. W.F. Benedict, Y.-K.T. Fung, and A.L. Murphree. The gene responsible for the development of retinoblastoma and osteosarcoma. Cancer 1988; 62 (Suppl 8):1691–1694.
11. S.H. Friend, R. Bernards, S. Rogelj, et al. A human DNA segment with properties of the gene that predisposes to retinoblastoma and osteosarcoma. Nature 1986;323:643–646.
12. G. Klein. The approaching era of the tumor suppressor genes. Science 1987;238:1539–1545.
13. S.H. Orkin. Reverse genetics and human disease. Cell 1986;47:845–850.
14. J.W. Fountain, M.R. Wallace, M.A. Bruce, et al. Physical mapping of a translocation breakpoint in neurofibromatosis. Science 1989;244:1085–1087.
15. P. O'Connell, R. Leach, R.M. Cawthon, et al. Two NF1 translocations map within a 600-kilobase segment of 17q11.2. Science 1989;244:1087–1088.
16. J.K. Darby, J. Feder, M. Selby, et al. A discordant sibship analysis between beta-NGF and neurofibromatosis. Am J Hum Genet 1985;37:52–59.
17. M.J. Cline. Gene therapy: Current status. Am J Med 1987;83:291–297.

17

Genetic Counseling for Neurofibromatosis

Barbara Bernhardt, M.S., and Jane C. Halperin, M.S.

When a genetic condition such as neurofibromatosis (NF) is diagnosed in a child or an adult, a multitude of questions arise, any of which may eventually lead to referral for genetic counseling. Typical questions raised in a general genetics clinic or NF clinics are: Why me? Why did this condition occur? Have I done anything to cause this condition? How will it change my life? How can it be treated? Is there a cure? Will it occur in any other family members? What family planning alternatives are available?

A formal definition of genetic counseling, as published by the American Society of Human Genetics (1), is:

> a communication process which deals with the human problems associated with the occurrence, or the risk of occurrence, of genetic disorder in a family. This process involves an attempt by one or more appropriately trained persons to help the individual or family (1) comprehend the medical facts, including the diagnosis, the probable course of the disorder, and the available management; (2) appreciate the way heredity contributes to the disorder, and the risk of recurrence in specified relatives; (3) understand the options for dealing with the risk of recurrence; (4) choose the course of action which seems appropriate to them in view of their risk and family goals, and act in accordance with that decision; and (5) make the best possible adjustment to the disorder in the affected family member and/or to the risk of recurrence of that disorder.

Thus genetic counseling is multifaceted and involves family education regarding medical, genetic, and family planning issues. In addition, a genetic counseling session is the appropriate forum to begin to explore emotional and psychological issues which arise when a family member has NF. Unlike the usual experience when receiving medical services, genetic counseling does not result in a list of recommendations the patient is urged to follow. Instead, an individual or family member is encouraged to express feelings, ask questions, and seek help in defining available options.

REFERRAL FOR GENETIC COUNSELING

People may be referred for counseling by a variety of sources, including physicians, nurses, social workers, family members, or clergy. Some people refer themselves for counseling. Genetic counseling may be sought by a person who has NF or by parents or other relatives of the affected individual. Counseling may be requested just after NF is diagnosed or when a couple with a family history of NF is contemplating starting a family or having another child. Unfortunately, it may not be until a pregnancy is in progress that some couples are informed of their increased risk for giving birth to a child with a genetic disorder such as NF, and referred for genetic counseling.

Preliminary genetic counseling is often provided by the primary care physician, such as the family pediatrician, or an obstetrician. More specialized genetic counseling services are available at over 300 genetic centers throughout the United States. Most genetic centers are a part of university medical centers where sophisticated diagnostic and consultative resources exist, although an increasing number of sparsely populated areas are served by outreach programs. The majority of genetics clinics are staffed by a multidisciplinary group of professionals, which may include physicians trained in genetics (medical geneticists), genetic associates or counselors, social workers, or nurses. The disciplines represented will vary from clinic to clinic. NF specialty clinics or centers exist in medical centers across the country, providing diagnostic and medical care, counseling and support services, access to research projects, and educational programs. There is generally a charge for genetic counseling, ranging up to several hundred dollars. The charges incurred are sometimes, but not always, covered by health insurance. The specific organization of genetics clinics varies from setting to setting, but what transpires in genetic counseling can be discussed in general terms.

THE GENETIC COUNSELING SESSION

Typically, when a family is initially referred for genetic counseling, telephone contact may be made to obtain preliminary family history information, to discover the reason for referral, to discuss the expectations of those seeking counseling (the consultands), and to explain the genetic counseling process. Reasons for referral may include diagnosis, medical management, emotional support, counseling as to recurrent risk and reproductive options, or any combination of these. A consultand may be told which family member needs to be examined. If a couple is referred for counseling, both husband and wife will be encouraged to be present for the counseling session. When possible, pertinent medical records are collected prior to the genetics clinic visit.

At the time of the initial visit to a genetics clinic, medical records are reviewed, a complete family history is taken, and physical examinations may be performed on affected family members and, if indicated, on those at risk for being affected. Medical evaluations are important in order to establish an exact diagnosis, which may sometimes be made by physical examination alone, but which may also require consultation with other specialists. Information on the health of relatives and the presence or absence of similar symptoms may be exceedingly useful in making an exact diagnosis. In some cases, the findings are clearly present and diagnosis is medically obvious and straightforward. In a small number of cases, a final diagnosis may not be available by the close of the first session pending further case review. Lack of a precise diagnosis will preclude providing exact information regarding recurrence risk (the chance to have a child born with the disorder under question). For the majority of individuals seen in counseling for NF, an exact recurrence risk can be given.

In the counseling session, the genetic disorder and possible complications are described and available treatments are reviewed. Patients may be questioned about their prior understanding of the medical and genetic aspects of the condition in order to correct any misconceptions. The risk for future children of both affected and unaffected family members is outlined. Pregnancy options are reviewed and information is provided to help in making decisions about future pregnancies. Families are informed about community resources which might provide assistance to them, and of the availability of appropriate education and support groups, such as the National Neurofibromatosis Foundation (NNFF). Generally, a letter summarizing the points covered in the genetic counseling session is sent to both the family and the referring physician following the session.

Follow-up visits to the genetics or NF clinic are often necessary. Preliminary genetics counseling is often initiated just after a new diagnosis is suspected or confirmed, a time that is emotionally charged and not ideal for optimal family education. Because genetic counseling involves medical evaluation, explanation of genetics, introduction to new medical terminology, assimilation of information, and decision making, multiple visits to the clinic may be necessary. New breakthroughs in the areas of treatment, diagnosis, or prenatal detection may lead to further contact with the families served in the past by a particular clinic. Families are encouraged to contact the staff in the genetics clinic as new questions arise.

GENETIC COUNSELING IN NEUROFIBROMATOSIS

Individuals come to be diagnosed with NF, and eventually referred for genetic counseling, in two general ways: those that are unsuspecting of any medical condition and those that anticipate the presence of a medical condition. Clearly, this difference in expectations and degree of preparedness influences the initial perception of the diagnosis. It is often the case that upon routine medical checkup parents will be told that their child is suspected of having NF due to the presence of café au lait spots. Such news is clearly unexpected and unwelcome and may understandably trigger tremendous anxiety and fear. For others, the diagnosis may be the culmination of a search to find the answers to questions that have been plaguing them or to gain treatment to alleviate a symptom. Perhaps this search has been a long and arduous one involving considerable anxiety and expense. For some such individuals the diagnosis may be initially experienced as a relief after long periods of confusion or discomfort. While circumstances may vary, the constant and universal factor is that the period of diagnosis is always a time of stress.

Genetic counseling for NF follows the same general scheme as just outlined. Confirmation of diagnosis for all family members interested in counseling is vital. At the present time there is no laboratory test that can be utilized to secure a diagnosis of NF. Therefore such a determination can be made only by the presence of specific clinical findings upon examination by an experienced physician. There are times, however, when such an examination does not lead to a definitive diagnosis, but instead to a label of "NF suspect," meaning there is a reasonable suspicion that an individual may have NF but there are insufficient clinical findings to support this at the present time. The variability, both within and among families, which categorizes NF is a particularly important issue to discuss and one which presents a significant intellectual and emotional challenge to individuals and families coping with NF. Criteria for diagnosis of NF, variability, and medical management of the condition are reviewed in detail in Chapter 2 and will not be covered further here.

For teenagers affected by a condition such as NF, the appropriate age for genetic counseling will vary from child to child. Parents are generally in the best position to determine when their affected child is ready to learn about the genetics of NF. It is perfectly reasonable for the parent to explain the genetic facts if they feel comfortable doing so, or the services of the pediatrician or genetic counselor can be utilized.

In a genetic counseling situation involving NF, the recurrence risk is either very low, as in the case of unaffected parents whose child has NF caused by a new gene mutation, or 50%, as for the person with NF. A decision to have children is an intensely personal one and generally depends on many factors in addition to genetic ones. Genetic considerations include the magnitude of the recurrence risk and the real or perceived severity of the disorder. Interpretation of the severity of NF is subjective and is modified by the affected person's clinical manifestations and perception of how the condition has impacted on life-style, self-image, happiness, and future goals (2–5). Those being counseled must be reminded of the variability of the condition and of the fact that if the parent is mildly affected, this is *not* a guarantee that an affected child will not have severe complications. Oftentimes, partners may have differing interpretations of the severity of the condition, with the unaffected person downplaying the burden of the condition or vice versa. The counseling session provides a setting for the couple to discuss the condition and how they feel they would cope with, and feel about, an affected child.

Other nongenetic factors play an important role in the decision-making process. They include the number of children already present in the family and their health, expected family size, the intensity of desire for children, and various ethnic, religious, and socioeconomic considerations. Oftentimes, pressure from other family members may impact heavily on family planning decisions. Couples making important decisions about having children are encouraged to discuss their medical and genetic concerns with those people who will influence their decisions. This will sometimes lead to the suggestion that other family members be seen in the genetics clinic for education as well.

The acceptability of available reproductive alternatives will impact heavily on family planning decisions. Such alternatives, as outlined in the counseling session, may include artificial insemination by a donor, surrogate motherhood, adoption, prenatal diagnosis with selective pregnancy termination, no children or no further children, or having the desired number of children despite the genetic risk. The advantages and disadvantages of each of these options must be thoroughly reviewed before an informed decision can be made.

With recent advances in genetics the options for dealing with the recurrence risk of NF have increased. Current research involving the NF gene now allows prenatal diagnosis of the fetuses with NF by linkage analysis in some instances (reviewed in Chapter 16). Prenatal diagnosis is the name given to procedures that test the unborn fetus for the presence of a variety of medical conditions. Such testing would provide families with the option of terminating a pregnancy if the fetus is affected. Decisions along these lines are obviously very personal and complex. Prenatal diagnosis may not be an option for families with specific cultural, ethical, or religious objections to abortion. For those who accept the general concept of prenatal diagnosis, the possibility of terminating a pregnancy of a fetus that may be mildly affected, although there is no way of predicting severity, is unacceptable. For other families the availability of prenatal diagnosis may make childbearing possible by allowing them to proceed only with pregnancies that have been shown by linkage analysis to have a high likelihood of being unaffected. In families in which linkage analysis is not possible, the precise location and identification of the NF gene will improve the chances for prenatal diagnosis. We believe this direct test is still a few years away.

It is important for couples to consider the implications of all possible reproductive choices and to remember that reproductive attitudes may change as their life experiences change. Genetic counseling will provide a couple with the facts about a genetic condition present in the family, an enumeration of reproductive options and knowledge of resources available for future assistance. Genetic counseling will provide help and guidance, but decision making will be left to those seeking the counseling.

Genetic counseling is also important in aiding the family to make the best possible adjustment to the disorder. This may begin with the diagnosis. Recollections of individuals and families confirm that the diagnosis of NF is an emotionally charged event. The manner in which it is anticipated by the individual and handled by the physician constitutes a landmark in one's life, one which is not forgotten and one which may greatly affect the future adjustment to the condition.

Helping families to make the best possible adjustment to NF involves dealing with a variety of important issues in addition to childbearing decisions. The genetic counselor, ideally involved with the family from the time of diagnosis, is in a unique position to aid affected individuals and relatives by accessing resources and providing information and support.

Counselors often provide crisis intervention at the time of diagnosis or the occurrence of a serious medical complication. During these trying periods, feelings of grief, guilt, and anger are often coupled with a sense of confusion. There are so many questions without answers, so much frustration! Crisis intervention addresses these feelings in the following ways: one, reducing, when possible, the impact of the stressful event; and two, using the crisis situation to help people cope more effectively with their present problems and to provide guidance in facing future problems. Working with individuals to help them help themselves through difficult times builds self-confidence and restores a sense of control.

Individuals may need help dealing with many of the feelings that they are experiencing as a result of being affected by NF. Proper attention to feelings of guilt and anger may help individuals learn to channel this energy into constructive action. Reinforcing the fact that conditions such as NF are caused by factors beyond human control may be useful. People often need help in coming to grips with the fact that there is no satisfactory answer as to why this has happened to them.

Preoccupation with medical care and other issues associated with having NF may lead one to feel alone in dealing with problems that others do not have to face. Isolation can be a very real problem. The inability to seek a way out may seem equally real. This painful sense of isolation can become demoralizing. The genetic counselor can often provide support in helping individuals interact with others who have similar concerns or provide encouragement in developing other social contacts, such as going back to work or school.

Marital stress is often the result of each member of a couple developing their own style of coping with the occurrence of NF in the family. Differences of opinion on important decisions, economic pressures, reactions of friends and relatives, the needs of other children, and sheer exhaustion may all increase the level of tension. This degree of tension often discourages open communication between partners. While one may be "up" (coping, optimistic, ready to talk), the other may be "down" (depressed). This "up" and "down" combination may help a family cope from day to day as partners alternate in taking charge, but it does not create an environment conducive to sharing feelings. Reassurance that marital stress is common in families dealing with medical conditions should reduce feelings of surprise at experiencing such dissension. Families need not handle marital difficulties themselves. Genetic counselors can help couples to examine and share their feelings, to reevaluate unwritten rules and roles that guide their marriage, and to explore their expectations. Some situations may require more intense intervention. The genetic counselor can often refer such couples to professionals who are specifically trained to help them deal with these difficult issues.

Genetic counselors can often provide guidance in helping affected individuals to deal with others. Siblings, relatives, and strangers may all be involved to different degrees. Family members such as grandparents and siblings have their own reactions and feelings regarding the occurrence of NF in the family. Issues involving how one family member's condition impacts upon others can be quite delicate and crucial to future family interaction. Guilt and anger involving who is and is not affected may also require considerable attention. Families often need guidance in negotiating if and when to inform relatives of the condition. The genetic counselor can meet with the whole family or some members to help air their feelings and work toward compromises. For families requiring more intensive aid, referral to a specialist in family therapy can be made. Facing strangers may not be easy for those affected by NF. People often stare or ask questions, do not listen to answers, or show ignorance in ways that are hurtful. Affected individuals are often caught in a bind; they want their privacy and anonymity, but they may also want to share their experience in hopes of shaping others' attitudes. Working with a counselor, an individual can be correctly informed and taught to have a ready response to inquiries or receive support that they are entitled to protect their privacy. Particularly when one does not feel like explaining or being rude, ready answers often make the situation easier to get through.

Genetic counselors, by virtue of their training and experience with emotional issues associated with genetic conditions and their access to several individuals affected by the same disorder, are often uniquely qualified to offer group experiences. Group sessions provide information, emotional support, and opportunities for social interaction. Although talking to others facing similar problems does not make the problems go away, it may help to reduce feeling of isolation and teach ways of coping. Individuals may feel pressure by unaffected family members or friends to be positive about themselves and their medical status at all times. With others experiencing similar concerns, it is often possible to take time out to share even the worst fears and frustrations, knowing that they will be understood. Often people find satisfaction in providing solace or helpful information to others during group sessions.

SUMMARY

NF provides formidable challenges for those who are affected by it. The genetic counseling process is important to the process of adjustment to NF in a variety of ways. The genetic counselor in conjunction with physicians, nurses, clergy, social workers, therapists, and other health-care personnel provides a greater opportunity for as complete an adjustment to NF as possible. Emphasizing that all individuals, regardless of medical condition, are more like than unlike others is important. Confidence in the ability of individuals to make their own decisions once they are carefully informed, and in their strength to meet challenges and overcome their difficulties must always be the basis for genetic counseling.

REFERENCES

1. F.C. Fraser. Genetic counseling. Am J Hum Genet 1974;26:636–659.
2. I. Ambramovsky, L. Godmilow, K. Hirschhorn, and H. Smith, Jr. Analysis of a follow-up study of genetic counseling. Clin Genet 1980;17:1–12.
3. M.L. Griffin, C.M. Kavanagh, and J.R. Sorenson. Genetic knowledge, client perspectives, and genetic counseling. Soc Work Health Care 1976;2:171–180.
4. A. Lippman-Hand, and F.C. Fraser. Genetic counseling—The postcounseling period: I. Parent's perceptions of uncertainty. Am J Med Genet 1979;4:51–71.
5. D.C. Wertz, J.R. Sorenson, and T.C. Heeren. Clients' interpretation of risks provided in genetic counseling. Am J Hum Genet 1986;39:253–264.

SECTION III

PSYCHOSOCIAL ASPECTS

18

Impact of Neurofibromatosis on the Adolescent

Barbara Wellman, M.S.W.

The period of adolescence, from about the age of 13 to 18, may be a time of turmoil and stress for both the child and the parents, whether or not the child has neurofibromatosis (NF). It requires particular attention from both parents and professionals. An adolescent is no longer a child and is not yet an adult. With the exception of early infancy, adolescence is the time when the most rapid physical, emotional, and intellectual growth and development take place. Adolescence can be thought of as a process—of preparing to become an adult, and of discovering the answer to "Who am I?"

The hallmarks of adolescence are self-consciousness, self-awareness, and self-centeredness. During this period, a teenager must confront and resolve the confusions and contradictions presented by the complex array of biological, social, and legal definitions of adulthood in American society. The adolescent must discover, understand, and come to terms with a rapidly changing physical, emotional, and intellectual self. It takes great effort to become less dependent on parents and adults in general, to outgrow dependence on parental authority and nurturing, to learn to assume personal responsibility for impulses and actions, and to form emotional attachments outside the family. Adolescents must select a value system, a life-style, and life work that will provide not only a livelihood, but also a sense of importance, self-worth, and self-fulfillment.

All adolescents, with or without health problems, experience some awkwardness, doubt, and uncertainty while moving from childhood to adulthood. Adolescence has been described as the time of promise, fulfillment, and emancipation, and the sense of having something "wrong" with one's body presents a cruel paradox. NF complicates the period of adolescence—for those with very mild manifestations as well as for those with more serious problems. This chapter will review a few of the major impacts that NF may have on the adolescent, focusing on special needs and how parents and professionals may help to make this important period of life easier.

PHYSICAL APPEARANCE

The adolescent places extreme importance on outward appearance. He or she is acutely aware of even slight imperfections in physical makeup. The teen with NF will likely feel self-conscious because of café au lait spots or skin tumors, let alone other more disfiguring aspects of the disorder.

Adolescence is the most difficult time in an individual's life to appear different. The existence of social norms for physical beauty and for what is desirable in terms of physical makeup results in special problems for those who do not see themselves as measuring up. The teen wants to look like his or her peers, and their support and approval are critical. NF, with its visible signs, may make an individual appear different from others. Some teens with NF have indicated that their peers have reacted with avoidance or teasing. The adolescent with NF is faced with physical deviations that extend far beyond the common defects of adolescence—having pimples or crooked teeth, or being too fat or too thin. Parents must be doubly aware that their child is dressing or cutting his or her hair, or making up her eyes, for their peers and no one else. Within the bounds of parental values of decency, parents must be willing to let the teen go with the crowd. Having clothes or a haircut that "fits" can overcome some of the anxiety generated by looking different.

MEDICAL CARE

There is an increased sense of privacy as a child moves into adolescence. This is reflected in the teen's attitude toward medical care and thus represents a serious problem for parents and caregivers. As questions and concerns about one's body increase, so does reluctance to admit these concerns. Some youngsters continue to confide in their parents, others shut them off. Learning to respect this need for privacy while remaining sensitive and available is not an easy task. Parents and professionals alike need patience, tact, and a good sense of humor.

Adolescents tend to alternate between pampering their body and neglecting or abusing it. Often their declaration of independence is expressed in physical terms: "My body belongs to me to do to it as I wish." Medical orders and regimens are the equivalent of parental authority. Procedures related to a medical problem provoke resentment against intrusiveness, loss of independence, and lack of privacy, as well as forced submission to authority figures. This is also the time of increased modesty—his or her bodily privacy may have to be invaded as doctors and nurses have to inspect, examine, or manipulate the body. When parents or health professionals cannot get information from the teen, it is necessary to ask more and more questions which are met with increasing evasiveness and hostility. Being "bugged" can cause the teen to feel that he or she is not trusted or respected.

ADJUSTING TO NEUROFIBROMATOSIS

The adolescent with NF may react with outrage at the unfairness of having NF and may feel cheated. He or she needs accurate information about NF and opportunities to discuss and come to grips with his or her feelings. Parents need tolerance for anger and acting out. But an adolescent is still a child practicing to be an adult. There must be curfews and rules about using the car, or bringing friends to the house. Parents must stay in touch with behavior and consider asking for extra help from professionals.

The teenager must be helped by parents and professionals to understand NF in realistic and practical terms. He or she must be told the truth about any special problems. Knowing the truth helps the teenager to feel in charge. Listen to and evaluate what he or she says and does so you know if he or she is realistic. Keep channels open for the teen to ask questions and receive information. This is also the time when adolescents need specific, honest words to tell others about NF. Helping your teen to explain NF to friends, classmates, teachers, and other professionals usually helps to prevent unkind statements or actions. Most adolescents become quite sophisticated in their understanding of NF. They may take an intellectual view of the disorder, becoming absorbed in learning about its physiology, treatment, and relevant research. The teenager may benefit from being involved in the National Neurofibromatosis Foundation (NNFF), and, if available, local chapter activities. Always remind the adolescent that there are things being done to help those with NF—by family, doctors, and researchers—and that he or she can join in the effort.

A part of growing up is developing the ability to recognize one's shortcomings and assets and to live with them. The confidence to accept one's self as one really is and to believe that others can do the same comes with advancing adolescence. The teen with NF should be encouraged to pursue activities where he or she can achieve success and feel worthwhile. How parents and professionals act toward the adolescent is critical. If they do not treat him or her with respect, the teen will not develop a sense of worth or feeling of security.

NF is a special problem because it is a complex disorder that is progressive and lifelong. It calls for long-term acceptance of being different and of possible limitations at a time when the adolescent must be encouraged to assume increasing responsibility for required medical monitoring and treatment. Finding a doctor whom the teen can trust and respect, who is capable of treating NF but will also listen to questions and worries is of utmost importance. Parents make every attempt to respect their youngster's right to confidentiality. They should allow the teen to talk to the doctor privately while recognizing their need to keep informed of their teen's medical status and treatment needs. They should work with the doctor to find areas in which the teen can make decisions and function with some autonomy.

Hospitalization

Hospitalization during adolescence is particularly troublesome. More and more major medical centers have recognized this and are developing adolescent units to help the adolescent deal with loss of identity, privacy, and self-determination, as well as fear of abandonment, deformity, and even death.

A major conceptual milestone in adolescence is the development of a sense of time. Young children are not able to think clearly about their past or ahead for their future. They deal only with the present. The adolescent has the capacity to imagine the future and to sense one's mortality. This is why some teenagers may worry about their death, or at least may express concern about how NF will affect adulthood.

Genetic Counseling

With a hereditary disorder such as NF, the adolescent must learn about the risks of passing NF on to children. Handling this with the adolescent calls for great compassion and tact. Many parents find it helpful to seek professional guidance. The adolescent should be told that when the time comes to consider reproduction, there are genetic counselors and other professionals who can assist him or her and a future spouse to reach a personally meaningful decision.

Conclusion

It is common for parents of an adolescent with a health problem to behave toward their teen as if this was their last opportunity to baby their child. This leads to infantilization, permissiveness, and overprotection. Remember that your teenager needs you in a "standby" capacity. He or she needs to know that you are there and will help if needed. Through it all, remember that the teenager is still a teenager. The specific developmental patterns and needs of a teenager are not changed by NF. It helps to recognize that and to let the teen take on the world on his or her terms. NF is a part, not the whole, of the teenager's life.

Bibliography

For teenagers: Your stay in the hospital. Washington, D.C., Association for the Care of Children's Health, 1982. Available from Association for the Care of Children's Health, 3615 Wisconsin Ave N.W., Washington, D.C. 20016. A pamphlet to help teens prepare for and understand the hospital.

J. Howe. The Hospital Book. New York, Crown Books, 1981. A thorough guide about a stay in the hospital, suitable for children and young adolescents.

K. McCoy. The teenage survival guide: Coping with problems in everyday life. New York, Pocket Books, 1981. Written for teenagers, this is a discussion of issues important to the teen such as school, friends, family relationships, and coping with crisis.

K. McCoy and C. Wibbelsman. The teenage body book. New York, Pocket Books, 1978. Questions and answers for teenagers about their changing bodies.

E. Richter. The teenage hospital experience: You can handle it! Boston, Coward, McCann and Geoghegan, 1982. This book is a compilation of interviews of hospitalized teenagers and health professionals. It also includes a section on the rights of teenagers as patients.

19

Impact of Neurofibromatosis on the Family

Mary Ann Wilson and Felice Yahr, M.S.

Families in which neurofibromatosis (NF) occurs face a number of problems that can have a serious impact on their lives. Severe medical problems—among them tumors on nerves anywhere in the body, skeletal defects, loss of hearing or vision—can develop at any time. Psychological and social difficulties can be all-encompassing. Financial costs may be a considerable burden. While problems vary from one family to another, virtually every family experiences unending anxiety about what NF may do to them, and when.

The Impact of the Diagnosis

How the individual or family learns the diagnosis of NF may set the tone for the impact of the disorder on the family. The diagnosis is generally made during a visit to a physician, who looks for the common characteristics of NF. These include café au lait spots, tumors, scoliosis, and Lisch nodules on the iris of the eye. When the diagnosis is determined, some physicians tend to give an overly optimistic view of NF, telling families not to be concerned. Although it is true that most people with NF have mild or moderate cases, a family needs to be prepared for what may lie ahead. At the other extreme, a physician might place a medical textbook with photographs of people severely affected by NF in front of the individual or family and say, "This is what you (or your child) has." The individual can be so traumatized that it may take years to get over the shock. At that point, all else that the physician says may not register. It is hoped that the physician will provide a careful and balanced explanation of the possible manifestations of NF, emphasizing the variability and unpredictability of the disorder so that the family can begin to place NF in perspective. Offering basic material on NF such as National Neurofibromatosis Foundation's (NNFF's) information brochure is also helpful at this time.

As more information about NF is disseminated through the media, many people have literally diagnosed themselves or a family member from radio and

TV programs or newspaper articles featuring NF. Although learning the diagnosis in this way is better than remaining in the dark, it can be a harsh experience.

For example, a 30-year-old woman called a local NNFF chapter following a television program featuring adults with NF. After confirming that café au lait spots are a sign of NF she put down the phone, counted the spots on her body, and then ran to check her baby before coming back on the line. Her fear was all too evident, as was her anger at her physician and members of her family for not telling her sooner that she had NF.

Learning about NF before entering adolescence seems to have a positive effect on adjustment. When a person with NF grows up with the knowledge of having the disorder, he or she seems to accept the condition more easily and be better able to cope with its consequences. Just as a youngster becomes accustomed to bodily changes, he or she can observe the changes (if any) brought on by NF and learn to live with them. Then NF is a matter of fact instead of a constant surprise.

When the diagnosis is made in adulthood, the effect can be quite different. Adults may fear that the careers they have chosen will now not be feasible, or that marriage or plans for a family are in jeopardy. Young adults, who often have feelings of uncertainty, may find the diagnosis particularly difficult to accept. The possibility—or sometimes the reality—of disfigurement and medical problems which might impair their life-style can be devastating for some young people.

Perhaps the hardest time for an individual to learn that he or she has NF is after the birth of a child with the disorder. This happens when a parent who has a case so mild that it was never diagnosed is found to have the disorder after a more severely affected child is diagnosed. Such a situation can evoke strong feelings of guilt, anger, and even denial, which may take a long time to work through. Other family members often bear the brunt of these emotions. One father with NF would not allow any material on NF to be in the house, and his teenage daughter who has symptoms of NF has never been told. The professional assistance of a social worker, psychologist, or psychiatrist may be needed in such situations. This does not imply that there is a need for long-term therapy or that the individual has psychiatric problems.

When the diagnosis of NF is first made, agonizing questions sometimes arise, such as:

- Was it my fault?
- Did I eat properly?
- Did my body provide an unhealthy environment for the genes?
- Why me and/or my family?

Answers to some of these questions are known. People with NF can be assured that having the disorder or transmitting it to a child is not their fault. NF is not caused by poor eating habits. It did not occur because of an unhealthy environment in their bodies. NF occurs only if an individual has an NF gene, and this happens purely by chance. (These points are discussed more fully in other chapters in this handbook.) No one knows how this gene causes the disorder. These answers will come from research that is being conducted at numerous medical centers in this country and abroad, where researchers are attempting to discover the cause of NF and how to control its manifestations.

TELLING A CHILD ABOUT NEUROFIBROMATOSIS

If a child is involved, further questions arise:

- When should I tell my child?
- How should I tell my child?
- How much should I tell them?
- Should I tell them at all?

Telling the child that he or she has NF depends largely on the child. If he or she is old enough to ask questions, he or she is old enough to be given answers. As a general rule, children probably do not need to be given more information about the disorder than they ask for. A *Handbook for Kids* and a *Handbook for Parents*, available from the NNFF, are highly recommended.

Telling the child also depends on the seriousness of the manifestations. If the child has a mild case, the information offered could serve for coping with the present situation. For example, if a child has scoliosis, a parent might wish to explain what NF is doing to the body, and why a brace must be worn. The child could be encouraged to discuss the situation openly at school so that it is a fact of life like glasses or braces on teeth. Preparing children with answers to possible questions that their friends and classmates may ask helps them to cope with NF and build self-confidence.

It is important that parents let children with NF know that they can come to them at any time with questions or just to express feelings about having NF, explaining it to their friends, or for such special needs as going to the doctor when they are not sick.

THE FAMILY'S ATTITUDE

The family atmosphere into which a child with NF is born can have an important bearing on the individual and the family. An overprotective atmosphere might lead to an unnecessary emphasis on the disorder in the family life and create a lack of self-confidence in the child. Constant "watching" of the family member with NF seems to be a universal behavior on the part of parents and other family members, such as grandparents or aunts and uncles. Each relative has his or her own checklist of areas such as tumor growth, skeletal changes, or possible coordination problems that they feel compelled to observe. Gradually shifting responsibility to watch for changes to the growing child can be helpful to all concerned. As children get older and privacy becomes a very important factor in their lives, they can be encouraged to be on the lookout for any changes in their bodies and to communicate any observations to a parent and/or physician in order to obtain necessary treatment. In this way, the young person will develop a sense of control over his or her body.

Atmospheres of rejection, unusually high standards, or parental or sibling conflict may cause the person with a genetic disorder to feel like a burden to the family. The family's own perception of NF also can have an impact on the family. Is the person with NF viewed as a "handicapped" or "sick" individual? Is that person seen as "defective", or does the parent think of himself or herself as a "defective" person for passing on the disorder? Such attitudes are likely to create an atmosphere that fosters serious self-doubt in the affected individual.

On the other hand, a family atmosphere of mutual respect and acceptance encourages independence and a sense of self-worth. The family attitude to aim for might be, "You are a member of our family who can catch a cold, break an arm, clean up the kitchen, play soccer, ski, perform on stage, and go to college just like any other family member. You just happen to have NF and have to go to the doctor more often than the rest of us." An accepting attitude of this kind helps to instill confidence in the individual in coping with the disorder[1].

THE ELEPHANT MAN AND NEUROFIBROMATOSIS

During the height of the publicity surrounding the play and the movie "The Elephant Man," a young mother took her 9-year-old son to a pediatric neurologist and said, "My son's chest is becoming shaped like a barrel, his head is much larger than last year, and there is something the matter with his right leg." After the doctor examined the boy, he said, "His head has not grown out of proportion to his growth rate. He is fine." The mother then knew that she was seeing physical changes that were not there and that her son was not going to look like the Elephant Man.

As discussed in Chapter 1 of this handbook, Joseph Merrick, or the Elephant Man, as he was called, probably did not have NF after all, but another disorder called Proteus syndrome. Nevertheless, NF has been linked to the Elephant Man for many years, which has created an image of the most severe and disfiguring manifestations that families, particularly young people, may find very difficult to handle. Inappropriate or not, family members who are watching the person with NF may think of the Elephant Man and see physical changes that are not actually developing.

THE UNCERTAINTY OF NEUROFIBROMATOSIS

Perhaps the most difficult aspect of NF for families to cope with is its uncertainty. Families need help in learning to live with the fact that NF is varied and unpredictable. It may be mild; it may be severe; any of a wide range of manifestations may develop at any time. The empathetic physician, aware that this can have a profound effect on the family, avoids extremes in offering guidance. He or she realizes that for the individual with very mild manifestations of NF and no medical problems, it is all to easy to "sweep it under the rug" and even deny having it. The physician, therefore, does not offer more reassurance than is warranted. The family, the doctor knows, needs to be prepared for possible changes. If symptoms intensify, perhaps during puberty, early intervention or treatment—whether it is bracing for scoliosis or surgery on tumors beginning to cause discomfort—may be needed to ward off severe problems later.

Families may find it helpful to realize that there may be peaks and plateaus in the course of NF, and that this allows regrouping of psychological, financial, and physical resources for the next medical problem, if it comes.

NEUROFIBROMATOSIS'S IMPACT ON SIBLINGS AND OTHER RELATIVES

When several family members have NF, there seems to be more understanding among family members and less of a sense of isolation and fear. If only one person in the family is affected, more difficulties may arise. Often brothers and sisters of the affected individual, grandparents, or anyone "on the outside looking in" have a difficult time in keeping the disorder and its effects into perspective. Siblings who do not have NF are often concerned about the possibility of the symptoms developing in them later in life, or about their grandchildren having the disorder. The brothers and sisters of the affected individual may intellectually understand that if a person does not have NF, then that person cannot pass it on, and that it does not skip generations; however, emotionally, the concern may remain. Upon hearing that his younger sister was diagnosed as having NF, a young teenager made a decision to not ever get married or have any children even though he did not have the disorder.

Unaffected siblings, parents, children, grandparents, and spouse need support along the way, too. They may feel guilty that they are not affected with the disorder. They may have difficulty in accepting the family member with NF—whether it is a parent or sibling—and not wish to have anything to do with the affected person. They may resent being saddled with too much responsibility for their affected relative or for having to stand up for him or her. They may feel rejected by their parents who must spend endless time and energy on their affected child[(2)].

Impact on the family can also be in terms of broken dreams and changed plans—which might not even have been verbalized. A parent who learns early in their child's school career that he or she has learning disabilities experiences disappointment that the child cannot follow in their educational footsteps. A mother may grieve over a normal child that was not born to her.

FAMILY DECISIONS

At times, tough decisions have to be made by individual family members and by the family as a unit. Adults who have NF may have to make significant decisions about marriage and having children. The choice of profession and employment is a major decision in which the family may be called upon to participate. The following questions may be asked in preparation for seeking employment:

- Is the job located near or in an area with sophisticated medical facilities that are familiar with NF?
- Will this mean uprooting the family?
- Dare I tell about having a potentially disfiguring medical condition?
- Is there comprehensive medical insurance that includes coverage for a preexisting condition?

Douglas R. Fox of the Multiple Sclerosis National Capital Chapter offers the following advice derived from his own experience in the job market[3]:

- If you don't have a marketable skill, get one through education, job retraining, or whatever is necessary.
- Be comfortable with yourself.
- Accept [NF]—don't let [NF] rule you; you are the boss.
- Disclose the fact that you or a family member has [NF] when *you* feel the need, either externally or within yourself.

Parents of a child or children with NF are often faced with another set of tough decisions, such as:

- How often do we let our children be "put on exhibit" for teaching medical personnel at teaching hospitals? Do we have to exhibit them at all? Could they benefit in the long run from allowing this?
- How do I know whether or not the child has a learning disability?
- How often is a physical checkup necessary?
- How often should the child have a computed tomography (CT) scan or other medical tests?
- Is recommended surgery really necessary?

A discussion of the medical questions listed above will be found in other chapters of the handbook. In general, the key watchword for families with NF is preparedness—preparedness for the unpredictable. And the best way to be prepared is to be armed with as much accurate, up-to-date information about NF as possible.

At various times there are "crisis points" (adapted from D.D. Cowell, unpublished lecture, Wash., D.C., 1986) that a lot of people with long-term conditions, including individuals with NF and their families have:

- When the diagnosis is made or comprehended
- When surgery or medication is necessary
- When there are side effects of the treatment
- Waiting for "success" of the treatment
- Re-entry into a regular routine
- Setback due to recurrence of problem or new problem
- Search for additional and/or alternative treatment
- In some cases, being faced with death

The Financial Impact of Neurofibromatosis

For some families the financial burden of medical expenses may be largely born by insurance. Others experience great difficulty in getting insurance coverage, so that finding the money for medical care becomes an overriding concern. In any case, such costs as the first visit to a physician's office, transportation and lodging when visits to distant specialty medical centers are required, time off from work, or child care may not be covered. Over a long period of time, these expenses can take their toll and have a major impact on the family's financial status. Much as a family may wish to do everything possible for a child, or other relative, with NF, the realities of the financial burden can give rise to stress, hardship, and even resentment, if only on an unconscious level.

When the Problems Are Too Great

Individuals with more severe cases of NF, and their families, are not always able to summon up the emotional and physical strength required to cope with the problems with disorder can cause. Disfigurement, social isolation, loneliness, and fear of serious medical complications can be burdens too great for some families to carry. It is urgent in such situations that families receive the assistance they need.

Sources of Help

The intensity of the impact that NF has on the family depends largely on the strength of the family's support system. The closeness of the family itself seems to provide the greatest support over a sustained period of time. For some, a deep religious faith is equally important. Friends, neighbors, and associates provide invaluable support by babysitting, preparing food, giving time off for doctor's appointments, etc., and also by being willing to listen when difficult situations arise.

Genetic counselors and social workers can help families with specific suggestions for obtaining information about NF-related situations, and about financial, psychotherapeutic, and other support services.

The NNFF and its chapters across the country not only provide up-to-date information about the disorder, local physicians who are familiar with NF, and appropriate medical facilities, but also offer contact with other NF families who are willing to discuss similar concerns.

The value of talking with other NF families cannot be overestimated. The sense of isolation seems to melt away. When talking with other parents or individuals affected by similar manifestations of NF, families may glean "helpful hints" in coping with the disorder, doctors, the health system, the educational system, and other family members, all of which can be invaluable in realizing that specific things can be done in dealing with the disorder, and that the family can survive! Although the manifestations and the severity of NF vary widely, the underlying anxiety of not knowing what it going to happen or when is a common bond among all NF families. Finding others who share this bond brings comfort and strength to each family.

CONCLUSION

A clear message from the NNFF is *hope*. Families affected by NF are working together through the Foundation to make the hope of finding the cause and an effective treatment for symptoms of NF a reality. They volunteer many hours to raise funds for the NNFF Research Fund, from which grants and fellowships are awarded annually to researchers for the study of NF. They participate in NF research projects that further understanding of the disorder. They have greatly enhanced awareness of NF in the medical community, the general public, and Congress by telling their personal NF stories. It is families in the NNFF sharing with other NF families who can provide the unique understanding and unique contribution to all who are affected by NF.

REFERENCES

1. B. Fairfield. Understanding the family drama: Guidelines for counseling strategies. Perspect Genet Counsel 1983;5(2):9–11.
2. J.O. Weiss. Psychosocial Stress in Genetic Disorders: A Guide for Social Workers. *Social Work in Health Care*, 1981; 6(4):14–18.
3. D.R. Fox. A Crucial Job-Hunt Question: Should I Tell? *Inside Multiple Sclerosis*, 1985; 3(3):24–27.

BIBLIOGRAPHY

J.O. Weiss, B.A. Bernhardt, and N.W. Paul, eds. Genetic disorders and birth defects in families and society: Toward interdisciplinary understanding. New York, March of Dimes Birth Defects Foundation, 1984.

J.O. Weiss, et al., eds. Genetics support groups: Volunteers and professionals as partners. New York, Maternal and Child Health and March of Dimes Birth Defects Foundation, 1986.

20

Psychosocial Aspects of Appearance in Neurofibromatosis

Sarah A. Ellis, Ph.D.

Neurofibromatosis (NF) may bring many sufferings to its victims, and among the most poignant is the burden of a changed or disfigured appearance. So basic is the mental image of our bodies to our total sense of self that any change, even for the better, is hard to integrate. Dealing with an altered appearance demands a painful self-confrontation and re-examination of personal values to regain equanimity. In addition to the psychological struggle, there is social stress from the reactions of others to abnormal appearance. In the last 20 years psychologists have explored the impact of physical appearance on an individual's environment and have documented the effect that looks have on people's lives (1). The loss of good looks and normal appearance is no trivial matter. Professionals need a sensitive awareness of this to help patients in their efforts to attain a new equilibrium and a satisfying life.

Psychological Adjustment

The development of a body image is of central importance to our functioning within a social and cultural context. This image is the mental representation or perception of our body at any moment in time. Our sense of reality and sense of identity as separate persons are rooted in bodily experiences. As infants see and touch outside objects and parts of their bodies, they gradually differentiate between inner and outer, between self and the outside world. Along with a cognitive plan of their bodies, they acquire a sense of spacial relations and orientation. Gradually the images of the separate parts are integrated into a whole, and this becomes the basis of a sense of continuity of the self. In time, the body image comes to include feelings, evaluations, and attitudes toward the self acquired from other people's reactions. Thus the body image is central to the self-image.

The basic integration process occurs in the toddler period, a time when children are very sensitive to separation and vulnerable to fears about the loss of beloved parents and other security figures. Later in life, alteration or loss of body parts can re-awaken these primitive fears. Concern about body alteration appears in many children's stories, for example, "Alice in Wonderland," "Pinocchio," and the "Frog Prince." In fact, the myths of all cultures are full of transformation themes, often involving punishment for wrongdoing or the capricious spite of some supernatural being. Bodily changes brought on by disease threaten our emotional security at a deep level. For people affected with NF, the proliferation of tumors, particularly on the face, is not simply an insult to vanity, but an assault on the security of physical integrity and on the ongoing sense of identity and self-esteem.

SOCIAL ADJUSTMENT

The stress of disfigurement is social as well as psychological, for a person's appearance has a powerful and pervasive impact on how he or she is treated by others. Paying close attention to the faces of others is instinctual behavior: studies of newborn babies show that they gaze longest at patterns that have the configuration of a human face. Throughout life we are constantly aware of the appearance of others for what it will communicate about moods, intentions, expectations, and reactions to ourselves. We attend to people's expressions, gestures, and bodily attitudes. The face and hands are central to communications, but all parts of the body contribute. The communicative importance of this mutual monitoring is clear when you consider how much you know about people and interpersonal situations that is never verbalized.

Our sensitive awareness of each other's bodies ensures that even a minor distortion will attract attention and make its owner feel self-conscious and exposed. Any visible damage to the face in particular is liable to cause a pervasive sense of shame and loss. The curiosity, pity, and aversion the sufferer meets in the eyes of others can disrupt interpersonal relations and result in social withdrawal and loneliness.

PHYSICAL BEAUTY AS A CULTURAL VALUE

In our society normal physique and attractive appearance are strong cultural values. This is obvious from TV ads, the plethora of beauty products on drug store shelves, etc. However, the present high emphasis on physical attractiveness conflicts with our religious and democratic ideals. Traditionally, Americans have cherished the concepts of equal opportunity for all and of character and hard work as the basis of success. We say, "Don't judge a book by its cover," and "Beauty is skin deep." The conflict between our traditional values and the emphasis on beauty and health makes us highly uncomfortable. Our guilt and embarrassment are aroused in encounters with people who have a visible disfigurement. The social awkwardness adds to their distress. The notion that a person's physical attractiveness has a significant and pervasive effect on the quality of his or her life is unwelcome.

A sampling of circumstances in which studies have indicated that the attractive receive preferential treatment will give a picture of the surprising power of the stereotype. Attractive adults are at an advantage in securing jobs. If they go for counseling, they are viewed as less psychologically disturbed and more likely to improve. They are more likely to receive help from strangers. Essays of college students were more favorably evaluated by peers if they believed the writer to be attractive. Having an attractive companion enhances a person's social prestige.

The impact of attractiveness begins at an early age. A number of researchers have explored how attractive and unattractive children receive differential treatment from adult caretakers and other children. It appears that attractive children develop in an atmosphere far more welcoming and supportive: for example when teachers were given identical descriptions along with a picture of an attractive or an unattractive child, they systematically rated the attractive children, both boys and girls, more favorably. They were more likely to place an unattractive child in a class for the mentally retarded, predicted less academic success for them, more psychological disturbance, and more difficulty in peer relations. When serious, the transgressions of attractive children were evaluated less severely and the children viewed as less likely to have an enduring tendency toward antisocial behavior.

All in all, the attractiveness research demonstrates a robust stereotype that attractive people are better, more competent, and desirable. Of course, real life is far more complex than a stereotype allows for. If an individual's self-concept is indeed the product of the treatment he or she receives from others, then the attractive should have high self-esteem while unattractive or disfigured people should feel far less satisfaction with themselves. Some researchers have found attractive people to be more confident, but the expected advantage of the attractive person is not clear. Ellen Berscheid and her associates (2) found no significant relationship between the physical attractiveness of a group of men and women and their own body image or satisfaction with their nonphysical attributes. Furthermore, there is no evidence that attractive people are happier.

In the social climate set by our emphasis on physical beauty and health, people with facial and bodily disfigurement suffer continuous social stress. A facial deformity in particular cannot be hidden. It constitutes an ever-present obstacle to being comfortably accepted by others until familiarity with the afflicted person can partially outweigh the strangeness, embarrassment, or outright hostility often felt in the presence of people perceived as different or abnormal. They are frequently stared at, rejected, and discriminated against. Along with the unremitting negative attention they must endure in daily life, they have fewer options vocationally and socially. When they marry, they often feel that they must settle for any willing partner. Many internalize the devalued image reflected by society and become depressed and reclusive.

When a child is not merely unattractive, but facially disfigured, his or her appearance may have a strong negative impact on school authorities, as anyone who works regularly with such children can attest. Children with deformities as can occur in NF may encounter resistance to placement in regular classes; the school's rational is that their appearance will upset other children. Because of appearance, they may be assumed to be retarded. Families and friends of such children are well aware of how severely they can be stigmatized in school (3).

THE FEAR OF LOSS OF HEALTH

Visible changes from a disorder such as NF present a physical threat as well as a psychological and social one. Health as well as beauty is a strong cultural value among modern people. In folktales good health is usually associated with virtue, illness with sin and punishment. The ugly are often wicked, and the wicked are scourged with bodily ills. Such ideas influence us in an unconscious way and many lead people who are ill or disfigured to feel that their condition is a punishment for wrongdoing. Children, normally egocentric in their thinking, tend to see themselves as causing their own misfortunes. In adulthood, the legacy of childlike thinking about causation that we all retain tends to evoke a sense of responsibility for our illnesses, and their visible effects. With feelings of guilt associated with disease, the sight of an obviously ill person can arouse anxiety in others and make them avoid him or her, sometimes without being aware that they are doing so.

From the start of life the body image is a central part of the sense of identity (4). Normally, bodily changes come slowly enough to be integrated, but the rapid changes brought by illness can make a person feel strange to himself, lost and disoriented. The loss of familiar looks is a grievous blow to self-esteem. A sense of deterioration in one aspect of appearance may spread to the body image as a whole, and from there to other aspects of the self, so that disabled people may lose confidence in their abilities and the general acceptability as persons. As a disability becomes more visible, the sufferer must struggle harder against feelings of inferiority and alienation. Since appearance is particularly associated with feeling sexually attractive, a person who feels that his or her appearance is deteriorating may withdraw from a lover or spouse. The partner is afraid of hurting the ill one, so there is a danger of mutual silence with loss of contact and emotional support.

Furthermore, a change in appearance is a sign of the illness itself—a signal to the patient and those around him or her of its existence and advance. People who are ill, after all, do not necessarily look ill; people with heart conditions, for example. Those developing disfiguring changes are forced into a confrontation with the fact of the illness and cannot deny or overlook it. This means the loss of an important defense. All of us use denial to deal with threatening or painful circumstances we can do little about. This kind of selective inattention is constructive in that it protects our peace of mind and leaves us free to put our energy into dealing with things we can do more about. For people with an incurable illness, this poignant confrontation may render them more vulnerable to anxiety and depression. Of course, many factors will influence how an individual copes with chronic illness and the degree to which he or she can make peace with it, but to lose denial is to lose a helpful respite from the struggle (5).

ADJUSTING TO AN ALTERED PHYSICAL APPEARANCE

Living constructively with a disfiguring illness presents its victims with a difficult challenge. However, despite the hard social realities of life within a culture obsessed with physical beauty and health, people who are afflicted often show amazing courage, resilience, and resources in making their lives rich and full.

Primary to attaining equilibrium is the development of a value system that subordinates beauty to more attainable and enduring goals. It needs to be based on a concept of individual worth as a person, not as an object or a commodity. Strength and pride in overcoming adversity can be expressed in helping others in distress. In her follow-up studies of facially disfigured patients, Frances Macgregor (6) found that many of them worked in the helping professions. The growth of the self-help movement of recent years attests to the psychological benefits of reaching out to others to share problems and solutions and of becoming an advocate for one's own interests in the community at large. Work and other activities providing self-affirmation play an important role for people fighting a stigmatizing condition.

In interpersonal situations first meetings remain a problem, but most facially disfigured people learn gradually to navigate the formation of new friendships, allowing the other person time to get used to the unfamiliar physical appearance. A flexible use of psychological coping strategies, including the use of denial and the avoidance of aggravating situations at times, is needed since one cannot fight adversity all the time (7,8).

Very important, too, is the emotional support of family and friends who validate one's worth. When there is a basic self-respect, a disfigurement of some part of the body need not contaminate a person's entire view of his or her looks. Also, one can enjoy one's physical self in many other ways besides as an object of admiration. For example, one need not be a bathing beauty at the beach to enjoy the sun and wind on your skin and the coolness of the ocean.

SUMMARY

The competitiveness in our society and our way of evaluating our qualities by comparison with others rather than by what they can do for ourselves reduces pleasure in life for all of us. If we think about appearance less in terms of standards that we ought to meet, the changes in appearance due to illness, like those due to aging, need not be a cause for shame or inferiority, but simply one aspect of the person. Particularly as we grow older, a heavy emphasis on beauty and health needs to give way to more enduring human qualities, such as courage, humor, and compassion. Thus we affirm our awareness of the value and dignity of human beings and of their right to respectful and humane treatment no matter how they look.

REFERENCES

1. G.R. Adams. Physical attractiveness research: A developmental social psychology of beauty. Hum Dev 1977;20:217–239.
2. E. Berscheid. Physical attractiveness. In L. Berkowitz, ed. Advances in experimental social psychology. Baltimore, Williams and Wilkins, 1974, pp. 157–215.
3. J.M. Goin and M.K. Goin. Changing the body. Baltimore, Williams and Wilkins, 1981.
4. S.M. Kalick. Toward an interdisciplinary psychology of appearance. Psychiatry 1968;41:243–253.
5. R. Lazarus. Positive denial: the case for not facing reality. Psychol Today 1979;12:44–60.
6. F.C. Macgregor. After plastic surgery. New York, Praeger Publishers, 1979.
7. F.C. Macgregor. Transformation and identity. New York, Quadrangle, New York Times Book, 1974.
8. B.A. Wright. Physical disability: A psychological approach. New York, Harper and Bros., 1960.

SECTION IV

APPENDICES

APPENDIX A

The National Neurofibromatosis Foundation

Peter R.W. Bellermann, Executive Director

The National Neurofibromatosis Foundation (NNFF) was established in 1978 as a means of stimulating clinical and basic research on neurofibromatosis (NF), and enhancing public and professional education about the disorder. Today the Foundation sponsors and manages a broad spectrum of programs as follows:

Research

The NNFF supports basic research designed to determine the cause and cure for NF. Such support is provided through 1-year research grants and postdoctoral, 2-year *Young Investigator Awards.* Support is based on recommendations from the Foundation's Research Advisory Board. The Board peer-reviews all applicants and consists of leading scientists and clinicians from all parts of the United States and several foreign institutions. Applications are solicited annually and should be submitted no later than April of each year.

Research Newsletter

The NNFF publishes a quarterly Research Newsletter in an effort to chronicle and disseminate the most significant research developments in NF. The Research Newsletter has a subscriber list of about 1500 in the United States and abroad.

Clinical Care

The NNFF's Clinical Care Program is designed to oversee the development of specialized clinical care centers in the United States and to develop diagnostic standards and protocols. The Clinical Care Program functions through the NNFF's Clinical Care Advisory Board. The members of the Clinical Care Advisory Board have assumed particular areas of oversight as follows:

1. Therapeutic claims
2. Diagnostic criteria, screening, and follow-up
3. Socioeconomic issues
4. Data base and information management
5. NF clinics/referral centers
6. Ethical issues

SYMPOSIA

The NNFF conducts symposia for physicians, health-care specialists, and interested lay public. The symposia are designed to broaden the understanding of NF in the medical and lay communities, to facilitate active interchanges among specialists on their research activities, and to disseminate general information of interest to specialists and the lay public.

PUBLIC EDUCATION

The NNFF works to promote public awareness of NF in the United States. Toward that end, the Foundation creates public education programs. It produces and disseminates educational materials in film and video form; booklets for patients, families, and children; and public service announcements for broadcast on radio and television.

PATIENT SERVICES

The NNFF is a clearinghouse for information on NF. It also provides referral services to NF specialists and clinical care facilities. The Foundation maintains a library of NF publications and sells books, periodicals, and miscellaneous informational materials published elsewhere.

The Foundation also publishes and disseminates the following publications, the use of which is recommended in conjunction with professional medical care:

1. *Neurofibromatosis: Information for Patients and Families*
2. *Neurofibromatosis: A Handbook for Parents*
3. *Neurofibromatosis: A Handbook for Kids*

Neurofibromatosis Newsletter

The NNFF publishes a quarterly newsletter for use by the general public. The newsletter has a circulation of about 22,000 in the United States and abroad. The newsletter provides NF information to the lay public on such topics as Foundation programs, research, clinical issues, fundraising, public education programs, and chapter activities.

Chapter Development

As a grassroots organization, the NNFF functions through its chapters across the United States. The chapters are the key to fundraising, patient services, and creating awareness in their areas. The chapters are usually staffed by volunteers, many of whom have NF. Chapter activities include solicitation of memberships, managing special events, publication of newsletters, holding support group meetings, and public education activities.

* * * *

For additional information please contact:
National Neurofibromatosis Foundation
141 Fifth Avenue, Suite 7-S
New York, NY 10010
(212) 460-8980 (NY State)
(800) 323-7938

The National Neurofibromatosis Foundation, Inc.

Chapters

California Chapter
Diane E. Melone
President
1606 Del Dayo Drive
Carmichael, CA 95608
916-482-3418

Colorado Chapter
Tim Gardiner, President
PO Box 2393
Evergreen, CO 80439
(h) 303-674-2074
(o) 303-670-3408

Connecticut Chapter
c/o Jodi Rucquoi
Yale NF Clinic
333 Howard Avenue
New Haven, CT 06510
203-785-2660

Florida Chapter
C. Daniel Holmes
President
2460 Royal Oaks Drive
Tallahassee, FL 32308
904-893-8610

Georgia Chapter
Shela Baird, President
2518 Mill Ridge Circle
Lawrenceville, GA 30244
404-978-1415

Illinois Chapter
Beverly & Lewis Oberlander
Co-Presidents
1418 Rose Blvd.
Buffalo Grove, IL 60089
312-259-1315

Indiana Chapter
Lila Seelen, President
4132 Alahambra Drive
Anderson, IN 46013
317-642-0176

Iowa Chapter
Karen Bedard, President
1924 Mulberry St.
Waterloo, IA 50703
319-235-7500

Kentucky Chapter
Eleanor Van Pelt
President
5102 Princewood Place
Louisville, KY 40216
502-447-8946

Louisiana Gulfcoast Chapter
Geneva Landry
President
572 Oakwood Drive
Gretna, LA 70056
504-366-9440

Massachusetts Chapter
Bill and Rita Needel
Co-Presidents
68 Samoset Avenue
Quincy, MA 02169
617-472-0582

Michigan Chapter
Richard Mette, President
244 Birch Hill
Rochester, MI 48064
313-651-8026
answering service
313-351-4350

Missouri Chapter
Phillip L. Lilley
President
1810 Dougherty Estate Drive
Manchester, MO 63021
Missouri Neurofibromatosis Line
314-391-7872

New Jersey Chapter
Donna Oettinger
President
271-B Reichelt Road
New Milford, NJ 07646
201-265-2354

New York State Chapter
Susan Novak, President
RD 2 Mountainview Rd.
Box 70
Putnam Valley, NY 10579
914-528-9121

Ohio Chapter
Dolores Goldfinger
President
3709 Donegal Drive
Cincinnati, OH 45236
513-891-0725

Oregon Chapter
Bob Peterson
President
9920 N. Jersey
Portland, OR 97203
503-286-0084

Pennsylvania Chapter
Joyce Demain
President
238 Birch Avenue
Pittsburgh, PA 15228
412-563-2954

Rhode Island Chapter
Joyce A. McElhaney
President
21 Hoxsie Road
West Kingston, RI 02892
401-539-2550

Utah Chapter
John C. Carey, M.D.
Acting President
Department of Pediatrics
University of Utah Medical Center
Salt Lake City, UT 84132
801-581-6956

Washington State Chapter
Mr. Kim Herman
President
P.O. Box 25883
Seattle, WA 98125
206-746-1970

MEDICAL BOARDS

Medical Director

Allan E. Rubenstein
Medical Director NNFF
Mount Sinai School of Medicine
New York, NY 10029

Research Advisory Board

Co-chairmen

Richard Bunge, M.D.
Washington Univ. School of Medicine
St. Louis, MO

Robert Martuza, M.D.
Massachusetts General Hospital
Harvard Medical School
Boston, MA

Members

Barry G.W. Arnason, M.D.
The Pritzker School of Medicine
University of Chicago
Chicago, IL

Ira Black, M.D.
Cornell University Medical College
New York, NY

John C. Carey, M.D.
University of Utah Medical Center
Salt Lake City, UT

Dr. Thomas Caskey
Baylor College of Medicine
Institute for Molecular Genetics
Houston, TX

Dr. Francis Collins
The University of Michigan
Medical Center
Ann Arbor, MI

David E. Comings, M.D.
City of Hope
National Medical Center
Duarte, CA

Roswell Eldridge, M.D.
Clinical Neurogenetics, NES
NINCDS-National Institutes of Health
Bethesda, MD

Kenneth Fischbeck, M.D.
University of Pennsylvania
School of Medicine
Philadelphia, PA

Robert J. Gorlin, D.D.S.
University of Minnesota
Minneapolis, MN

James F. Gusella, Ph.D.
Massachusetts General Hospital
Harvard Medical School
Boston, MA

Judith Hall, M.D.
University of British Columbia
Vancouver, B.C., Canada

David E. Housman, Ph.D.
Massachusetts Institute of Technology
Center for Cancer Research
Cambridge, MA

William G. Johnson, M.D.
Columbia University
College of Physicians & Surgeons
New York, NY

Anna T. Meadows, M.D.
University of Pennsylvania
Medical School
Philadelphia PA

John J. Mulvihill, M.D.
National Cancer Institute
Clinical Epidemiology Branch
Bethesda, MD

James Patrick, M.D.
Baylor College of Medicine
Institute for Molecular Genetics
Houston, TX

David Pleasure, M.D.
University of Pennsylvania
Medical School
Philadelphia, PA

Bruce Ponder, M.D., Ph.D.
Cambridge University
Cambridge, England

Nancy Ratner, M.D.
University of Cincinnati
School of Medicine
Cincinnati, OH

Allan Roses, M.D.
Duke University
Durham, NC

Roger Rosenberg, M.D.
Univ. of Texas Health Science Center
Dallas, TX

Allan E. Rubenstein, M.D.
Mount Sinai School of Medicine
New York, NY

Lucien J. Rubinstein, M.D.
Univ. of Virginia School of Medicine
Charlottesville, VA

R. Neil Schimke, M.D.
College of Health Sciences and Hospital
The University of Kansas
Kansas City, KS

Dr. Bernd Seizinger
Neurogenetics Laboratory
Massachusetts General Hospital
Harvard Medical School
Boston, MA

James Weston, Ph.D.
University of Oregon
Eugene, OR

Dr. Raymond L. White
University of Utah Medical Center
Salt Lake City, UT

Honorary Member

John Holt, M.D.
Ann Arbor, MI

Clinical Care Advisory Board

Co-chairmen

John C. Carey, M.D.
University of Utah Medical Center
Salt Lake City, UT

Bruce Korf, M.D., Ph.D.
Children's Hospital/Boston
Harvard Medical School
Boston, MA

Members

Dr. Arthur Aylsworth
University of North Carolina
Chapel Hill, NC

Alvin Crawford, M.D.
University of Cincinnati
Medical Center
Cincinnati, OH

David Dunn, M.D.
University of Indiana
Indianapolis, IN

Carol Greene, M.D.
University of Colorado Health Sciences Center
Denver, CO

Dean MacEwen, M.D.
LSU School of Medicine
New Orleans, LA

Prof. Joan Marks
Sarah Lawrence College
Bronxville, NY

Reed E. Pyeritz, M.D., Ph.D.
The Johns Hopkins Hospital
Baltimore, MD

Allan E. Rubenstein, M.D.
Mount Sinai School of Medicine
New York, NY

Ann Spence, M.D.
University of Southern California
Neuropsychiatric Institute
Los Angeles, CA

Peter R.W. Bellermann
National Neurofibromatosis Foundation
New York, NY

APPENDIX B

Neurofibromatosis Clinics and Centers

The following is a revised list of NF Clinics in North America. It contains centers which responded to a survey conducted by the National Neurofibromatosis Foundation (NNFF) and contains only those centers which stated that they had an NF clinic which met the criteria established by the NNFF. In addition to these facilities, most of the genetic centers in North America are involved in the care of NF patients even though some may not have designated themselves as NF patients clinics. (A complete list of genetic centers is available from the March of Dimes.) This list will be updated on a regular basis. The criteria of being listed as a clinic are available through the National Neurofibromatosis Foundation.

John C. Carey, MD
Bruce Korf, MD
Co-chairmen
Clinical Care Advisory Board
The National Neurofibromatosis Foundation

David Dunn, MD
Chairman
CCAB Clinics and Centers
Committee

ALABAMA
University of South Alabama
Gulf Coast Region Neurofibromatosis Clinic
Wladimir Wertelecki, M.D.
Dept. of Medical Genetics
Room 214 CC/CB
Mobile, AL 36688
205-460-7500

ARKANSAS
University of Arkansas for Medical Sciences
Genetics Clinic
Laura Keppen, M.D./Linda Fair
4301 W. Markham Street
Little Rock, AR 72205
501-370-2966

ARIZONA
The Genetics Center of Southwest Biomedical Research Inst.
NF Clinic
Judith Allanson, Director
6401 E. Thomas Rd.
Scottsdale, AZ 85251
602-945-4363

Phoenix Children's Hospital
Allen M. Kaplan, M.D.
909 East Brill Street
Phoenix, AZ 85006
602-239-4855

CALIFORNIA
Cedars-Sinai Birth Defects Center
John M. Graham, Jr., M.D.
Cathy Charman, R.N.
444 S. San Vicente Blvd.
Suite 1001
Los Angeles, CA 90048
213-855-2211

Children's Hospital of Los Angeles
NF Center
Warren E. Cohen, M.D.
Division of Medical Genetics
PO Box 54700
Los Angeles, CA 90054-0700
213-669-2178

Northern California NF Clinic at Children's Hospital/Oakland
John P. Johnson, M.D.
747 52nd St.
Oakland, CA 94609
415-428-3550

Los Angeles County
University of Southern California Medical Center
Genetics Clinic
Atsuko Fujimoto, M.D.
Genetics Division, 1G-24
1129 North State St.
Los Angeles, CA 90033
213-226-3816

University of California/Irvine
Maureen Bocian, M.D./
Ann Walker, M.A.
Division of Human Genetics
Dept. of Pediatrics
UCI Medical Center
101 City Drive South
Orange, CA 92668
714-634-5789

COLORADO
University of Colorado Medical Center
Eva Sujansky, M.D./
Vivian Wang, M.S.
4200 East 9th Avenue, Box B-160
Denver, CO 80262
303-270-8742

CONNECTICUT
Yale University School of Medicine
Yale NF Clinic
Margretta R. Seashore, M.D./
J. K. Rucquoi, M.S., Directors
Department of Human Genetics
333 Cedar St., 305 WWW
New Haven, CT 06510
203-785-2660

University of Connecticut Health Center
Francis J. DiMario, Jr./
Robert M. Greenstein
Co-Coordinators
Neuro Genetics Clinic
Farmington Ave.
Farmington, CT 06032
203-679-3535

DELAWARE
Alfred I. Du Pont Institute
NF Program
Susan B. Stine, M.D./
Linda Nicholson, M.S., M.C.
P.O. Box 269, 1600 Rockland Road
Wilmington, DE 19899
302-651-4234

FLORIDA
University of Florida
College of Medicine
Dept. of Pediatrics/Div. Genetics
Charles Williams, M.D./
Lavanya Marfatia, M.S.
Box J-296
J. Hillis Miller Health Center
Gainesville, FL 32610
904-392-4104

University of Miami Medical School
NF Center
Mislen Bauer, M.D.
Dept. of Pediatrics
6125 SW 31 Street
Miami, FL 33155
305-665-9717
305-666-6511, Ext. 2385
and
North Broward Medical Center
Mislen Bauer, M.D./
Fram Kartz, M.S. (Coordinator)
201 East Sample Road, Suite 321
Pompano Beach, FL 33064
305-786-7346

University of South Florida Medical Center
NF Clinic
Boris G. Kousseff, M.D.
Director of Medical Genetics
Joanne Meares, L.P.N.
Clinic Coordinator
Box 15-G
Tampa, FL 33612
813-974-3310

Nemours Children's Clinic
Charlotte Lafer, M.D./
Suzanne Russo, M.S.
P.O. Box 5720
Jacksonville, FL 32247
904-390-3726

GEORGIA
Medical College of Georgia
Genetics Clinic
David B. Flannery, M.D.
Division of Medical Genetics
BG-121
Augusta, GA 30912
404-721-2809

ILLINOIS
Michael Reese Medical Center
NF Clinic
Mildred Schwartz, Jr., M.D.
2915 South Ellis-3KK
Chicago, IL 60616
312-791-4233

The Children's Memorial Hospital
NF Clinic (only children 0-16)
Robert Listernick, M.D.
Division of General and
Emergency Pediatrics
2300 Children's Plaza
Chicago, IL 60614
312-880-3832

INDIANA
Indiana University NF Clinic
David Dunn, M.D.
Neurology Dept.
1001 West 10th St.
Indianapolis, IN 46202
317-630-6103

IOWA
University of Iowa NF Clinic
Mary Waziri, M.D.
Dept. Peds./Div. Genetics
T304 University Hospital
Iowa City, IA 52242
319-356-4890

KANSAS
Kansas University Medical Center
Genetics—NF Clinic
R. N. Schimke, M.D.
39th & Rainbow
Kansas City, KS 66103
913-588-6043

KENTUCKY
University of Louisville,
Child Evaluation Center
Laura Profumo, M.S.W.
334 E. Broadway
Louisville, KY 40202
502-588-5331

LOUISIANA
Tulane Hospital
NF Clinic
Diane Africk, M.D.
Dept. of Neurology
1415 Tulane Ave.
New Orleans, LA 70112
504-588-5231

MARYLAND
Johns Hopkins Hospital
Neurofibromatosis Clinic
Reed E. Pyeritz, M.D., Ph.D.
Blalock 1008
600 North Wolfe St.
Baltimore, MD 21205
301-955-3122

Johns Hopkins Hospital
Pediatric Genetics Clinic
David Valle, M.D./
Linda Cooper, M.S.
Blalock 1008
600 North Wolfe St.
Baltimore, MD 21205
301-955-3071

National Institutes of Health
Interinstitute Medical Genetics Clinic
Sandra Schlesinger, Coordinator
Bldg. 10, Room 9C436 NIH
Bethesda, MD 20892
301-496-1380

MASSACHUSETTS
Franciscan Children's Hospital
& Rehabilitation Center
Murray Feingold, M.D.
National Birth Defects Center
30 Warren St.
Brighton, MA 02135
617-787-5958

The Children's Hospital, Boston
The Children's Hospital NF Program
Bruce Korf, M.D., Director
Ms. Leanne Haskin-Heady
Coordinator
300 Longwood Avenue
Boston, MA 02115
617-735-6394

Massachusetts General Hospital
NF Clinic
Robert L. Martuza, M.D., Director
15 Parkman St. ACC 312
Boston, MA 02114
617-726-3776

New England Medical Center
Birth Defects Clinic
Sydney Gellis, M.D.
Box 303
750 Washington St.
Boston, MA 02111
617-956-5451/956-5454

MICHIGAN
Henry Ford Hospital NF Clinic
Lester Weiss, M.D.
Medical Genetics and Birth Defects Center
2799 W. Grand Blvd.
Detroit MI 48202
313-876-3188

University of Michigan Hospital
NF Center
Francis S. Collins, M.D., Ph.D.
Division of Medical Genetics
4714 Medical Science II Bldg.
Box 0618
Ann Arbor, MI 48109-0618
313-747-3414
313-763-2532

MINNESOTA
University of Minnesota Hospital & Clinic
NF Clinic
Richard A. King, M.D., Ph.D.
Box 485 UMHC, 420 Delaware St. SE
Minneapolis, MN 55455
612-624-0144

MISSISSIPPI
University of Mississippi Medical Center
Neurogenetics Clinic
Robert Currier, M.D.
2500 North State St.
Jackson, MS 39216
601-984-5500

MISSOURI
Cardinal Glennon Children's Hospital
NF Clinic
Behrooz Akbarnia, M.D./Director
Liz Beckman, R.N., M.S.N., Coordinator
1465 S. Grand
St. Louis, MO 63104
314-577-5600, Ext. 6017

NEVADA
Neurofibromatosis Clinic of Nevada
Francis Paul Grenn, M.D.
3201 South Maryland Pkwy #600
Las Vegas, NV 89109
702-735-6164

NEW HAMPSHIRE
Dartmouth Medical Schoold
Dartmouth-Hitchcock Medical Center
NF Clinic
Melanie McDermet, M.S.
Clinical Genetics and Child Development Center
Dept. Maternal and Child Health
Hanover, NH 03756
603-646-5479

NEW JERSEY
Monmouth Medical Center
Neurocutaneous Syndrome Program
Susan Trecate, R.N., B.S.N.
Child Evaluation Services/ Pediatric Neurology
307 Third Avenue
Long Branch, NJ 07740
201-870-5216

NEW YORK
Children's Hospital of Buffalo—
SUNY/Buffalo
Michael E. Cohen, M.D.
Dept. of Neurology
Children's Hospital
219 Bryant St.
Buffalo, NY 14222
716-878-7530 Dr. Luther Robinson
716-878-7840 (Dir: Dr. Cohen)

Columbia-Presbyterian Med. Center
Babies Hospital
Genetics Clinic
Kwame Anyane-Yeboa, M.D./
Phyllis Taterka, M.S.
3959 Broadway, Room 202
New York, NY 10032
212-305-6731

Mount Sinai Hospital
NF Clinic
Allan E. Rubenstein, M.D./
Jane Halperin, M.S.
One Gustave Levy Place
New York, NY 10029
212-722-1784

NY Medical College
Westchester Medical Center
NF Clinic
Stanley Rothman, M.D.
Valhalla, NY 10595
914-285-8157 or 8158

North Shore University Hospital
NF Clinic
Anne Shields, C.S.W.
NSUH 300 Community Drive
Manhasset, NY 11030
516-562-4610

OHIO
University of Cincinnati
Dept. of Family Medicine
Family Practice Center
Andrew T. Filak, Sr., M.D.
234 Goodman St. ML 782
Cincinnati, OH 45267-0782
513-872-7594

University of Cincinnati College of Medicine
NF Clinic
Peter Dignan, M.D./
Patricia Stowens, R.N. (Coordinator)
Children's Hospital Medical Center
Elland & Bethesda Aves.
Pavillion Bldg 2-52C
Cincinnati, OH 54229-2899
513-559-4471

Cleveland Clinic
NF Center, Desk A120
A. David Rothner, M.D.
9500 Euclid Avenue
Cleveland, OH 44195-5045
216-444-5514

Wright State University
Ambulatory Care Facility
Richard C. Juberg, M.D., Ph.D.
Col. Glenn Highway
Dayton, OH 45435
513-873-3400

OKLAHOMA
University of Oklahoma
Children's Memorial Hospital
Genetics, Endocrinology & Metabolism
Adolpho Garnica, M.D.
PO Box 26901
Oklahoma City, OK 73190
405-271-4401
405-271-6764 (Dr. Garnica)

Children's Hospital of Oklahoma
Dept. of Pediatrics, Room 2B275
Neurogenetics Clinic
G. Bradley Schaefer, M.D.
940 NE 13th
Oklahoma City, OK 73104
405-271-3468

OREGON
Oregon Health Sciences University
Clinical Genetics Program
Child Development & Rehabilitation Center
Ellen Magenis, M.D.
CDRC P.O. Box 574
Portland, OR 97207
503-279-8344 (Clinic)
504-279-5289 (Dr. Magenis)
and
Eugene Office, CCD:
Kathi Marymee, Genetic Associate
Regional Services Center
Clinical Services Bldg.
901 East 18th
Eugene, OR 97403
503-686-3577

PENNSYLVANIA
Children's Hospital of Philadelphia
NF Clinic
Elaine H. Zackai, M.D.
34th St. and Civic Center Blvd.
Philadelphia, PA 19104
215-596-9800

Western Pennsylvania Hospital
Medical Genetics Clinic
Angela E. Lin, M.D.
4800 Friendship Ave.
Pittsburgh, PA 15224
412-578-7350

RHODE ISLAND
Rhode Island Hospital
NF Clinic
David Meryash, M.D./
Dianne Abuelo, M.D.
Co-Directors
593 Eddy St.
Providence, RI 02902
401-277-5685/277-8361

SOUTH CAROLINA
Greenwood Genetic Center
Robert A. Saul, M.D.
1 Gregor Mendel Circle
Greenwood, SC 29646
803-223-9411

TENNESSEE
Vanderbilt University
Genetics Clinic
John Phillips, M.D./Janet Ulm, M.S.
T-2404 Medical Center North
Nashville, TN 37232
615-322-7601

TEXAS
Children's Medical Center
NF Clinic
Michael Blaw, M.D./
Golder Wilson, M.D.
1935 Motor Street
Dallas, TX 75235
214-920-2744

UTAH
University of Utah Genetics Program
John C. Carey, M.D.
Dept. of Pediatrics
University of Utah School of Medicine
Salt Lake City, UT 84132
801-581-4943

WASHINGTON, D.C.
Children's Hospital National Medical Center
NF Clinic
Clinical Genetics Dept.
Kenneth N. Rosenbaum, M.D./
Jill Fonda Allen, M.S.
111 Michigan Ave. NW
Washington, DC 20010
202-745-2187

WISCONSIN
Children's Hospital of Wisconsin
NF Clinic
William B. Dobyns, M.D./
Jurgen Herrmann, M.D.
9000 W. Wisconsin Avenue
P.O. Box 1997
Milwaukee, WI 53201
414-266-2927

CANADA
Children's Hospital of Western Ontario
Joanne Sutherland, Genetics Associate
Box 5375
800 Commissioners Rd.
East London, Ontario
N6A4G5 CANADA
519-685-8140, Ext. 2424

The Montreal Children's Hospital
NF Clinic
June Ortenberg, M.D./
Vazken M. Der Kaloustian, M.D.
2300 Tupper Street
Montreal, Quebec
H3H1P3 CANADA
514-934-4427

Toronto Sick Children's Hospital
418 Kingswood Rd.
Toronto, Ontario
M4E3P3 CANADA

APPENDIX C

GLOSSARY

Acoustic neuroma—Benign tumor of the eighth cranial nerve (acoustic or hearing nerve) which causes hearing impairment (also called acoustic neurinoma or acoustic schwannoma).

Allele—Specific form of a gene. Each individual has two copies of every gene, one inherited from each parent. The particular forms of the gene inherited from each parent is referred to as an allele. Neurofibromatosis is due to an alteration of one of the two alleles at the neurofibromatosis gene locus.

Amniocentesis—Method of prenatal diagnosis in which a small amount of amniotic fluid which bathes the fetus is removed for genetic study. Usually performed at 16 to 20 weeks of gestation.

Angiogram—Means of visualizing blood vessels by x-ray taken after injection of dye into the vessel.

Anticonvulsant—Medication used to treat or prevent seizures.

Audiogram—Test of hearing acuity.

Autosomal dominant inheritance—Only one gene of a pair needs to be altered (mutated) for expression of a trait or disorder. A person who carries such a gene has a 50% chance of passing it on to any of his or her children. Neurofibromatosis is an autosomal dominant disorder.

BAER (brainstem auditory evoked responses)—Test of the brain pathway involved in hearing.

Bilateral—Affecting, or simply present on, both sides.

Biopsy—Surgical removal of tissue for examination for diagnostic purposes.

Café au lait spots—Light brown flat spots, variable in shape and size, commonly present on the skin of people with neurofibromatosis. Their presence constitutes an important sign that a person may be affected with neurofibromatosis.

Carcinoid—Hormone-secreting tumor found in many parts of the body, such as the gastrointestinal tract or lung. Rarely found in association with neurofibromatosis type 1.

CT scan—Computer processed x-ray which allows soft tissues inside the body to be visualized (also called CAT scan or computerized tomogram).

Cataract—Opacity of the lens of the eye. A specific type of cataract (presenile subcapsular) is seen in the eye in people with neurofibromatosis type 2.

Central neurofibromatosis—Another name for neurofibromatosis type 2.

Cerebral astrocytoma—A brain tumor containing cells derived from the glial cells (astrocytes or "star-shaped" cells) of the nervous system, which may be benign or malignant.

Cerebrospinal fluid (CSF)—Fluid which bathes the brain and spinal cord.

Chemotherapy—Treatment of person with malignant tumor by chemical agents.

Chorionic villus sampling—Method of prenatal diagnosis in which a small piece of fetal placenta is removed for genetic study. Can be performed in the first third of pregnancy.

Chromosomes—Structures located in the cell nucleus which contain genes determining hereditary characteristics.

Congenital—Present at birth.

Diplopia—Double vision, sometimes resulting from impairment of eye movements.
DNA—Deoxyribonucleic acid, chemical substance of which genes are made.
Dominant—See **Autosomal dominant inheritance.**
Dysplasia—Abnormal development of a part of the body.
EEG—Electroencephalogram, used to examine electrical activity of the brain for diagnosis of seizures and other problems of brain function.
EMG—Electromyogram, used to test for impairment of muscle function.
Evoked potentials—Methods for examining the electrical activity in the nervous system associated with perception of visual images or sounds. Used to assess the nerve pathways involved in vision or hearing.
Exophthalmos—Bulging forward of the eye, sometimes seen in individuals with neurofibromatosis type 1 who have a defect in sphenoid bone and/or orbital plexiform neurofibroma.
Expressivity—Degree to which a genetic trait is manifested.
Fibroblast—Cell type which is found in connective tissue throughout the body and is commonly used in medical tests and research which require analysis of "typical" cells grown in culture. These cells are not known to be abnormal in people with neurofibromatosis.
Fibroma—A tumor composed mainly of fibrous or connective tissue.
Gene—Basic unit of heredity.
Genotype—Particular combination of alleles occupying a gene locus in an individual.
Glaucoma—Increased pressure within the eyeball, which may occur in individuals with neurofibromatosis type 1 having a plexiform neurofibroma of the orbit.
Glioblastoma—A type of malignant brain tumor.
Glioma—A type of brain tumor.
Heterozygote—Individual who possesses different alleles at a gene locus on each of a pair of homologous chromosomes.
Homozygote—Individual who possesses the same allele at a gene locus on each of a pair of homologous chromosomes.
Hormone—Chemical substances secreted by glands in the body which serve particular roles.
Hydrocephalus—Presence of increased spinal fluid pressure within the ventricles of the brain.
Hypertrophy—Increase in the size of a part of the body.
Hypothalamus—Part of brain responsible for control of hormone secretion, appetite, and other "automatic" functions.
Kyphoscoliosis—Spinal deformity combining sideways curvature and hunching forward of the upper part of the spine.
Leukemia—Malignancy involving white blood cells, found rarely in association with neurofibromatosis type 1.
Linkage analysis—Method of mapping genes in relation to one another along the chromosome.
Lisch nodules—Small clumps of pigment on the iris of the eye, often seen in people with neurofibromatosis.
Macrodactyly—Enlargement of a digit.
Malignancy—Tumor growth that has tendency to spread through the body.
Marker gene—Gene which is closely linked to a locus of interest and which can be used to track the inheritance of that locus through a family.
Mast cell—Type of cell which is widely distributed throughout the body and particularly prevalent in neurofibroma tissue. This cell type secretes substances which may affect the behavior of other cells nearby. It has been implicated in the pathogenesis of neurofibromatosis, but such a role has not been proved.

Megalencephaly—Enlargement of the head.
Meiosis—Process of cell division which occurs exclusively in germ cells and functions to reduce the chromosome number from 46 to 23 in this cell lineage.
Melanosome—Structure inside melanocytes which contains pigment. Giant melanosomes are seen within pigment cells in a café au lait spot.
Meningioma—A benign tumor of the covering of the brain or spinal cord.
Mitosis—Process of cell duplication.
MRI scan—Magnetic resonance imaging, a new technique for visualizing soft tissues inside the body.
Mutation—A permanent, transmissible change in the genetic material, usually a single gene.
Myelin—The substance that forms an "insulating" sheath around many nerve fibers.
Myelogram—A means of examining the structures within the spine, including the spinal cord, employing x-ray visualization of the spine after injection of dye into the space which surrounds the spinal cord.
NCV—Nerve conduction velocity, test used to determine whether nerve function is impaired.
Nerve growth factor—Substance produced by certain tissues in the body which supports the growth and differentiation of certain types of nerve cells. These nerve cells, and some other cells, have receptors on their surface for nerve growth factor.
Neural crest—An embryonic structure which contains many of the cell types that tend to grow abnormally in neurofibromatosis.
Neurilemma—The thin membrane which spirally enwraps the myelin layers of myelinated nerves.
Neuro—Denotes relationship to a nerve or nerves, or to the nervous system.
Neurofibroma—A tumor of peripheral nerves caused by abnormal proliferation of Schwann cells and/or fibroblasts.
Neurofibromatosis—A disorder characterized by developmental changes in the nervous system, skin, bones, and often other tissues. The most distinctive features are the occurrence of multiple benign soft tumors (neurofibromas) and patches of skin pigmentation (café au lait spots).
Neurofibrosarcoma—Malignant tumor of nerve sheath (also called malignant schwannoma).
Neuroglia—Cells which support nerve cells (also known as glia, astrocytes, oligodendrocytes).
Neurons—Electrically active cells of the nervous system responsible for controlling behavior and body functions.
Noonan syndrome—Dominantly inherited disorder characterized by short stature, congenital heart disease, and distinctive appearance. Features of Noonan syndrome have been found in a small proportion of individuals with neurofibromatosis type 1.
Optic glioma—Tumor affecting the optic nerve which may occur in neurofibromatosis.
Optic nerve—Nerve which transmits visual information from the eye to the brain.
Orbit—Bony cavity of the skull in which lies the eyeball.
Penetrance—Proportion of individuals possessing a genetic trait who manifest specific features of the trait.
Peripheral—Situated away from the center or central nervous system.
Phenotype—Expression of a genetic trait.
Pheochromocytoma—Tumor of the adrenal gland which causes severe high blood pressure.
Pituitary—Gland located at the base of the brain which secretes hormones involved in growth, sexual function, and control of other endocrine glands.

Plexiform—Denotes a diffuse type of neurofibroma affecting a bundle or bundles of nerves.
Polymorphism—Genetic trait for which multiple alleles exist with appreciable frequency in the population.
Precocious puberty—Attainment of puberty abnormally early.
Proteus syndrome—Recently described disorder that causes overgrowth of parts of the body, as well as abnormalities of skin and bone. It has been suggested that The Elephant Man actually had Proteus syndrome rather than neurofibromatosis.
Pseudoarthrosis—A false joint. May result from fracture within long bone that does not heal in some people with neurofibromatosis.
Radiation therapy—Treatment of malignant tumor by exposure of the affected area to radiation, which kills tumor cells.
Recessive—Both members of a pair of genes need to be altered in order to have expression of the trait or disorder.
Recombination—Process whereby homologous chromosomes exchange segments during meiosis.
Restriction enzyme—Enzyme which cleaves DNA at a specific base sequence.
Restriction fragment length polymorphism—Difference in base sequence near a cloned fragment of DNA which occurs in some individuals and alters the ability of a particular restriction enzyme to cut the DNA. Used as the basis of tracking genes through families.
Retinoblastoma—Tumor of the retina of the eye, not found in association with neurofibromatosis. Molecular genetic studies of retinoblastoma have been valuable in elucidating genetic mechanisms of tumor formation.
Rhabdomyosarcoma—Malignant tumor of muscle cells, found rarely in association with neurofibromatosis type 1.
Sarcoma—Malignant soft-tissue tumor.
Schwann cell—The cell which provides the myelin that insulates peripheral nerves.
Schwannoma—Type of tumor composed of Schwann cells.
Scoliosis—An appreciable lateral deviation from the normally straight vertical line of the spine.
Segmental neurofibromatosis—Occurrence of features of neurofibromatosis confined to a specific part of the body. Thought by some to represent a mutation of the neurofibromatosis type 1 gene in some but not all cells of the body.
Seizure—Abnormal electrical discharge of brain tissue, often resulting in abnormal body movements or behaviors.
Slit lamp—Device used by ophthalmologists to examine the structures at the front of the eye. Necessary for proper examination for Lisch nodules.
Southern blot—Method of determining the molecular weight corresponding to a particular sequence of DNA in an individual after DNA from the individual is cleaved with a restriction enzyme.
Sphenoid—Skull bone that forms a portion of the back of the orbit. Sometimes abnormally formed in people with neurofibromatosis, resulting in deformity of the orbit.
Spinal fusion—A means of surgical treatment of scoliosis.
Spontaneous mutation—A mutation occurring without apparent external influence.
Sporadic trait—Occurring in a single individual in a family, with no prior family history.
Tibia—Long bone in front of lower part of leg (shin bone), sometimes bowed in people with neurofibromatosis.
Transgenic mouse—Mouse into which a foreign gene has been inserted during embryonic development; used for research studies of the effects of the inserted gene on the animal.

Tumor—Any swelling of a tissue; does not neccessarily connote malignancy or cancer.
Ventricles—Cavities within the brain which are filled with cerebrospinal fluid.
Vertebra—Bone of the spinal column.
Vertigo—False sense of motion, which occurs when the vestibular nerve or apparatus is not functioning correctly.
Vestibular nerve—Cranial nerve that conveys information about sense of balance to the brain. This is the portion of the eighth cranial nerve which usually gives rise to acoustic neuromas.
von Recklinghausen neurofibromatosis—Another name for neurofibromatosis type 1, the peripheral form of neurofibromatosis.
Wilms tumor—Childhood tumor of the kidney, found rarely in association with neurofibromatosis type 1.

Index